Essentials of
ESTHETIC DENTISTRY

Smile Design Integrating Esthetics and Function
VOLUME TWO

Essentials of ESTHETIC DENTISTRY

Smile Design Integrating Esthetics and Function

Volume Two

Edited by

Jonathan B. Levine DMD

Founder; Program Director and Clinical Assistant Professor

Jonathan B. Levine & Associates; New York University College of Dentistry CE

New York, USA

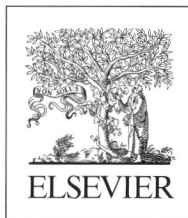

Edinburgh   London   New York   Oxford   Philadelphia   St Louis   Sydney   Toronto

ELSEVIER

© 2016 Elsevier Ltd. All rights reserved.

No part of this publication may be reproduced or transmitted in any form or by any means, electronic or mechanical, including photocopying, recording, or any information storage and retrieval system, without permission in writing from the publisher. Details on how to seek permission, further information about the Publisher's permissions policies and our arrangements with organizations such as the Copyright Clearance Center and the Copyright Licensing Agency, can be found at our website: www.elsevier.com/permissions.

This book and the individual contributions contained in it are protected under copyright by the Publisher (other than as may be noted herein).

ISBN 9780723435556

Notices

Knowledge and best practice in this field are constantly changing. As new research and experience broaden our understanding, changes in research methods, professional practices, or medical treatment may become necessary.

Practitioners and researchers must always rely on their own experience and knowledge in evaluating and using any information, methods, compounds, or experiments described herein. In using such information or methods they should be mindful of their own safety and the safety of others, including parties for whom they have a professional responsibility.

With respect to any drug or pharmaceutical products identified, readers are advised to check the most current information provided (i) on procedures featured or (ii) by the manufacturer of each product to be administered, to verify the recommended dose or formula, the method and duration of administration, and contraindications. It is the responsibility of practitioners, relying on their own experience and knowledge of their patients, to make diagnoses, to determine dosages and the best treatment for each individual patient, and to take all appropriate safety precautions.

To the fullest extent of the law, neither the Publisher nor the authors, contributors, or editors, assume any liability for any injury and/or damage to persons or property as a matter of products liability, negligence or otherwise, or from any use or operation of any methods, products, instructions, or ideas contained in the material herein.

Printed in China

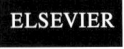

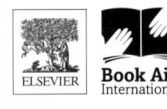

For Elsevier:
Content Strategist: Alison Taylor
Content Development Specialist: Clive Hewat
Project Manager: Anne Collett
Designer/Design Direction: Miles Hitchen
Illustrator: AEGIS Media

CONTENTS

	Contributors	vii
	Foreword	viii
	Series Preface	xi
	Preface	xii
Chapter 1	Esthetic diagnosis: a three-step analysis Jonathan B. Levine and Sivan Finkel	1
Chapter 2	The psychological assessment of the patient Sylvia S. Welsh	45
Chapter 3	Integration of function and esthetics Jeffrey McClendon and Jonathan B. Levine	53
Chapter 4	Clinical photography in esthetic dentistry Nicholas A. Hodson	89
Chapter 5	Periodontal factors Kia Rezavandi	123
Chapter 6	Space management Anabella Oquendo and Steven David	151
Chapter 7	Clear aligner therapy Frank Celenza	183
Chapter 8	Anterior bonded restorations Jonathan B. Levine, Sivan Finkel and Adrian Jurim	215
Chapter 9	High-performance planning with digital design Newton Cardoso and Paulo Battistella	275
	Index	301

CONTRIBUTORS

Paulo Battistella MDT CDT
Founder and CEO
Studio Paulo Battistella
São Paulo
Brasil

Newton P. B. Cardoso DDS MS PC
Adjunct Assistant Professor,
Department of Cariology and Comprehensive Care
Newclinic; New York University College of
Dentistry CE
São Paulo
Brazil

Frank Celenza DDS PC
Specialist in Periodontics and Orthodontics,
Private Practice
New York
USA

Steven B. David DMD
Clinical Professor; Former Director Advanced
Program in Esthetic Dentistry for International
Dentists; Private Practice
New York University College of Dentistry,
David, Hirsch, & David
New York
USA

Sivan Finkel DMD
Co-owner; Clinical Instructor and Education
Co-Director
The Dental Parlour NYC; New York University College
of Dentistry CE
New York
USA

Nicholas Hodson BDS BSc PhD FDS RSCEng(Rest)
Senior Lecturer and Honorary Consultant in
Restorative Dentistry
University of Central Lancashire
Preston
UK

Adrian S. Jurim MDT
Owner of Jurim Dental Studio, Inc
New York University College of Dentistry CE
New York
USA

Jeffrey L. McClendon BS Chemistry DMD Dentistry
Clinical Instructor Department of Cariology and
Comprehensive Care
New York University School of Dentistry
New York City
USA

Anabella Oquendo DDS
Clinical Assistant Professor and Program Director of
the Advanced Program for International Dentists in
Esthetic Dentistry
New York University
New York
USA

Kia Rezavandi BDS MSc MRD RSC(Eng)
Specialist in Periodontics
Private Practice
London
UK

Sylvia S. Welsh PhD
Clinical Associate Professor of Psychiatry
New York University Langone School of Medicine
New York
USA

FOREWORD

In the past decade, technology and innovations in the dental field have given dental professionals the opportunity to create esthetic restorations by mimicking nature. The esthetic demands and expectations of patients have risen with the impact of social media, which has made it easy to access information about new technologies and a lot of different esthetic cases. Today, patients are more willing to have restorations that copy the form, colour, surface texture and function of healthy and esthetic-looking natural teeth. This leads us to observe and imitate natural teeth and smile design not only from functional and morphological perspectives, but also structurally, optically and, more importantly, in harmony with the face.

In any dental treatment, diagnosis has prime importance, since many steps will be planned and constructed on the basic cause of the problem. Then it will be time for treatment planning. It is very obvious that, whether you work in a solo office or in a group practice, team work is absolutely essential. The importance of working as a team is that you will be able to achieve the most efficient treatment planning. There are different factors that may influence the treatment planning, including formal education, clinical experience, continuing education, books and journals followed, exchange of information, working within a good team and, finally, the common sense of the dentist. On the other side, there is the patient, who has to be satisfied with the results of the treatment. In addition to all of the above, the patient's expectations, mentality, commitment, time and financial conditions will also be taken into consideration while planning the treatment.

As we can clearly see, the way to 'excellence' is not easy, especially when the esthetic treatment should be executed using a minimally invasive approach. This definitely requires an understanding of the patient's expectations and a great team effort between the general dentist, the specialists and the laboratory involved. Only then can we can truly talk about a successfully completed esthetic case.

This select group of master clinicians and ceramists exemplifies many years of practical knowledge and presents invaluable and diverse perspectives. This book covers all of the necessary details mentioned above. And what makes this textbook special is that the authors base their discussions on being minimally invasive, hence the importance of the treatment planning, as well as sharing many different treatment planning modalities.

With the guidance of this book, dentists, specialists and ceramists will find it easier to take crucial decisions about the improved esthetics that will influence directly on their patients' lives. Readers will be most impressed with the overall organization of the text, the clarity of each chapter and the outstanding photography.

Nonetheless, my rationale for this foreword is not only my appreciation of the book but also my respect for Dr Levine (as the editor) and for all of the authors he has gathered for this book and their accomplishments.

Dr Galip Gurel DDS MSc

SERIES PREFACE

Esthetic dentistry is a complex subject and in many ways it requires different skills from those required for disease-focussed clinical care. The team that have created this series have shared a vision that a broad range of additional skills are needed.

The first volume provided useful, readily applicable information and sets the scene for those wishing to go further into ethetic techniques. It included techniques for smile makeovers using readily available procedures in general practice.

This volume covers the techniques applicable to more detailed patient assessment, advanced smile design and illustrates some of the more complex methods available to experienced clinicians where intervention is accepted.

Volume 3 which follows will provide in some ways an alternative approach to this present volume. While attitudes vary one increasing concern to many clinicians is the amount of tooth reduction and destruction carried out for esthetic change alone while the world moves towards MI, Minimal Intervention, in relation to oral and many other diseases. This series should be seen as a whole, challenging your thinking and approach to this growing subject area, particularly by showing different approaches to clinical situations. We no longer need to rely on a single formula to provide a smile make-over, selling only one treatment modality where both the dentist and their patients are losing out; the patient losing valuable irreplaceable enamel as well as their future options.

As the series progresses you can discover in greater depth the many clinical techniques to practice a range of effective procedures in esthetic dentistry.

Professor Brian J. Millar BDS FDSRCS PhD FHEA

PREFACE

When we set out to write another book on dental esthetics, I asked myself, is this what the dental education community really needs, another book on esthetics?

And then, I got to thinking. I thought about what is truly missing today for the practicing dentist, the ones who are in the trenches, with patients looking for new ways to improve their smile and maintain the health of their mouth. I took a step back and thought deeply about our challenges.

On one hand, we need to duplicate nature and use materials that are completely invisible when working in the esthetic zone. My team and I call this supernatural esthetics. On the other hand, we need to restore teeth conservatively, paying special attention to structure, function, and biology.

There are numerous challenges the clinicians face today and obstacles that prevent them from achieving great success for their patients and for their dental team. With the myriad of responsibilities that dentists have today – from running a business, to caring for his or her patients, to continually improving their talents and skills with additional education – I realized that we need to create an everyday guide for esthetic dentistry. Something that is easy to assimilate, with a goal of creating smile experts.

With the help of the Elsevier team, we have set the vision for this book. A practical guide for the clinician that looks at esthetics from both sides of the proverbial coin: beauty and function. We seek to create an integrated approach across the disciplines of dentistry, from communication and psychology, to periodontics and orthodontics, to esthetic techniques, all synthesized together for the restorative dentist. This approach will yield smile architects, with the right capabilities for successful esthetic outcomes every time.

We believe that it all starts with three C's: Communication, Collaboration, and Consistency. The clinician will know exactly where to begin and how to finish with great success. From simple to the most complex esthetic cases many esthetic failures occur because of lack of communication. Whether it is between the esthetic dentist and the patient, or with the technician or other specialists, we need to create a culture where open communication thrives between everyone involved. Once this happens, the patient feels heard, the esthetic dentist has direction, and the technician isn't guessing about color or incisal edge position. With this collaboration set into motion, success will follow success, and the necessary skills, check lists, protocols, and procedures will need to be developed and set into motion.

This volume focuses on the clinician's personal development. Our goal is to teach methods to develop consistency through checklists, protocols, and procedures in the practice. Clinical 'takeaway boxes' incorporated throughout the chapter highlight key data points, along with answers to potential FAQs that your patient might be asking.

As the old saying goes, "it all starts at the top". As a clinician, your role is to be a leader in the practice. Think about setting a *vision for your practice: whom you want to practice with, and what you want to do day in, and day out*. After you set this vision, map out a plan that will allow you to get there. Keep in mind, the quality of the people on your team, how well you communicate with one another, and how well you engage the patients of the practice, will ultimately determine everyone's collective happiness. The goal of this text is to help *you* achieve your vision, bringing *you* great personal satisfaction on the road to success.

Jonathan B. Levine DMD

CHAPTER 1

Esthetic Diagnosis: A Three-Step Analysis

JONATHAN B. LEVINE, SIVAN FINKEL

Introduction to the three-step analysis 2
The Esthetic Evaluation Form 3
Records. 27
The diagnostic wax-up. 33
The esthetic mock-up 36
Summary 40

'Beauty is in the eye of the beholder', it is said, and we have been hearing this old comment for many years. One person can love Renaissance art, for instance, while another favours post-modernism, and neither would be wrong. However, while the perception of 'beauty' is a subjective experience (flavoured by ethnicity, culture and an endless list of other factors), there are certain universal guidelines that transcend this subjectivity and provide us with factual, objective criteria as to what pleases the human eye. These fundamental esthetic standards can help us as clinicians to design and create 'beauty' in a quantitative, scientific and predictable manner.

Today – due in part to a convergence of trends in tooth-whitening, 'Extreme Makeover' style television shows and oral care companies spending millions on advertising – the smile has been solidified in our culture as a centrepiece of overall beauty. There is greater demand than ever before for elective, esthetically driven dentistry, which is a major shift from the atmosphere of just a few generations ago, when a trip to the dentist meant either a cleaning or the resolution of pain. Patients today, in addition to wanting clean, pain-free mouths, commonly seek rejuvenated, improved or completely transformed smiles. We as dentists must retool, redefine and reinvent ourselves to be not only competent clinicians, but 'smile experts'. Simply stated, we need to reimagine who we are today.

INTRODUCTION TO THE THREE-STEP ANALYSIS

As smile experts, we need to use objective, fact-based thinking to understand the esthetic demands of our patients. We must use a systemized and structured methodology to make sure no stone is left unturned and, through the data we have collected, propose a plan that will not only resolve the esthetic problems but will respect the critically important functional requirements of our patients' teeth as well. The approach can be broken down into three steps: **identify** the problems, **visualize** the customized solution (in three dimensions) and **choose** the appropriate technique to get there.

Historically the diagnostic approach has been to lead with structure–function–biology and only then to consider esthetics, which could easily result in a compromised esthetic outcome and an unhappy patient. What we are suggesting in this chapter is reversing the approach: considering the esthetics first (which is usually the patient's chief concern) and then studying the structure–function–biology[1] in the context of an ideal esthetic vision. By diagnosing cases in this new sequence we set ourselves up for success, optimizing communication from day one and ensuring that we meet the desires of our patients (Figs 1.1 and 1.2).

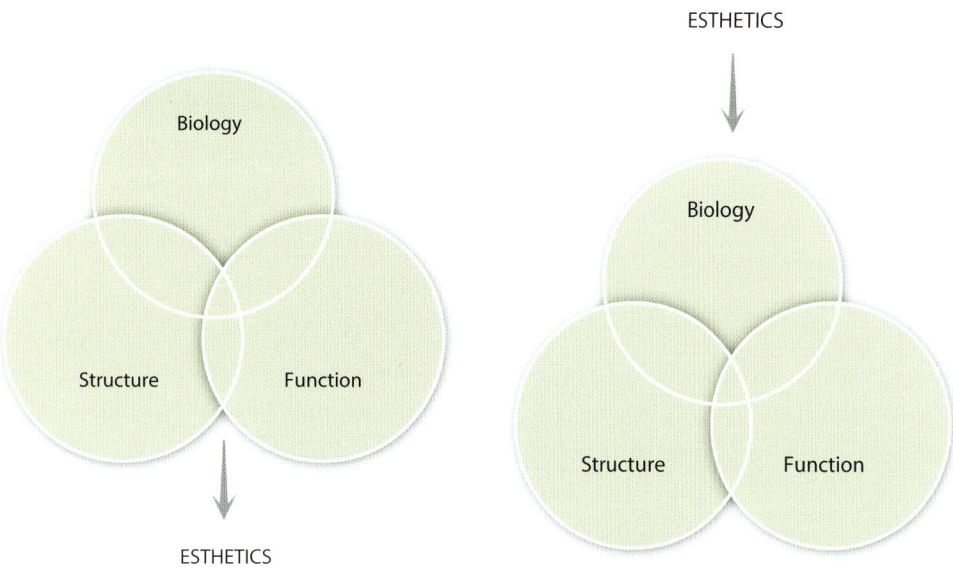

Fig. 1.1 Traditional thinking. **Fig. 1.2** New way of thinking.

Step two of the analysis is to perform a diagnostic wax-up on the mounted casts that is guided by the information from the Esthetic Evaluation Form. This allows us to visualize tooth shape, tooth position and soft tissue harmony as it relates to the three views of facial, dentofacial and dental esthetics.

Once the diagnostic wax-up is done, we then transfer a 'mock-up' of it into the patient's mouth. This offers our patient a preview of the visualized solution and is an opportunity for us to gather crucial feedback. By listening to the patient's opinion about the proposed tooth colour, shape and position, it is possible to avoid future communication mistakes.

CLINICAL TIP

Many failures are attributable to a breakdown of communication among the essential trinity of patient, dentist and technician, rather than a problem of a technical nature involving the restorations themselves.

The notes we take during this stage will be conveyed directly to the lab technician and, together with the dentist and patient, the three parties then become an empowered team (Fig. 1.3). We can now co-create our esthetic vision together.

THE ESTHETIC EVALUATION FORM

Dr Peter Dawson once said, 'If you know where you are and you know where you want to go, getting there is easy.' That statement alone is the key to tackling any case. In this section we will describe a systemized method for determining exactly 'where you are' at the outset of any esthetic case.

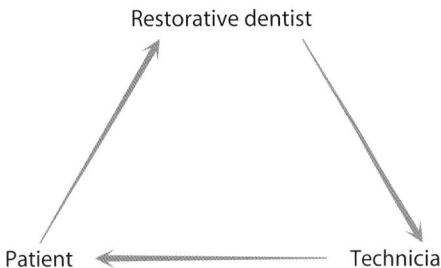

Fig. 1.3 Communication triangle: information flow.

As we know from other industries (i.e. technology, manufacturing and hospitality), a factual checklist approach to any process avoids errors, miscalculations and miscommunication. In our field, a checklist used at the esthetic consultation appointment will allow a clinician to move seamlessly through the diagnostic process, assessing both esthetics and function at the same time. Figure 1.4 is an Esthetic Evaluation Form that was originally created by the author (Dr J. Levine) in 1995 and has now gone through multiple revisions.

> **CLINICAL TIP**
>
> The key objective of the Esthetic Evaluation Form is to establish the incisal edge position and the gingival margin of the maxillary central incisor, two crucial landmarks around which the entire case will be designed.

As we move through the form, we study the smile in increasing detail and ask effective, open-ended questions to pinpoint the patient's true esthetic needs. Like a camera zooming in, we analyse facial esthetic elements first ('macro-esthetics'), follow this with a dentofacial assessment and, finally, study the dental view ('micro-esthetic' elements).

SECTION ONE: EFFECTIVE QUESTIONS

We begin by asking our patient the open-ended question, 'If there was anything you could change about your smile, what would it be?' This question is designed to elicit as much information as possible, as opposed to a closed-ended question such as, 'Do you like your smile?' which only gives the clinician a yes or no answer. We want the patient involved in the process and, by creating effective communication right from the beginning, the team (comprised of the patient, dentist and technician) can then begin to build a strong relationship that is focused on effective communication and, by default, success. We are guided by the 80:20 rule of listening, where we ask our effective questions and we listen 80% of the time.

Esthetic Evaluation Form ©

Patient _____ Examiner _____ Date _____

1. Effective Questions

:A: If there was anything you could change about your smile, what would it be?
_____
_____

:B: Do you like the visual image of "Straight, White, Perfect", "Clean, Healthy, Natural", or "White and Natural" looking teeth?
_____
_____

:C: History of Esthetic Change
_____
_____

:D: Previous Records – Do you have any photos of your smile, or any smile you like, to aid in aesthetic treatment planning?
   o Yes   o No

2. Facial Analysis

:A: Full Smile

1. **Interpupillary Line to Occlusal Plane**
   o Parallel
   o Canted right
   o Canted left

2. **Midline Relationship of Teeth**
   (Maxillary) **to Face** (Philtrum)
   o Coincident
   o Right of center
   o Left of center

3. **Relationship of Lips to Face**
   (Lip Symmetry)
   o Symmetrical
   o Left side higher
   o Right side higher

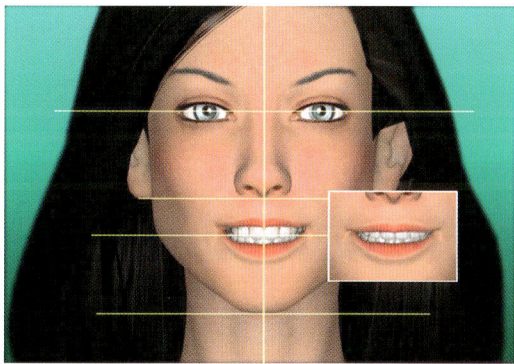

:B: Lips at Rest

1. **Upper Lip**
   o Full
   o Average
   o Thin

2. **Lower Lip**
   o Full
   o Average
   o Thin

3. **Lips**
   o Prominent
   o Retruded

4. **Tooth Exposure at Rest:**
   Maxillary _____ mm
   Mandibular _____ mm

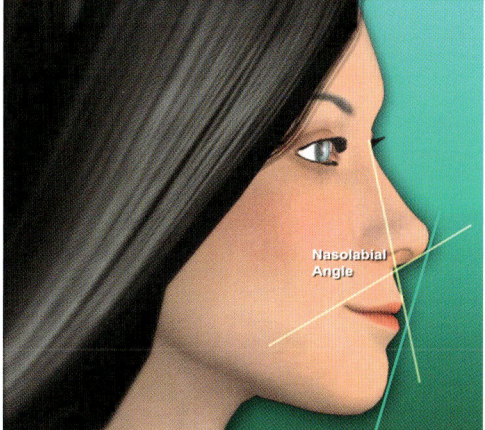

:C: Profile View: Facially – Directed Treatment Planning

1. **Nasolabial Angle**
   o Normal (approx. 90°)
   o Prominent Maxilla (< 90°)
   o Retruded Maxilla (> 90°)

2. **Ricketts' E-plane** (Drawn from tip of nose to chin)
   Upper Lip to E-plane _____ mm (ideally 4 mm)
   Lower Lip to E-plane _____ mm (ideally 2 mm)

3. **Profile Shape**
   o WNL   o Convex   o Concave

If maxilla is prominent, nasolabial angle is < 90°, or profile is convex, consider smaller, less dominant maxillary anterior restorations.

If maxilla is retruded, nasolabial angle is > 90°, or profile is concave, consider more dominant maxillary anterior restorations.

Esthetic Evaluation Form © Created by Jonathan B. Levine, DMD

Fig. 1.4 Esthetic Evaluation Form.

Continued

THE ESTHETIC EVALUATION FORM

3. Dentofacial Analysis – Vertical and Horizontal Components

:A: Upper Smile Line
o Average o High o Low

:B: Incisal Edges to Lower Lip
o Convex Curve o Straight o Reverse

:C: Tooth – Lower Lip Position
o Touching o Not Touching o Slightly Covered

:D: Full Smile – Number of Teeth Displayed
o 6 o 8 o 10 o 12

:E: Midline Location – Central Incisors to Philtrum
o Center o Right of Center o Left of Center

:F: Midline – Skewing to Left or Right
o Right o Left o Straight

:G: Bilateral Negative Space
o Normal o Increased

:H: Phonetics
1. **F** Sounds – Incisal edge of maxillary centrals on wet/dry line of lower lip?
   o Yes o No
2. **S** Sounds – Closest speaking space – clear sound?
   o Yes o No

4. Dental Analysis

:A: Starting shade
Maxillary _____
Mandibular _____

:B: Central Incisor Width/Height Ratio
o > 80%   o < 80%

:C: Proportion of Central/Lateral/Canine
Central Width: _____ mm
Lateral Width: _____ mm
Cuspid Width: _____ mm

:D: Occlusal Analysis

1. Complete Occlusion — Interferences: _____

2. Incisive Position — Interferences: _____

3. Left Working — Interferences: _____ Guiding teeth: _____

4. Right Working — Interferences: _____ Guiding teeth: _____

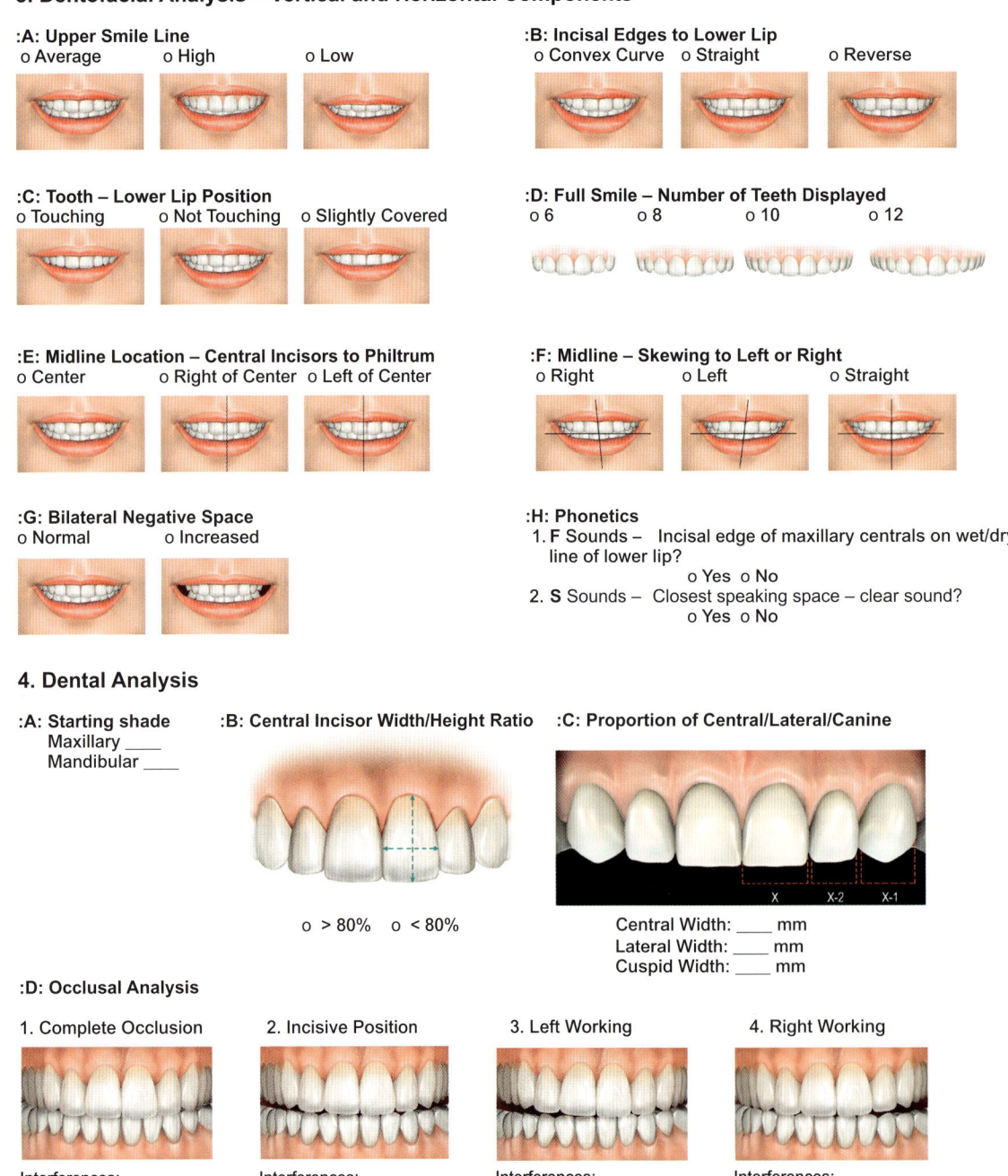

Esthetic Evaluation Form © Created by Jonathan B. Levine, DMD

Fig. 1.4 *Continued*

CHAPTER 1
ESTHETIC DIAGNOSIS: A THREE-STEP ANALYSIS

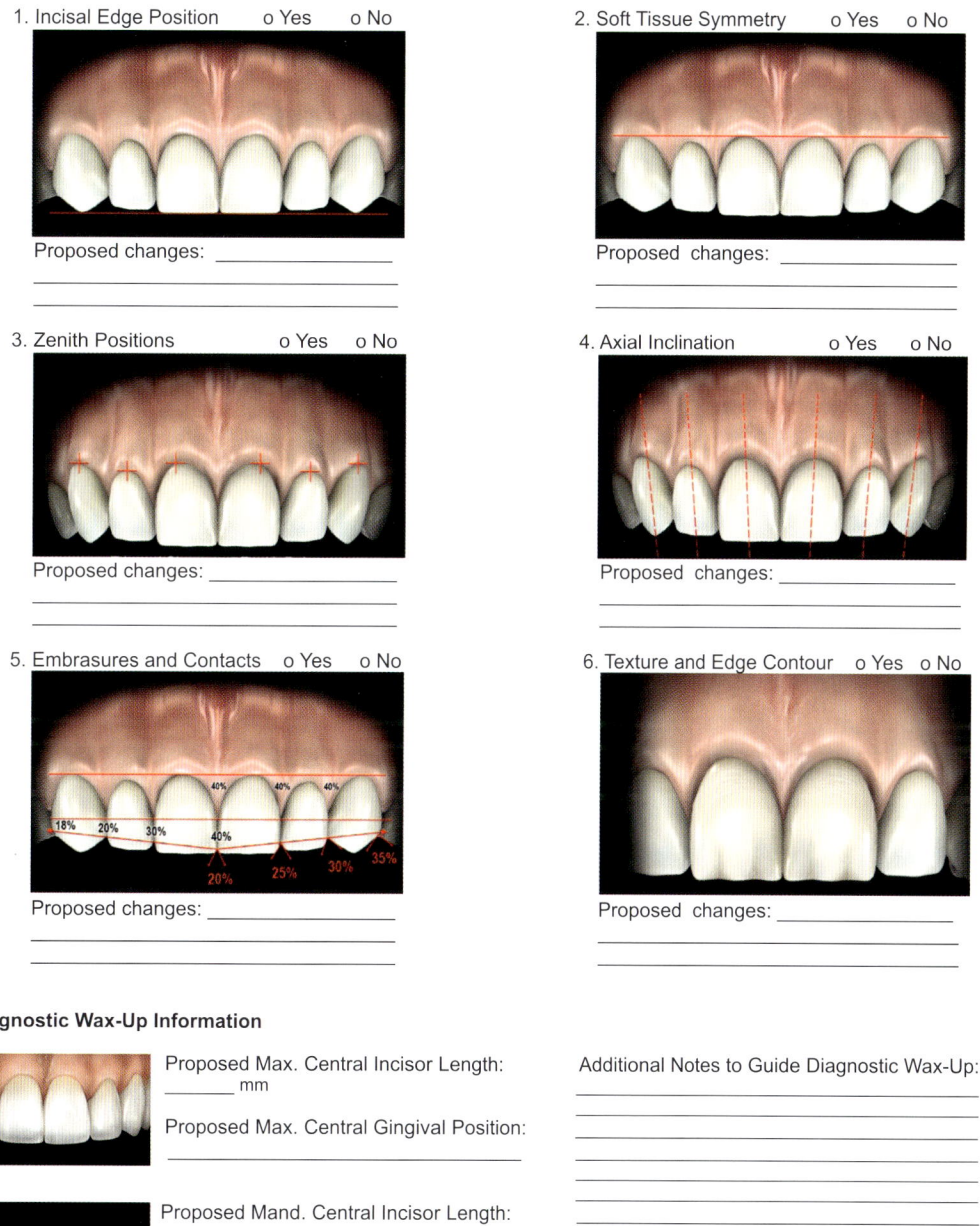

:E: Micro-Aesthetic Elements: Acceptable or Not?

1. Incisal Edge Position   o Yes   o No

   Proposed changes: _____

2. Soft Tissue Symmetry   o Yes   o No

   Proposed changes: _____

3. Zenith Positions   o Yes   o No

   Proposed changes: _____

4. Axial Inclination   o Yes   o No

   Proposed changes: _____

5. Embrasures and Contacts   o Yes   o No

   Proposed changes: _____

6. Texture and Edge Contour   o Yes   o No

   Proposed changes: _____

:F: Diagnostic Wax-Up Information

Proposed Max. Central Incisor Length: _____ mm

Proposed Max. Central Gingival Position: _____

Proposed Mand. Central Incisor Length: _____ mm

Proposed Mand. Central Gingival Position: _____

Additional Notes to Guide Diagnostic Wax-Up:
_____
_____
_____
_____
_____

Esthetic Evaluation Form © Created by Jonathan B. Levine, DMD

Fig. 1.4 *Continued*

Once the patient is able to tell the esthetic dentist what bothers them and what brought them into the office, an esthetic smile design question is asked to determine the degree of naturalness the patient desires. Because 'beautiful' means different things to different people, it is crucial to establish the patient's preference at this early stage. Therefore, we ask, 'Do you like the visual image of "straight, white and perfect", "clean, healthy and natural" or "white and natural"?'

'Straight, white and perfect' is defined as a symmetrical smile where the right and left sides are mirror images and all teeth are a very light shade and in perfect alignment. We like to offer a picture of the actress Halle Berry, someone everybody knows whose smile is a great example of this.

The 'clean, healthy and natural' category is defined as having the perfect imperfections of nature: slight rotations and/or setbacks of the lateral incisors, slightly irregular incisal edges and a more natural shade. The actress we refer to for this description is Sarah Jessica Parker.

The final category, a middle ground mentioned only after the first two have been described, is 'white and natural'. This implies natural tooth forms but in a light shade, exemplified by the smile of Julia Roberts. At the time of this publication, the majority of patients seem to prefer this final category as preferences have shifted away from the 'Hollywood' smiles of the 1990s towards a less artificial look. But again, beauty is extremely subjective and so the patient's desires need to be determined early on. The three types of smiles are summarized in Figure 1.5A–C.

We conclude this section by asking if there has been any previous esthetic dentistry done and, if so, what the patient's experience was like. To further understand the patient's concept of esthetics, we also ask whether there are any relevant photos of the patient (particularly useful in 'rejuvenation' cases) or of any other smiles they admire.

CLINICAL TIP

The importance of the questions in this section cannot be overemphasized, as the entire case will be designed according to the ideals of the patient and not those of the dentist or the laboratory technician.

SECTION TWO: FACIAL, DENTOFACIAL AND DENTAL ANALYSIS

The next step of the Esthetic Evaluation Form is to take a three-view approach to the smile, i.e moving from the facial view (full face) to the dentofacial view (teeth and lips) and only then assessing the dental view (retracted smile). Each view has important esthetic elements to review as we move through our diagnosis.

CHAPTER 1
ESTHETIC DIAGNOSIS: A THREE-STEP ANALYSIS

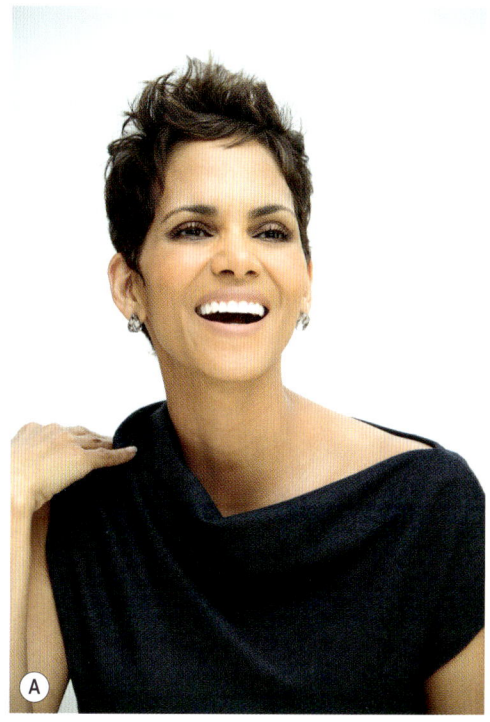

Fig. 1.5A The Halle Berry smile: 'straight, white and perfect'. Teeth are uniform in size and shape and have perfect edges, and the smile is symmetrical. Photograph by Vera Anderson. Getty Images Entertainment, Getty Images.

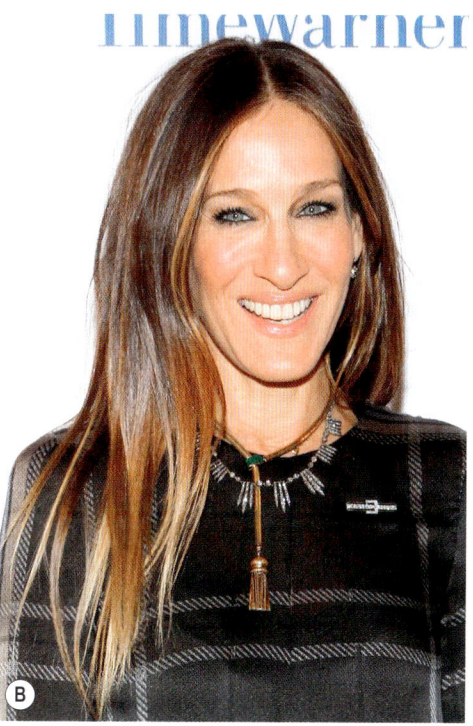

Fig. 1.5B The Sarah Jessica Parker smile: 'clean, healthy and natural'. Teeth are clean looking, but not too bright and white. They have slight imperfections, like a subtle rotation here and an irregular edge there. Teeth are not exactly the same shape. Photograph by Mireya Acierto. Getty Images Entertainment, Getty Images.

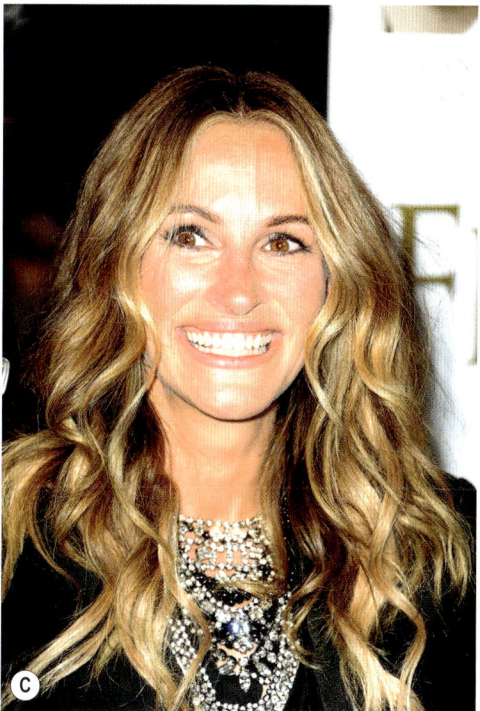

Fig. 1.5C The Julia Roberts smile: 'white and natural'. This is a combination of (A) and (B). The teeth are a bright white shade, but have slight imperfections. Photograph by Frazer Harrison. Getty Images Entertainment, Getty Images.

THE ESTHETIC EVALUATION FORM

Facial view: Macro-elements

The critical elements we look for in the facial view are balance and harmony, or a lack of tension in the composition of the face. We start by observing a frontal view with a full smile and then take two orthodontic measurements from the profile view with the patient in repose. The macro-esthetic elements are as follows:

1. The parallelism between the interpupillary line and the line corresponding to the occlusal plane (drawn between the cusp tips of the maxillary canines as shown in Figure 1.6). Here we are looking to determine any canting of the maxilla. Clinically, a length of floss can be used to visualize this.

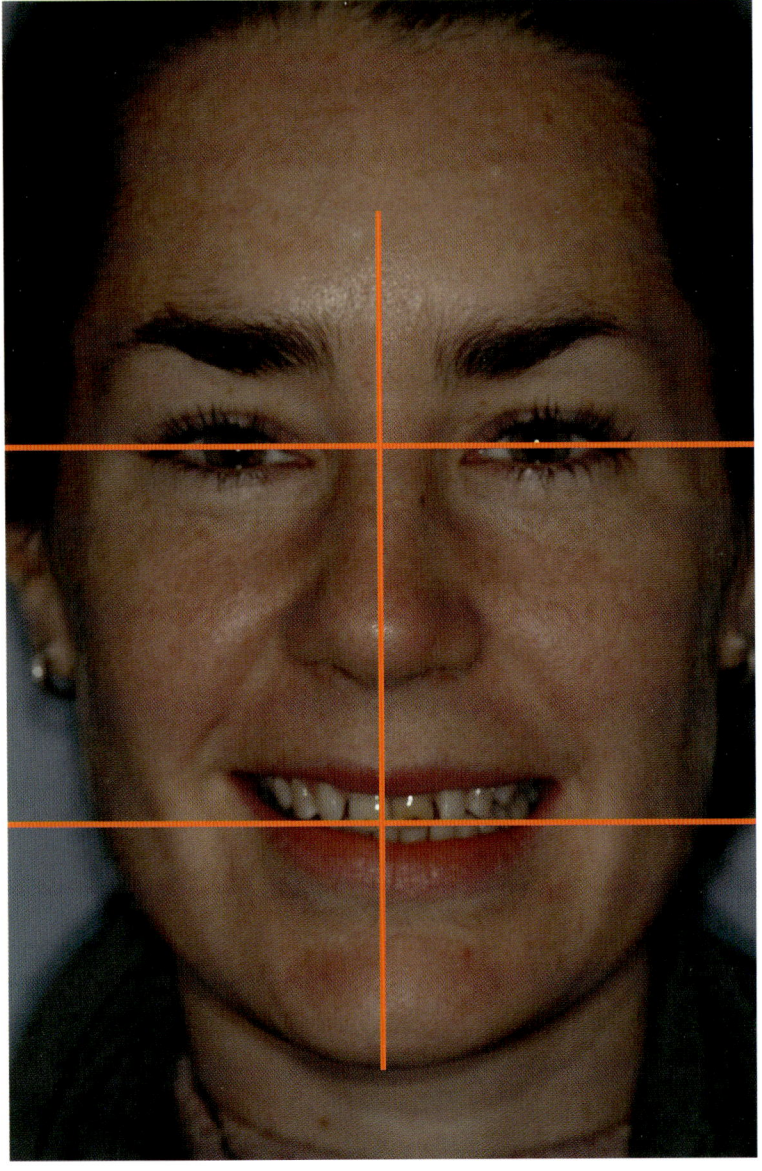

Fig. 1.6 The macro-esthetic elements.

2. The location of the facial midline in relation to the maxillary dental midline (Fig. 1.6). This too can be visualized clinically with floss.

3. Lip anatomy. This is viewed in terms of symmetry to the face and fullness of the upper and lower lips. We also assess how prominent or retruded the lips are, from a profile view. The degree of lip support helps determine if the case should be 'built out' facially or not.

4. Tooth exposure at rest. This is one of the most critical elements of facially directed treatment planning. As we know from Vig and Brundo's study[2], a woman at age 30 shows 3.4 mm of her maxillary central incisors with the lip at rest; at 60 years of age the maxillary centrals are no longer displayed and she shows approximately the same 3.4 mm of her lower incisors. A man shows 1.7 mm of the maxillary centrals at 30 years of age and that same amount on the lower arch at 60 years of age.[2] This decrease in maxillary central display is due to the loss of muscle tone over time, gravity and wear of the incisal edges. Lengthening the incisal edges of our patients' teeth will thus result in a more youthful appearance. To assess the amount of tooth display at rest, we ask our patients to relax their lips, say the word 'Emma' and then freeze (Fig. 1.7). In the Esthetic Evaluation Form this is the first step towards determining the existing incisal edge position of the tooth to the lips and face. The next thought should be, where is this edge located ideally?

5. Nasolabial angle (Fig. 1.8). This is an orthodontic measurement assessed from a profile view of the patient with the lips in repose.[3] Typically, we

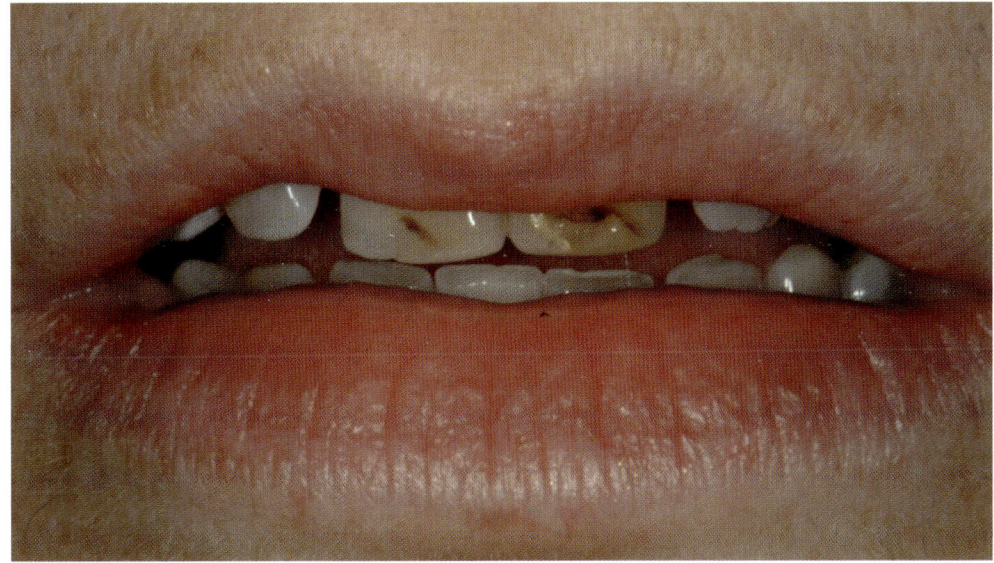

Fig. 1.7 Relax the lips, say 'Emma' and then freeze.

THE ESTHETIC EVALUATION FORM

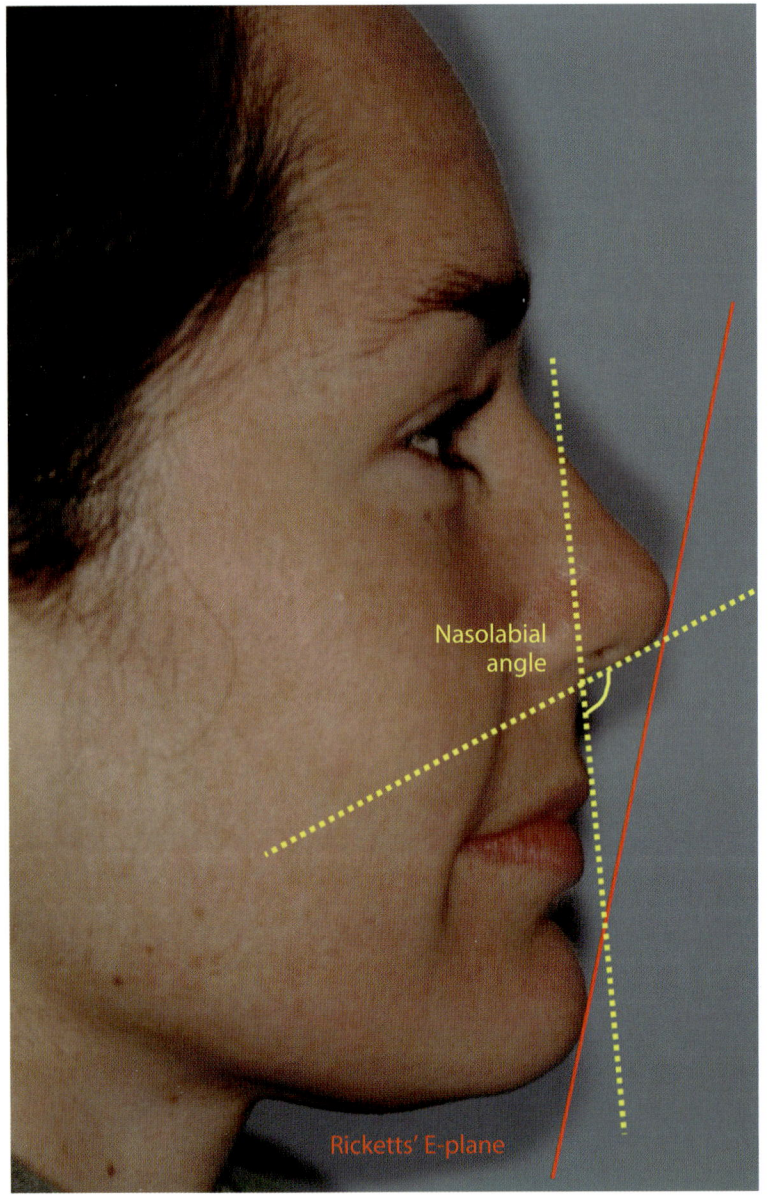

Fig. 1.8 The nasolabial angle.

strive for a nasolabial angle of 90°, and thus an angle of less than 90° (prominent maxilla) means the maxillary anterior restorations should be smaller and less dominant, while an angle of greater than 90° (retruded maxilla) means the patient can afford to have their maxillary anterior restorations 'built out'.

6. Ricketts' E-plane. A second orthodontic measurement, also assessed from a profile view, describes the imaginary line drawn from the tip of our patient's nose to the chin (Fig. 1.8). Clinically, we can utilize a length of floss held against these two facial landmarks and measure with a

CHAPTER 1
ESTHETIC DIAGNOSIS: A THREE-STEP ANALYSIS

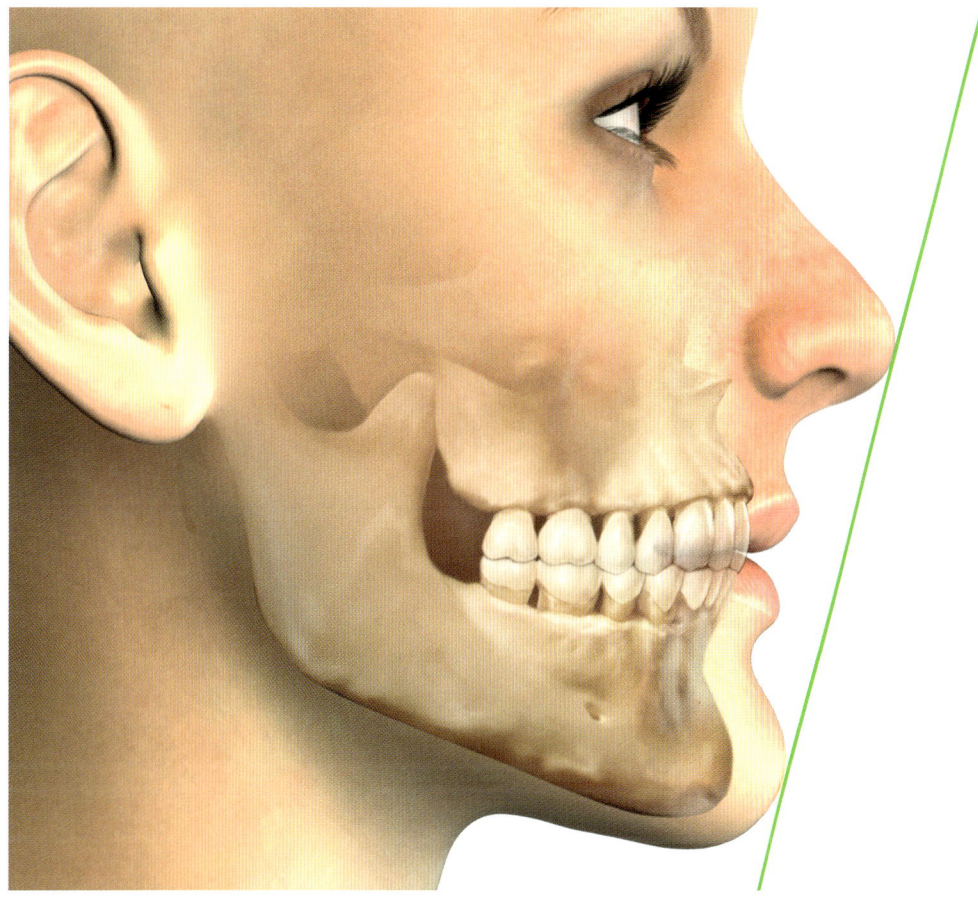

Fig. 1.9 A concave profile. This case can be 'built out' with changing tooth position and tooth size by increasing the length of the maxillary central incisors at the higher end of their range (10–12.5 mm).

periodontal probe. Ideally, the upper lip is 4 mm from the E-plane and the lower lip is 2 mm away. If the upper lip is greater than 6 mm from the plane then we consider this a concave profile (Fig. 1.9). If the lips are on the plane then there is more of a convex profile (Fig. 1.10). In nature, a maxillary central incisor can be anywhere from 10 mm to 12.5 mm long, and it is appropriate to design maxillary centrals towards the larger end of this range for the concave patient and towards the smaller end of this range for those who are more convex.[4,5] As a rule of thumb, for the convex patient with a high smile line, the length of the maxillary central should not exceed 10.5 mm.

Dentofacial view

This view (Fig. 1.11), comprising of the teeth and lips, deals with the vertical and horizontal components of the smile. We ask for a full, natural smile and assess the amount of gingival display (as a 'high smile line' case will be

THE ESTHETIC EVALUATION FORM

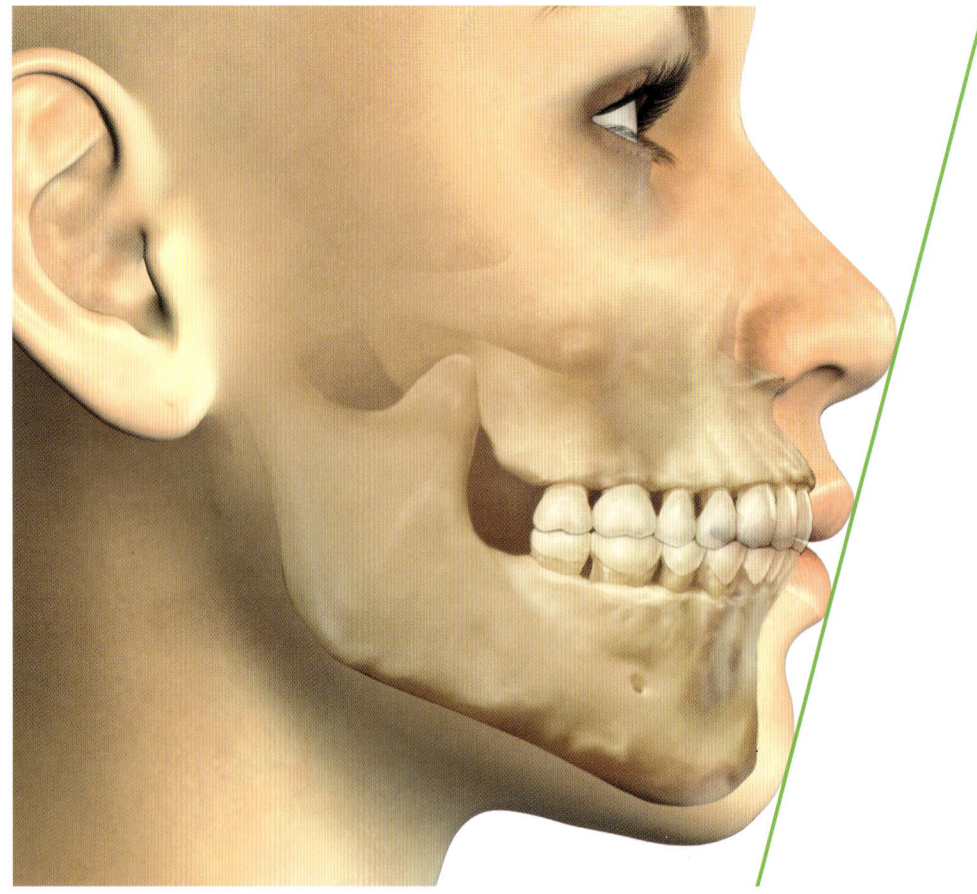

Fig. 1.10 A convex profile. In this case the shape and position of the teeth is downsized.

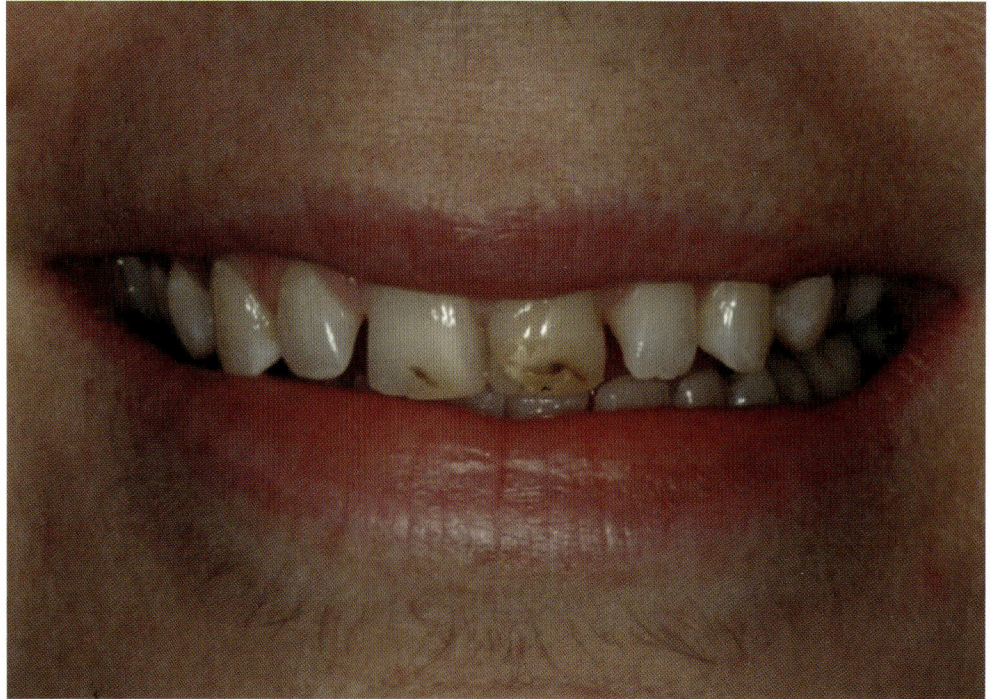

Fig. 1.11 The dentofacial view.

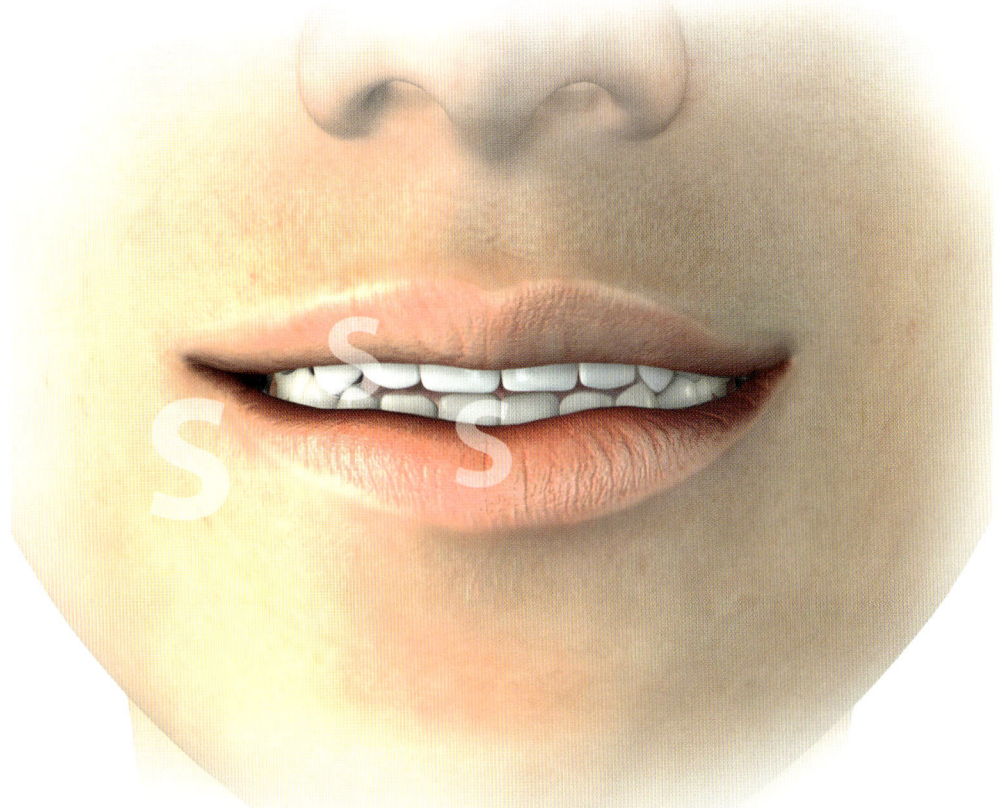

Fig. 1.12 Listen for any lisping as the patient pronounces 'S' sounds.

inherently more challenging). We observe the degree to which the incisal edges of the maxillary anterior teeth echo the curve of the lower lip, count how many teeth show in the smile and check for the presence of excessive negative space bilaterally.[6]

The position of the facial midline in relation to the maxillary dental midline is noted. We know from Kokich's study[7] that the midline can be 'off' up to 4 mm in either direction and will still be inoffensive to the layperson's eye. According to that same study, however, a midline cant is extremely noticeable to most people and thus a higher priority to correct.

Phonetics are addressed as well in this part of our diagnosis. We observe the closest speaking space and listen for any lisping as the patient pronounces 'S' sounds (Fig. 1.12). Next 'F' sounds are pronounced and we look for the incisal edge of the maxillary centrals to just brush against the wet/dry line of the lower lip (Fig. 1.13). The lip should not seem to 'reach' for that incisal edge (tooth too short) nor should the tooth 'trip over' the lower lip (tooth too long). Note that the 'F' sounds should be pronounced gently, as a forceful pronunciation will

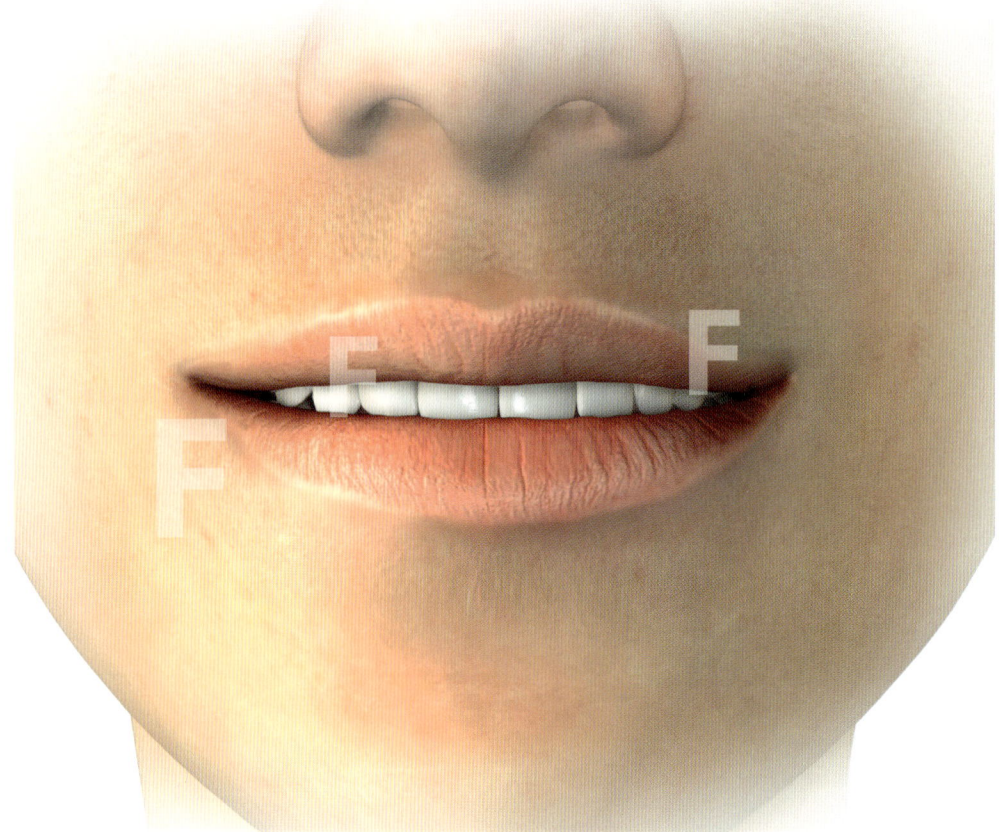

Fig. 1.13 'F' sounds are pronounced and we look for the incisal edge of the maxillary centrals to just brush against the wet/dry line of the lower lip.

recruit the muscles of the lips and give an inaccurate read. The letter 'E' should be pronounced as well, as this mimics a wide smile and is useful to observe.

Dental view: Occlusal analysis and micro-elements

With the dental view (Fig. 1.14) we begin by evaluating the patient's occlusion. We then assess the balance between the 'white zone' (the teeth) and the 'pink zone' (the gingiva) and consider 16 specific micro-esthetic elements.

The fundamentals of occlusion can be defined as a mutually protected occlusion. Simply stated, this means the front teeth separate the back teeth in all directions without interference ('anterior coupling')[8] and the back teeth support the front teeth in a vertical direction. This beautifully designed relationship works extremely well, as it minimizes premature contacts and interferences that would cause wear and trauma to the whole system. Any interference with complete occlusion, protrusive, and right and left working is identified with articulating paper and noted on the form. We also note which teeth provide guidance

CHAPTER 1
ESTHETIC DIAGNOSIS: A THREE-STEP ANALYSIS

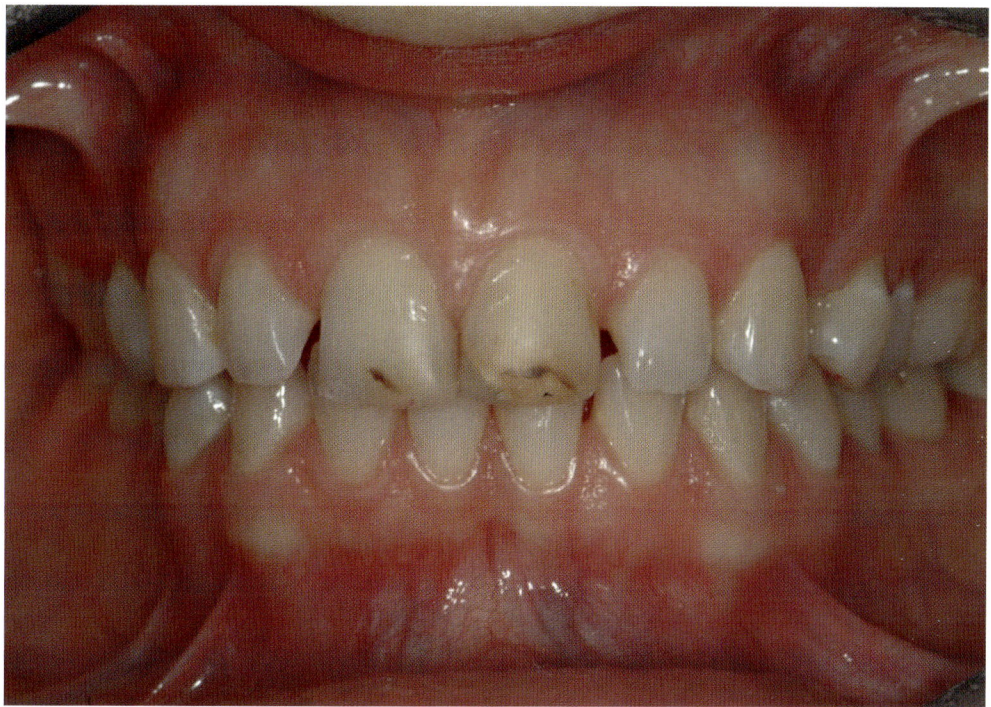

Fig. 1.14 The dental view.

in the working positions, whether it is canine guidance, premolar guidance or a 'group function' scenario.

Occlusion will be discussed at length in Chapter 3; however, as it relates to diagnosis it is important to remember that the palatal contour of the maxillary central incisor defines anterior coupling, the incisal edge defines phonetics and the facial surface defines esthetics (Fig. 1.15). All three surfaces must be considered, as oftentimes a veneer scenario becomes full coverage once the tooth's lingual contours are assessed.

MICRO-ESTHETIC ELEMENTS

We now turn our attention to the final section of the Esthetic Evaluation Form, the micro-esthetic elements. By analysing these elements we can clearly identify the necessary changes to be incorporated into our diagnostic wax-up:

- Incisal edge position. The position of the maxillary central's incisal edge as it relates to phonetics, function and esthetics. Remember once more that the position of the maxillary central incisor is the most critical aspect of the smile. Once we know where this tooth's gingival margin goes and where the incisal edge needs to be positioned then everything falls into place; the height of that tooth defines its ideal width (roughly 80% of the height, as we know from various studies) and simple biometric guidelines then provide

THE ESTHETIC EVALUATION FORM

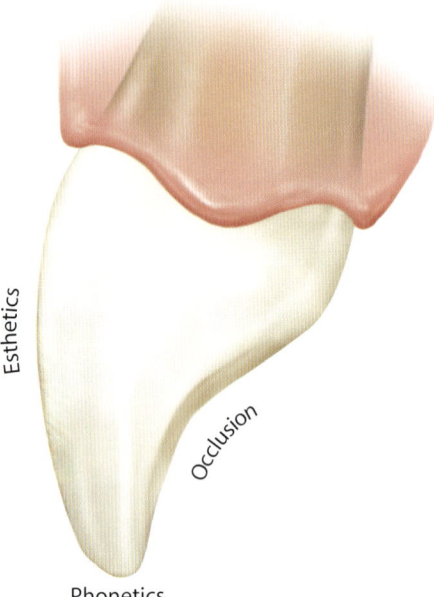

Fig. 1.15 The facial surface defines esthetics.

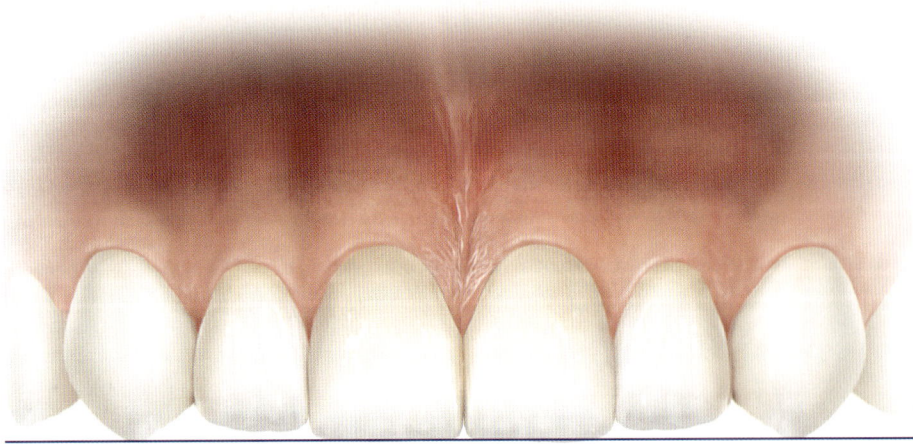

Fig. 1.16 Ideal incisal edge position.

the widths of the other teeth.[4,5] Ideally, the edges of the maxillary central incisors and the points of the canines lie on the same horizontal line, with the lateral incisors' edges set above this line (Fig. 1.16).

- Soft tissue symmetry. The gingival height of the maxillary centrals and canines should ideally be at the same level, with that of the lateral incisors being 1.0–1.5 mm below this line (Fig. 1.17). This is especially critical in the high smile line patient.[9]

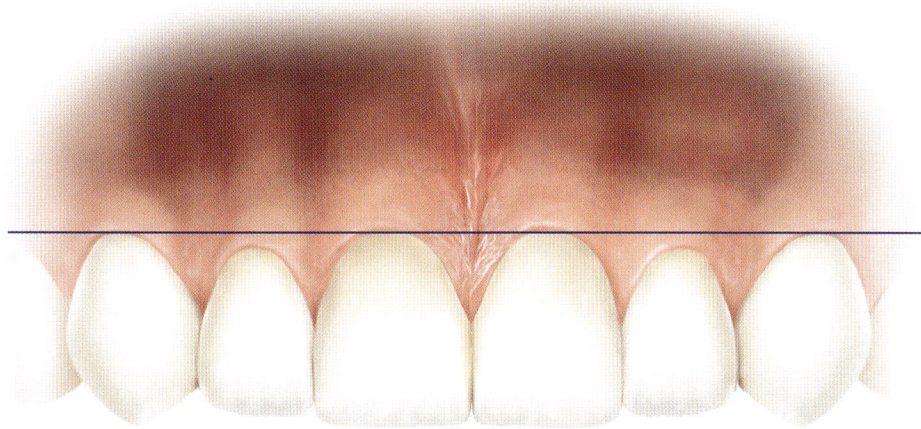

Fig. 1.17 Soft tissue symmetry.

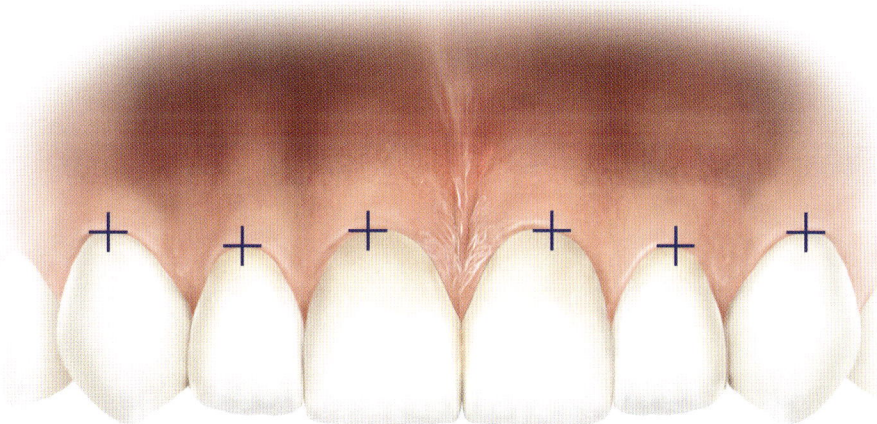

Fig. 1.18 Trigonal shapes.

- Trigonal shapes. The peak of the gingival seam is highest at the distal aspect of the maxillary central incisor, approximately 1 mm distal to the tooth's midline (Fig. 1.18). This is often described as a 'gull-wing' effect. The zenith point of the laterals and canines, however, should be centred mesiodistally.[10]

- Axial inclination. The six anterior teeth have their roots distally inclined, with the centrals being the closest to upright and the inclination increasing as we move distally (Fig. 1.19A,B).[9] This subtlety reflects the position of the underlying roots, as no two structures can occupy the same space.

- Tooth proportion. The width of the maxillary central incisor should be 75–85% of its height (Fig. 1.20).[4,6]

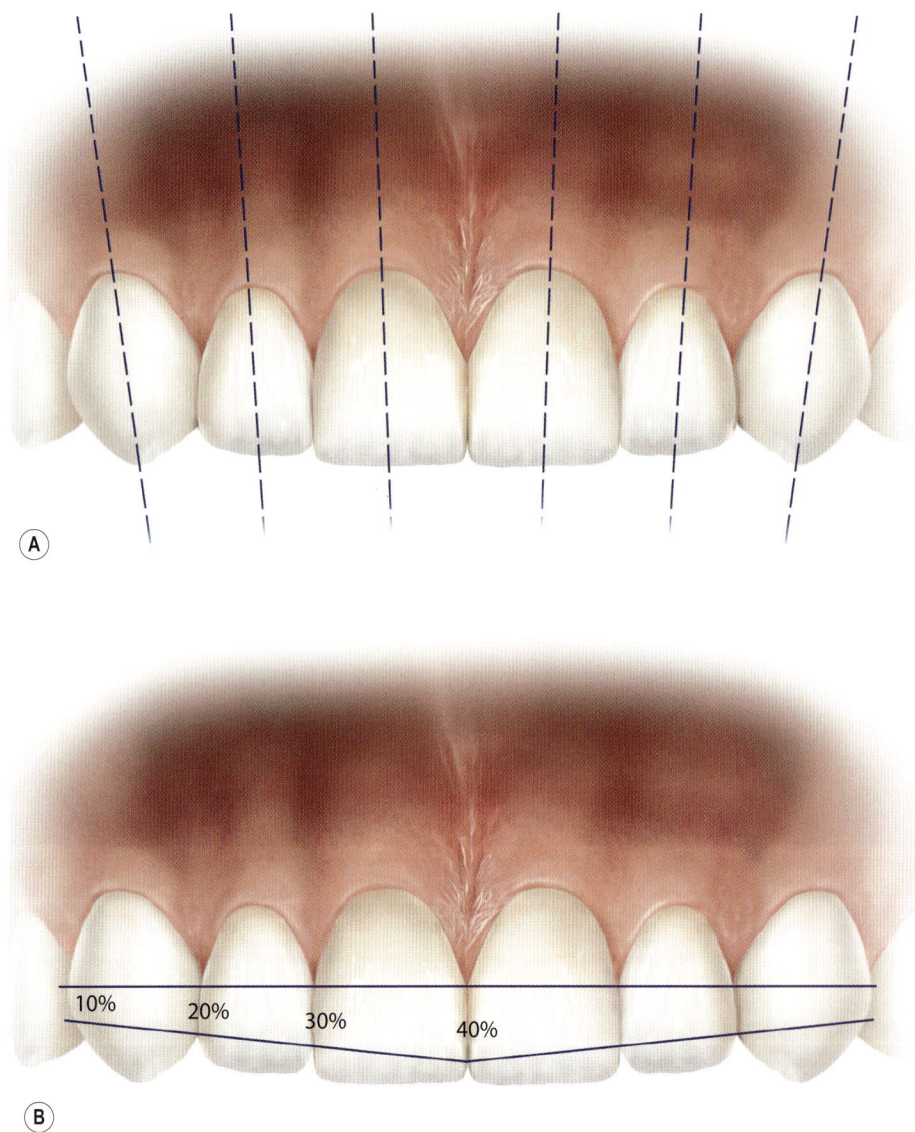

Fig. 1.19A,B Axial inclination.

CLINICAL TIP

One of our rules for the high smile line patient is never to exceed 10.5 mm for the height of the central incisor, as this would create an imbalance in the lower third of the face.

- Tooth-to-tooth proportion (Fig. 1.21). The latest biometric study from Dr Stephen Chu shows that if the central incisor's mesiodistal width is X mm, then the lateral should measure X–2 mm and the canine should be X–1 mm.[11] Note that X–1 should account for the entire mesiodistal width of the canine, versus the traditional golden proportion approach that only accounted for the mesial half of this tooth.

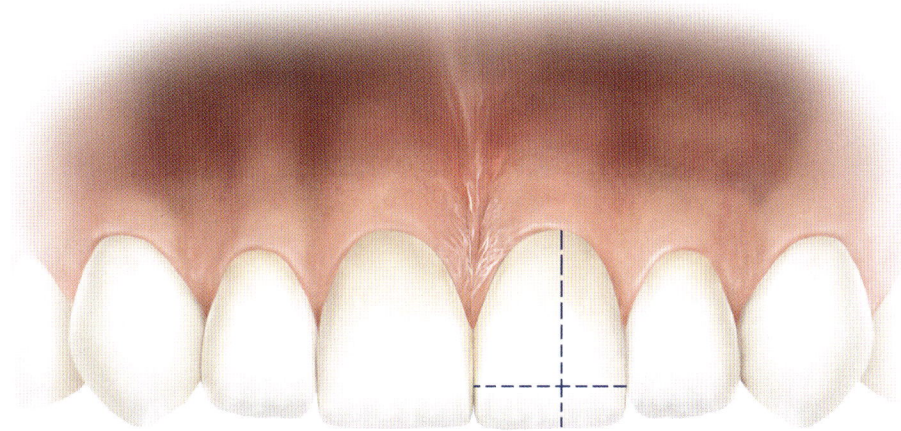

Fig. 1.20 Tooth proportion.

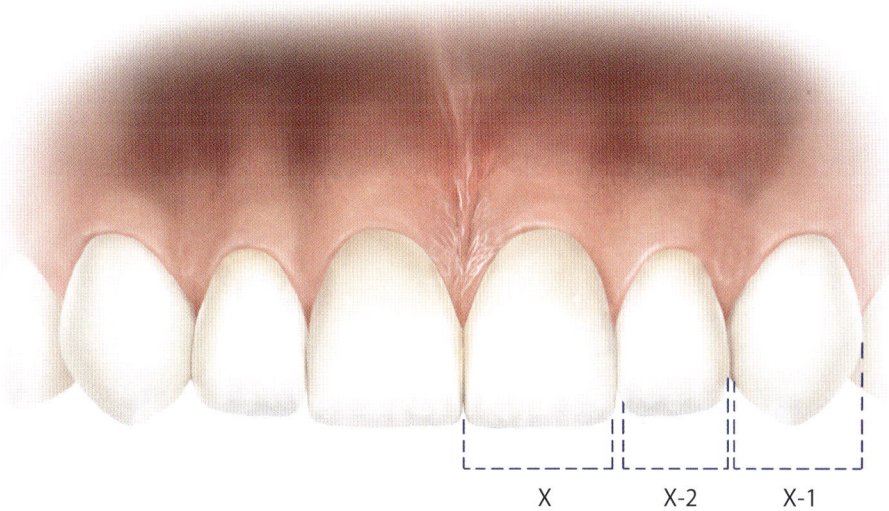

Fig. 1.21 Tooth-to-tooth proportion.

- Line angles (Fig. 1.22). The contour ridges, or line angles, give the outline form to the teeth. Adjusting the line angles of a tooth can make it appear wider or narrower.

- Height of contour (labial view). The height of contour should be distal to the midline at the gingival third (Fig. 1.23).

- Papilla proportions (Fig. 1.24). The papilla occupies 40% of the space from the contact area to the cemento-enamel junction of the central incisors and stays consistent in this volume from central to lateral to canine.[12]

THE ESTHETIC EVALUATION FORM

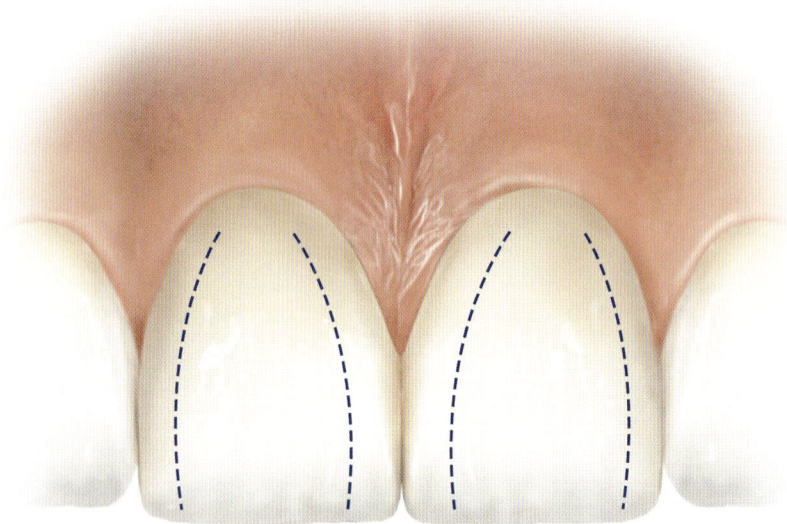

Fig. 1.22　Line angles.

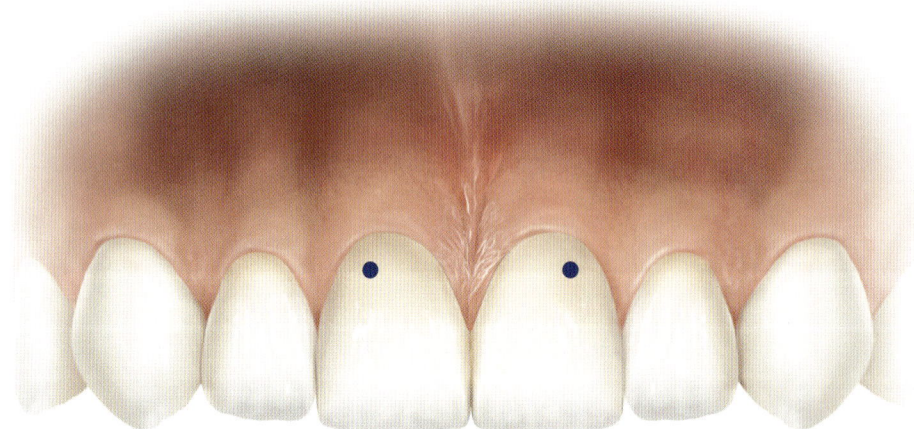

Fig. 1.23　Height of contour – labial view.

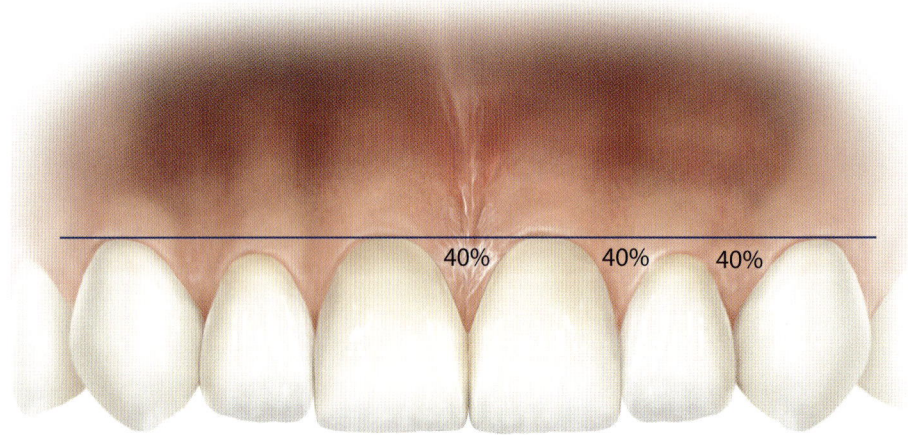

Fig. 1.24　Papilla proportion.

CHAPTER 1
ESTHETIC DIAGNOSIS: A THREE-STEP ANALYSIS

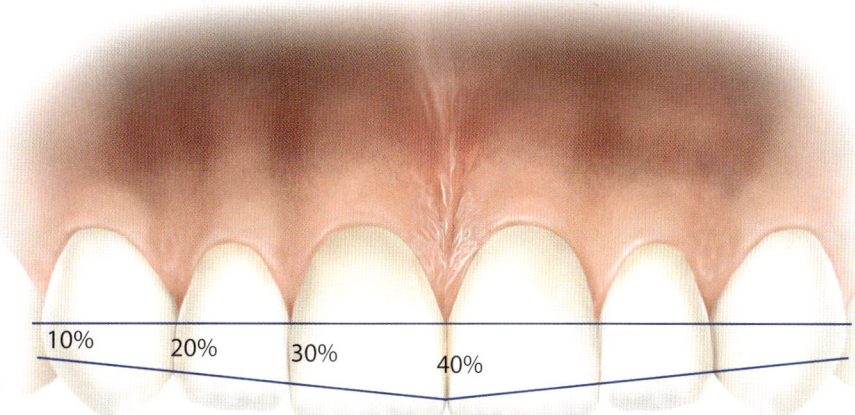

Fig. 1.25 Contact area.

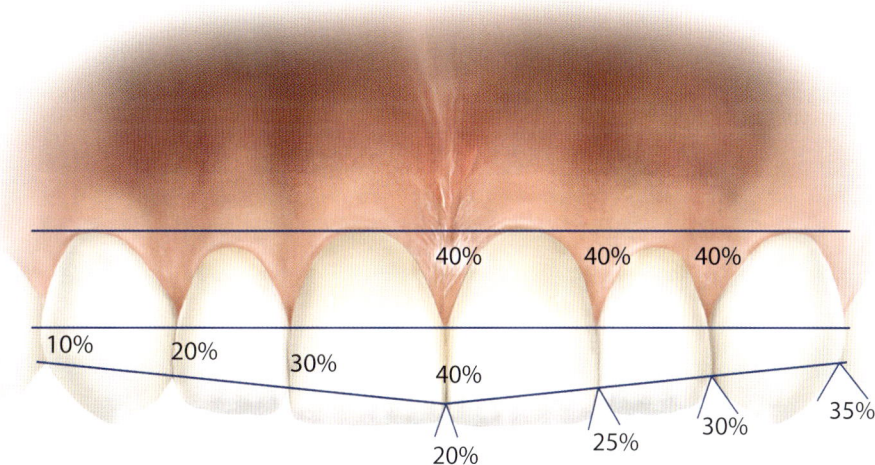

Fig. 1.26 Incisal embrasures.

- Contact area (Fig. 1.25). The contact area between the centrals starts at 40% of the height of the tooth and decreases to 30%, 20% and 18% as we go from the central to the lateral to the canine, and then to the distal of the canine.[13]

- Incisal embrasures (Fig. 1.26). Between the central incisors the embrasure space makes up 20% of the tooth's height. This increases to 25%, 30% and 35% as we move distally.[13] Abrasion and wear cause the incisal embrasures to disappear over time, and so recreating these embrasures will give our patients a more rejuvenated look.

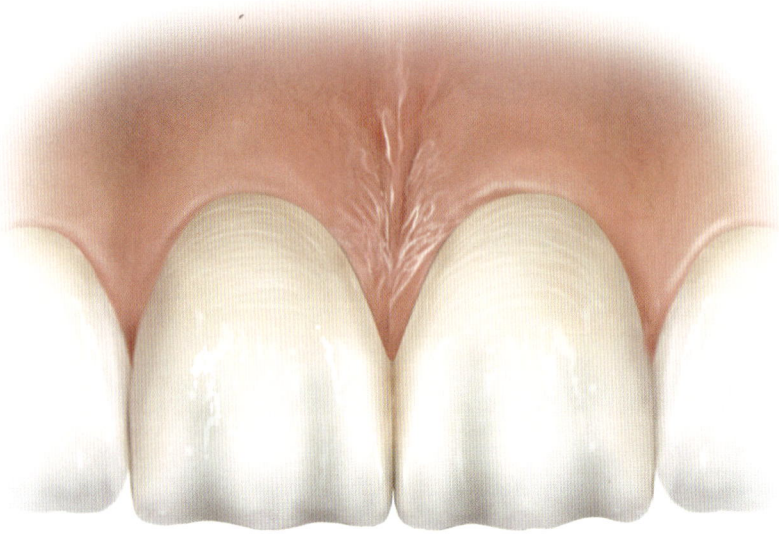

Fig. 1.27 Texture.

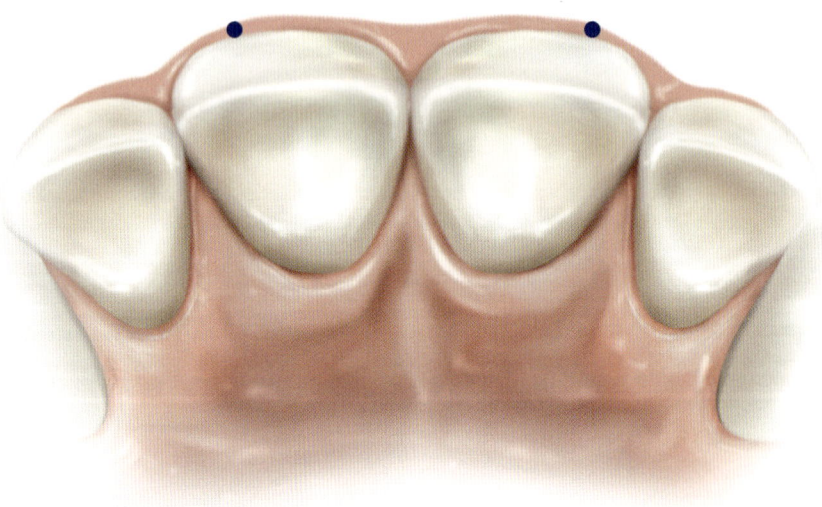

Fig. 1.28 Height of contour – incisal apical view.

- Texture (Fig. 1.27). This shows where the lobes of the tooth are formed in development and occurs in both a vertical and horizontal direction. It is an element that gives the tooth a more natural look and we must ask whether the patient desires this.

- Height of contour (incisal view) (Fig. 1.28). This vantage point shows that the maxillary central's height of contour is distal to the tooth's midline.

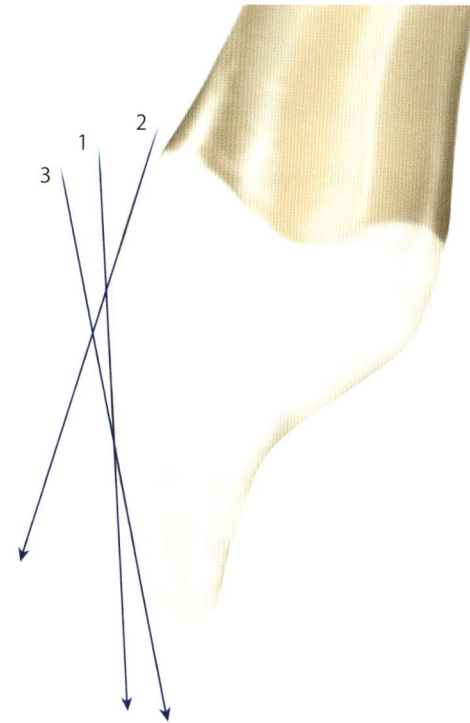

Fig. 1.29 Profile view.

- Profile view. This view shows that there are three planes of the tooth from the cemento-enamel junction, through the body of the tooth, to the incisal edge (Fig. 1.29).[6]

- Parallel of curves (Fig. 1.30). The contact points, incisal edges and lower lip should form three curves that echo one another harmoniously.[6,14]

- Incisal edge contour (Fig. 1.31). A 3-dimensional edge on the anterior tooth creates a natural appearance. The edges of worn anterior teeth have well-defined buccal and lingual incisal line angles, and these contours can be emphasized or minimized depending on our esthetic goals.

We indicate, on the form, whether each of these elements is acceptable or not in the existing dentition, and if not our planned improvements are described. By becoming comfortable in this language of micro-esthetics we can communicate meaningfully with our lab technician, and little is left to the imagination.

THE ESTHETIC EVALUATION FORM

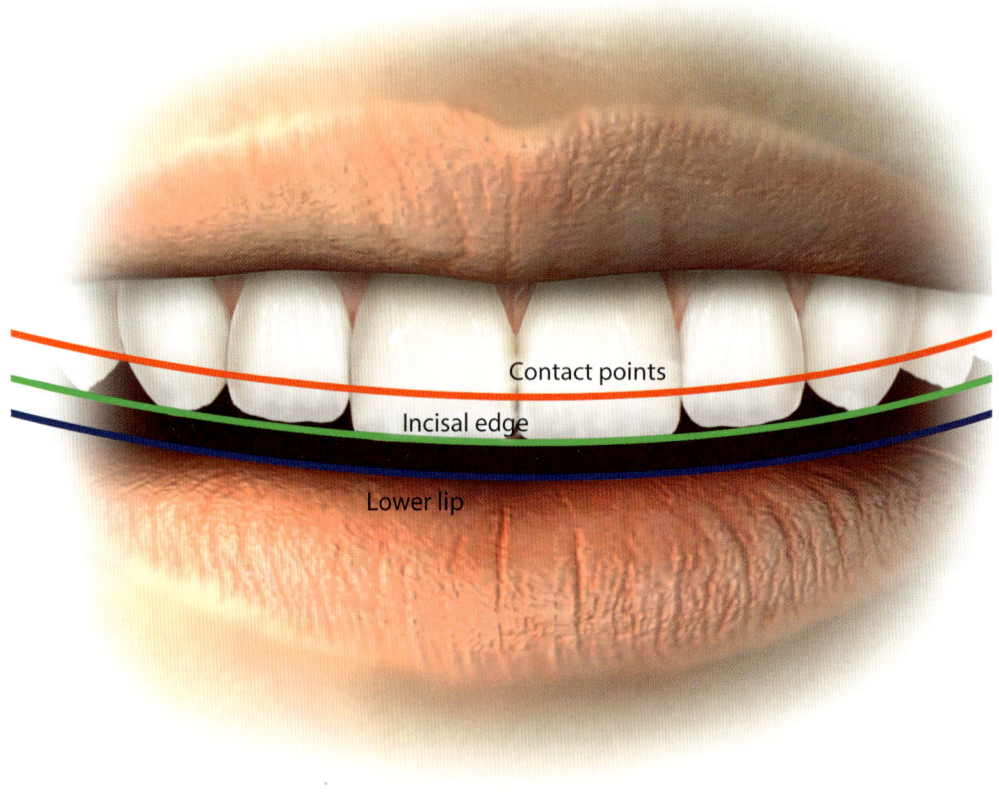

Fig. 1.30 Parallel of curves.

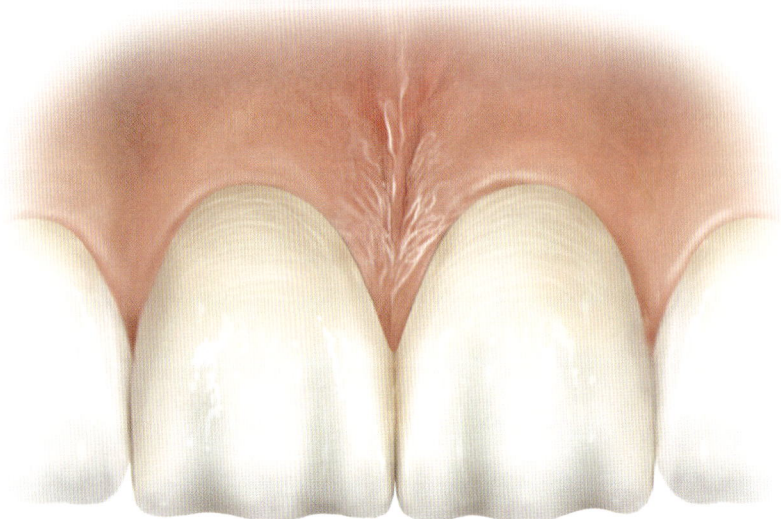

Fig. 1.31 Incisal edge contour.

RECORDS

Obtaining the patient's radiographs, diagnostic casts, interocclusal records and photographs is essential in helping us reach a proper diagnosis. These records should be thorough and accurate enough to diagnose and create a treatment plan for the entire case without having the patient present.

PHOTOGRAPHY AND VIDEO

A complete series of photographs can be taken before, during or after filling out the Esthetic Evaluation Form. In our opinion, however, it is beneficial to take all photographs after completing the form, as the clinician will be more aware of what each shot should capture. 'The eyes', as they say, 'don't see what the mind doesn't know.'

The following photographs should be obtained:

- Facial (Fig. 1.32A–C): full smile, normal smile and repose.
- Oblique facial (Fig. 1.33A–C): full smile, normal smile and repose.
- Lateral facial (Fig. 1.34A–C): full smile, normal smile and repose.
- Dentofacial:
  - Frontal (Fig. 1.35A–C): full smile, normal smile and repose ('emma')
  - Oblique: full smile, normal smile and repose (Fig. 1.36A–C).
- Dental (retracted views):
  - Retracted frontal and oblique (Fig. 1.37A–B)
  - Occlusal maxillary and mandibular (Fig. 1.38A–B).

In addition to photographs, the use of video can be very helpful to the clinician. Filming the patient talking, smiling and laughing naturally offers a dynamic view that can be very instructive to the dental esthetic team. A real or 'dynamic' smile is often much wider (and with a higher lip line) than a posed or 'static' smile. Engaging the patient in a short, relaxed video interview can evoke this truer smile, the smile around which the case should be designed.

Video is also particularly helpful in the assessment of phonetics. Slowing down a video is an excellent way to observe the position of the lips and teeth as 'S', 'F' and 'E' sounds are pronounced.

Just as with photographs and other records, sharing any videos with the technician will greatly help with the diagnostic wax-up and the second consultation with the patient.

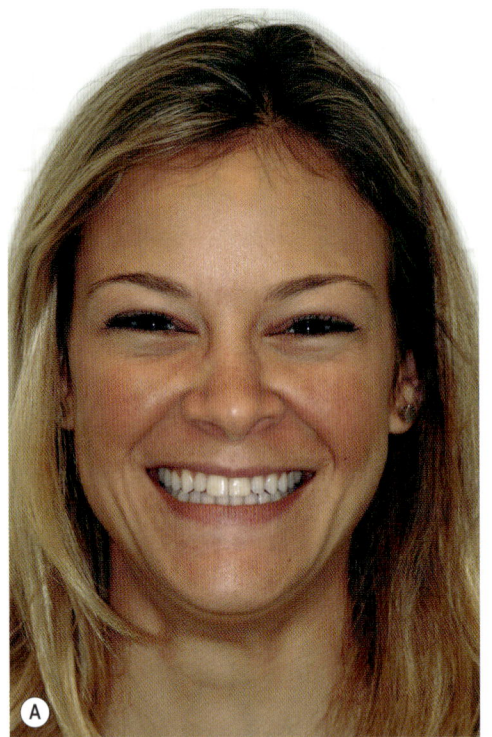
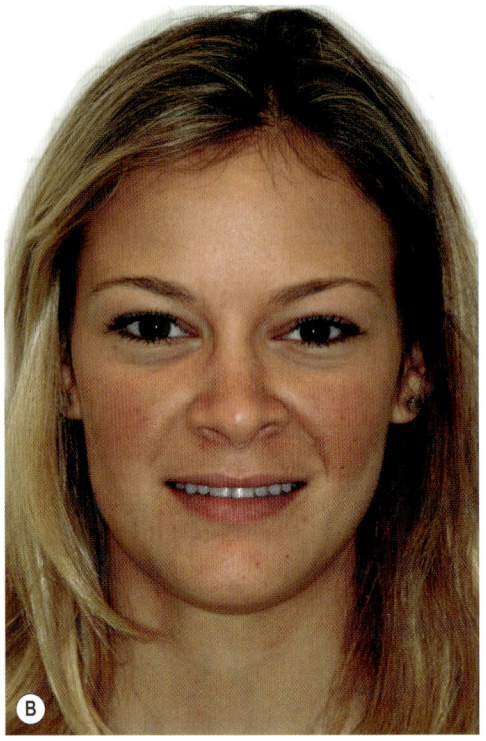
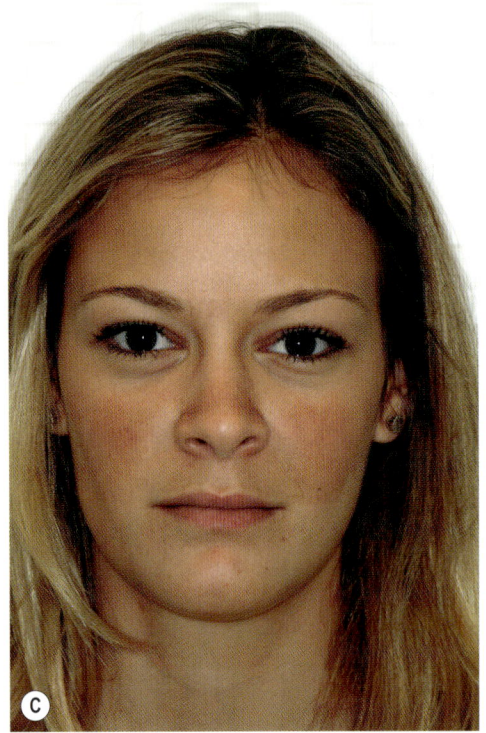

Fig. 1.32A–C Facial photos: (A) **full smile**, (B) **normal smile** and (C) **repose.**

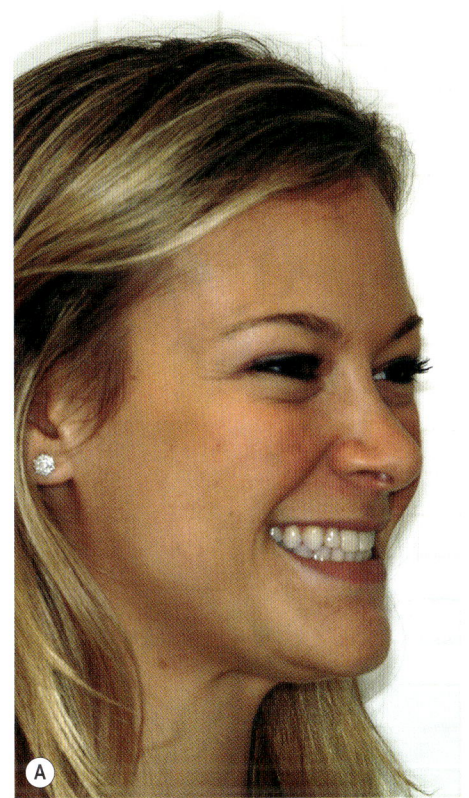
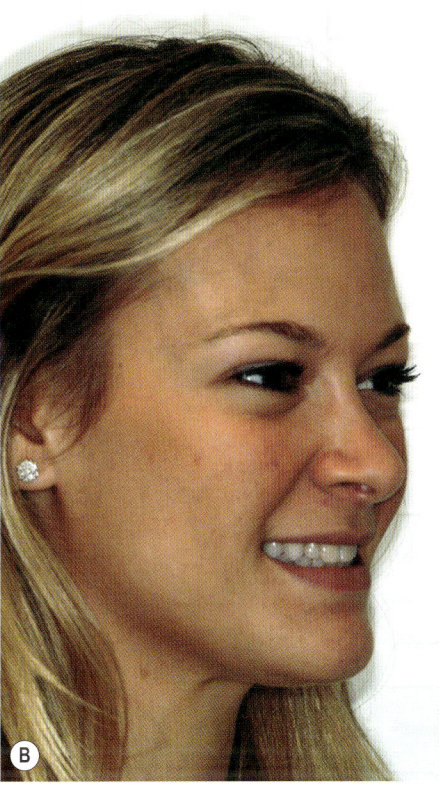
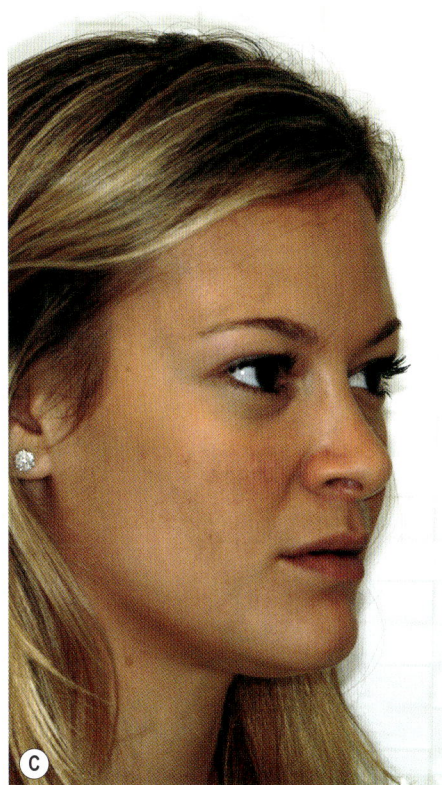

Fig. 1.33A–C   Oblique facial photos: (A) full smile, (B) normal smile and (C) repose.

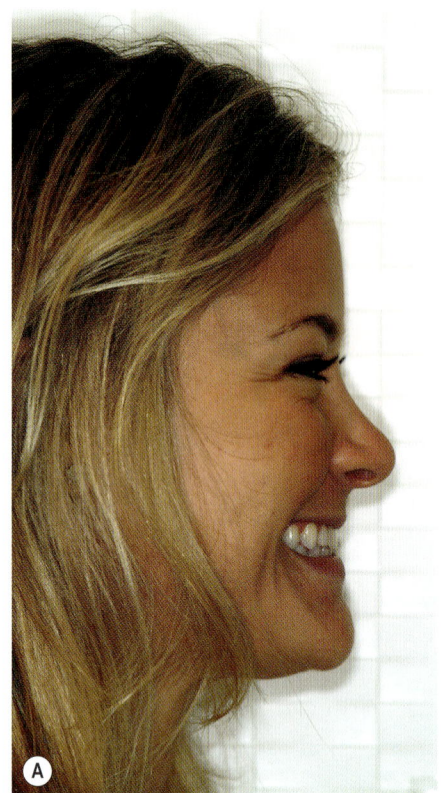
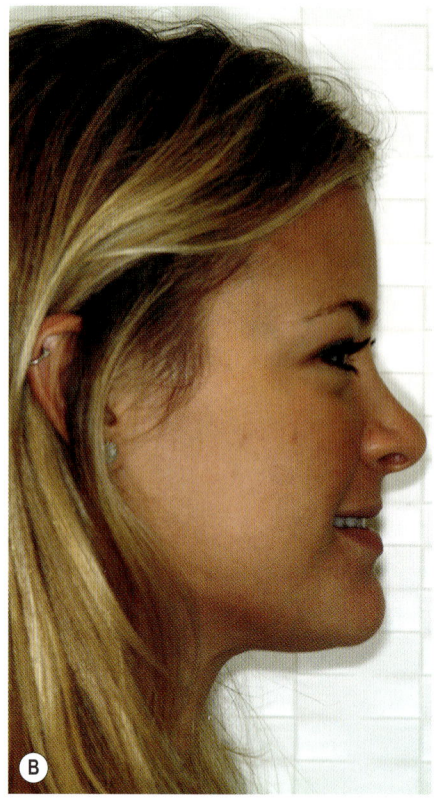
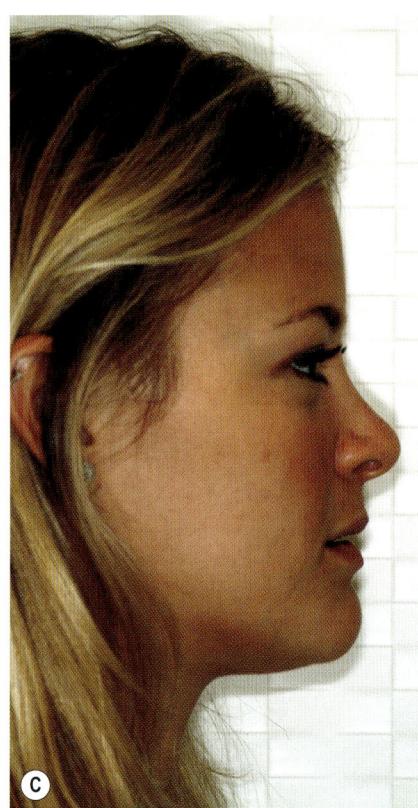

Fig. 1.34A–C Lateral facial photos: (A) full smile, (B) normal smile and (C) repose.

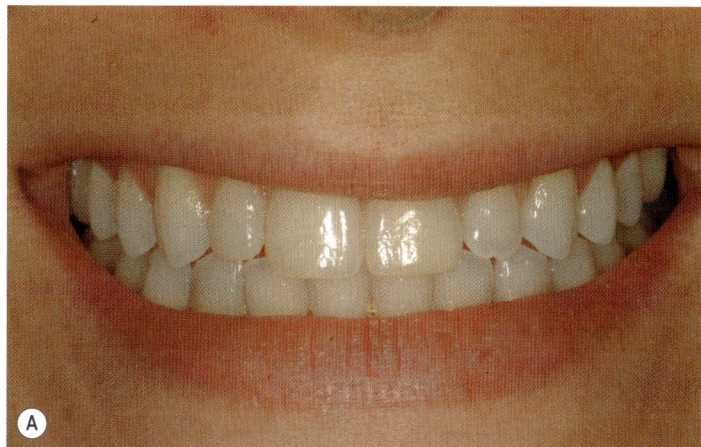
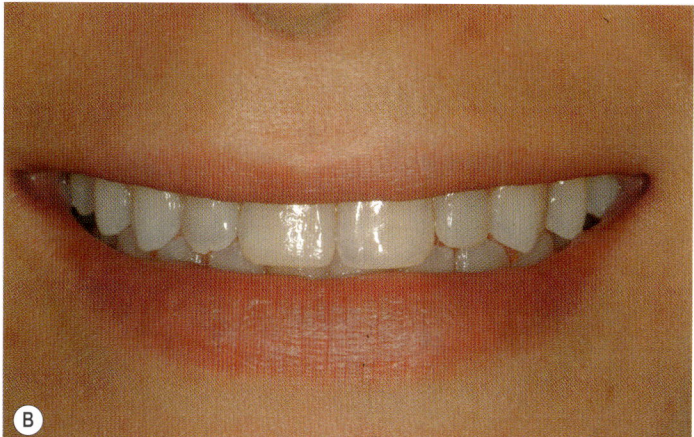
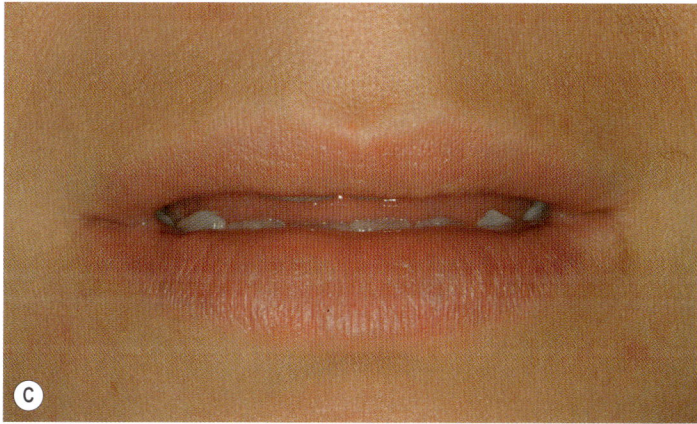

Fig. 1.35A–C   Frontal: (A) full smile, (B) normal smile and (C) repose ('emma').

DIAGNOSTIC CASTS

Once the Esthetic Evaluation Form has been completed we move to the next step: study casts mounted on an articulator, either in centric occlusion (CO) or centric relation (CR).

CLINICAL TIP

The decision to mount in CO or CR is made based on the presence of pathology. We analyse the occlusion for any signs of pathology (abfractions, worn incisal edges or occlusal areas, wear facets or cracks in the teeth) and if signs exist then the CR bite is obtained.

If there is no pathology then we register the habitual position of the mandible (centric occlusion). In either case a facebow is used to parallel the upper arch to the horizon and we find that in most cases a Kois Dentofacial Analyzer will suffice. This device was made for use with a Panadent articulator and is a simplified facebow that relates the maxilla to the true horizon by using levelling gauges (Fig. 1.39). This is a different approach from that of the traditional

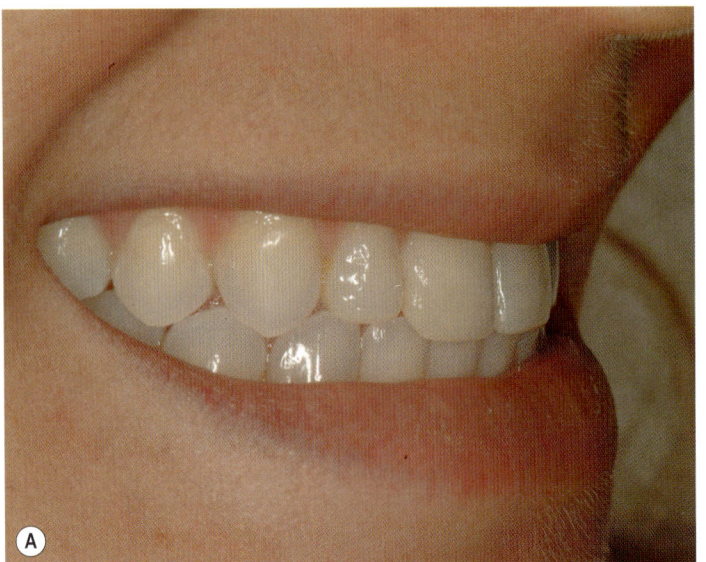
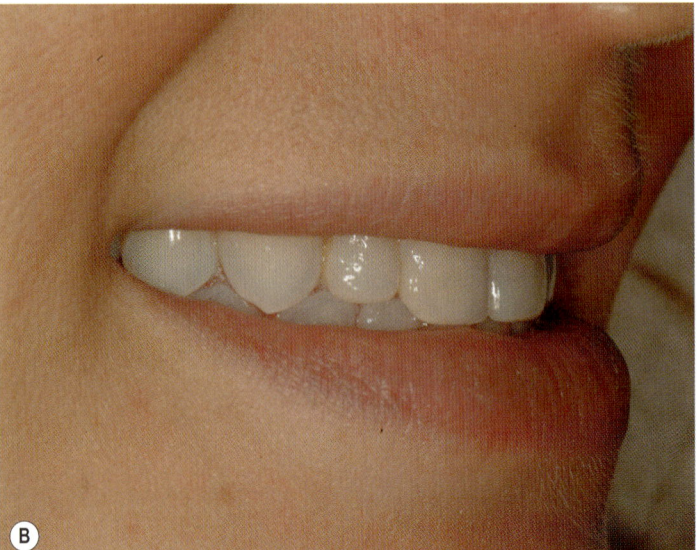
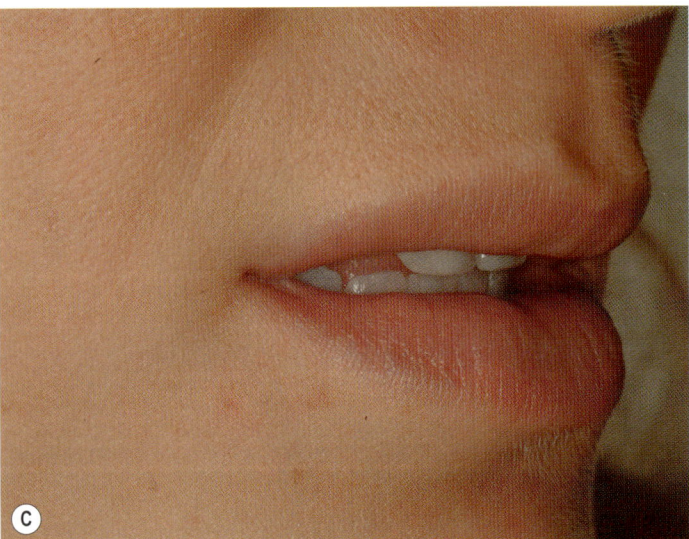

Fig. 1.36A–C Oblique: (A) full smile, (B) normal smile and (C) repose.

facebow, which is ear-mounted and assumes the line connecting the ears is level (whereas it is usually not). That being said, a traditional facebow is still indicated in certain particularly complex cases.

If we are recording the CO (habitual) position, then a traditional bite registration or even hand articulation for the maxillo-mandibular relationship is registered. If a CR position is being sought, then it is favourable to use a leaf gauge for an anterior stop and a Delar wax bite registration posteriorly, taken right before first tooth contact (Figs 1.40 and 1.41). The recommended leaf gauge technique is to remove leaves one by one, and at each increment checking for posterior contact with 15 μ *AccuFilm*. Once the first point of contact is identified, several

ESTHETIC DIAGNOSIS: A THREE-STEP ANALYSIS

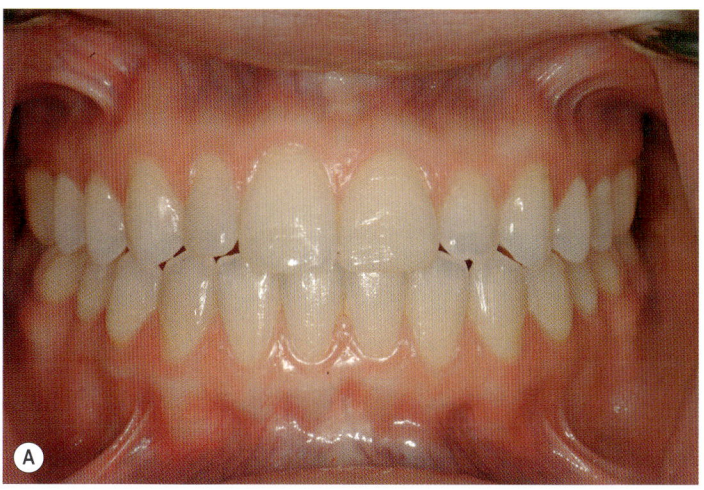 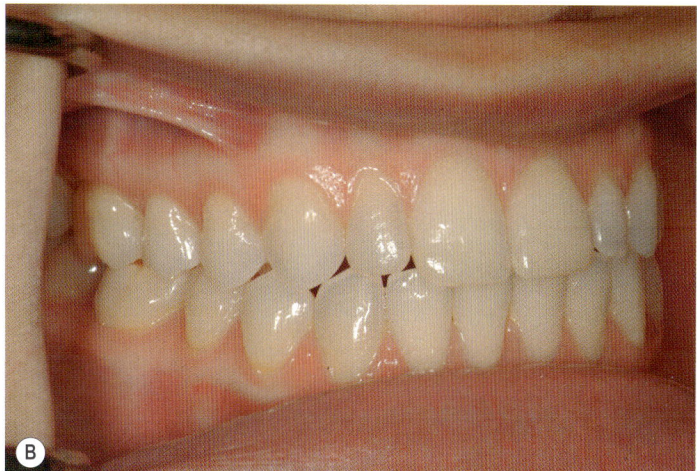

Fig. 1.37A,B Retracted: (A) frontal and (B) oblique.

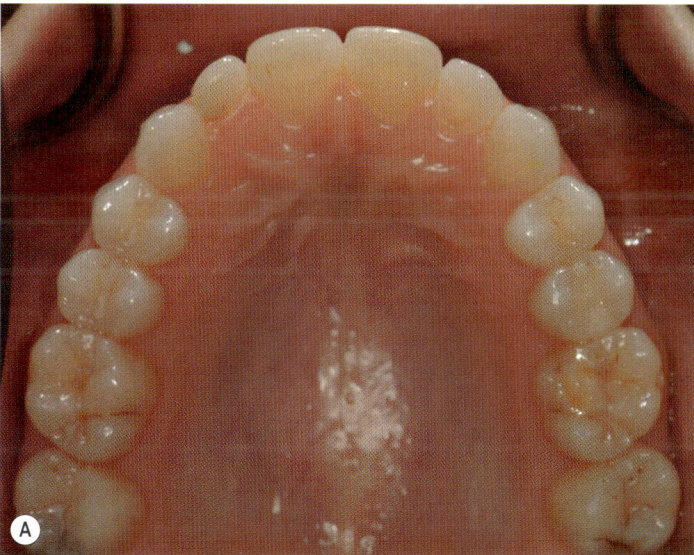 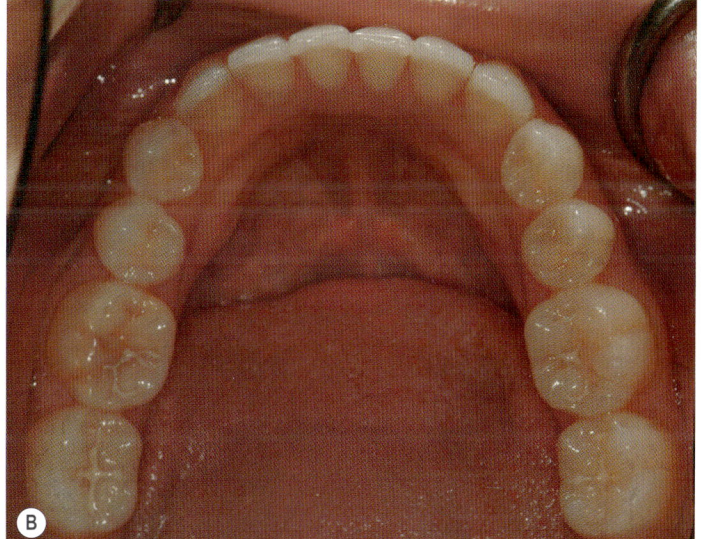

Fig. 1.38A,B Occlusal: (A) maxillary and (B) mandibular.

leaves are added back onto the gauge and the bite registration material is inserted.

Once the maxillo-mandibular relationship is recorded, the models are mounted. We are now ready for the diagnostic wax-up (Fig. 1.42).

THE DIAGNOSTIC WAX-UP

From the information gathered on our Esthetic Evaluation Form we know precisely where the gingival margin and incisal edge of the maxillary central incisor should be positioned. With the tooth's height known, the ideal width

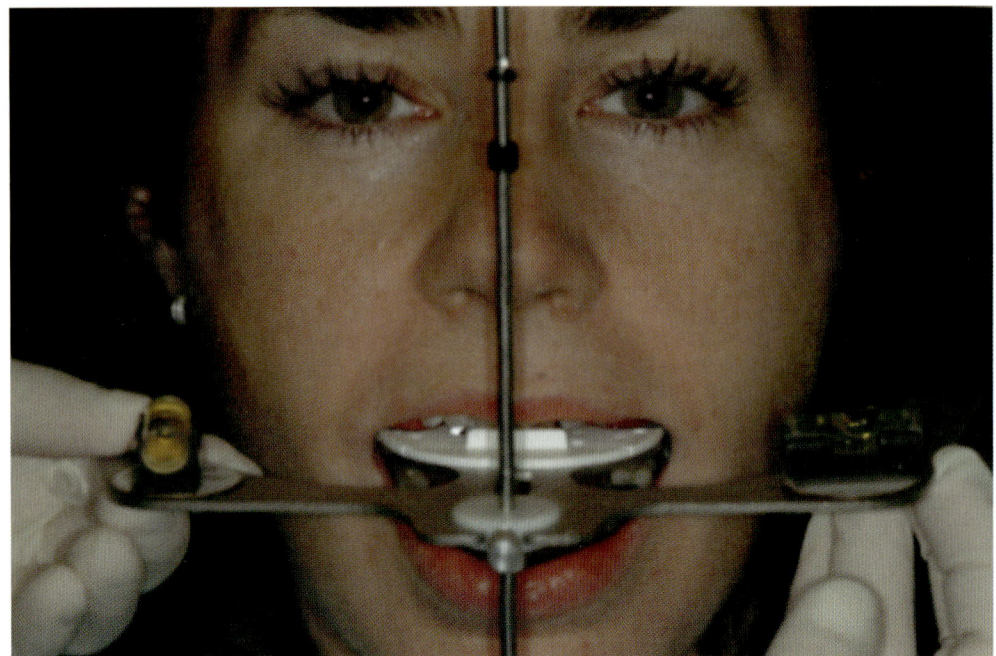

Fig. 1.39 The Kois Dentofacial Analyzer.

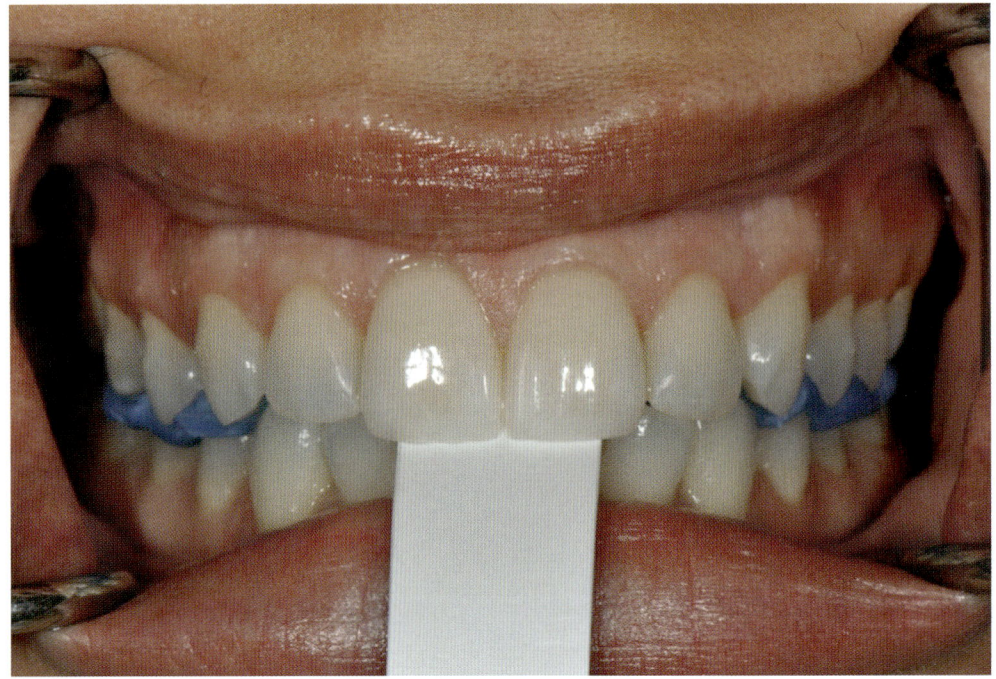

Fig. 1.40 A leaf gauge for an anterior stop.

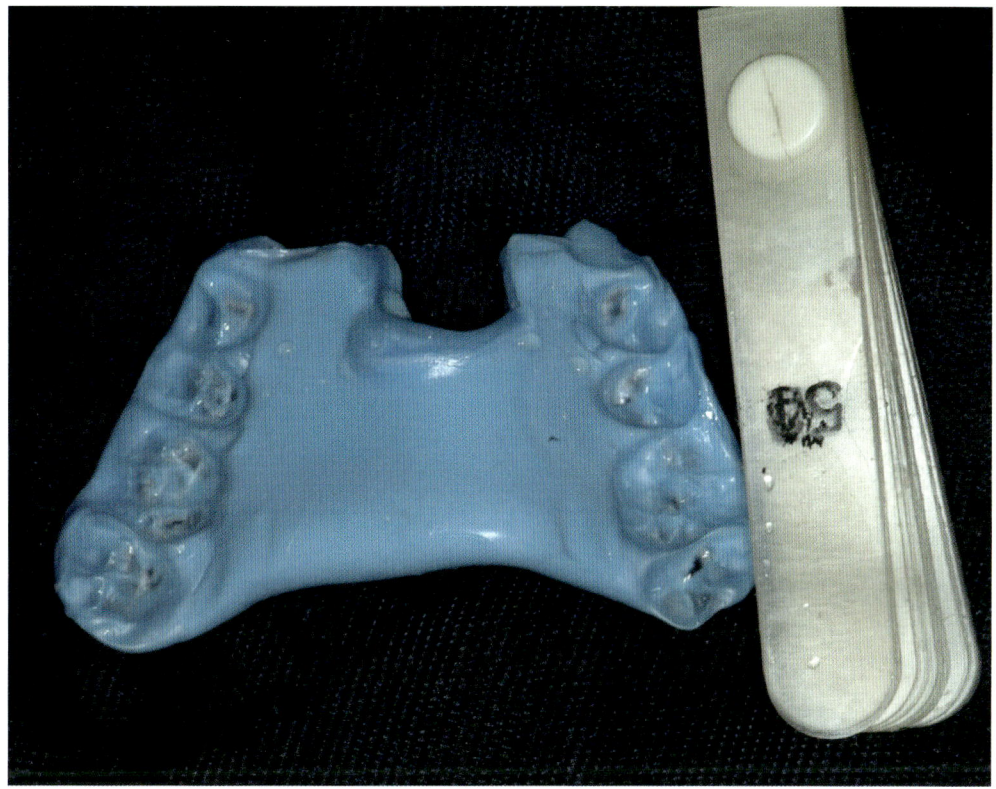

Fig. 1.41 A Delar wax bite registration (Almore International, Inc) posteriorly.

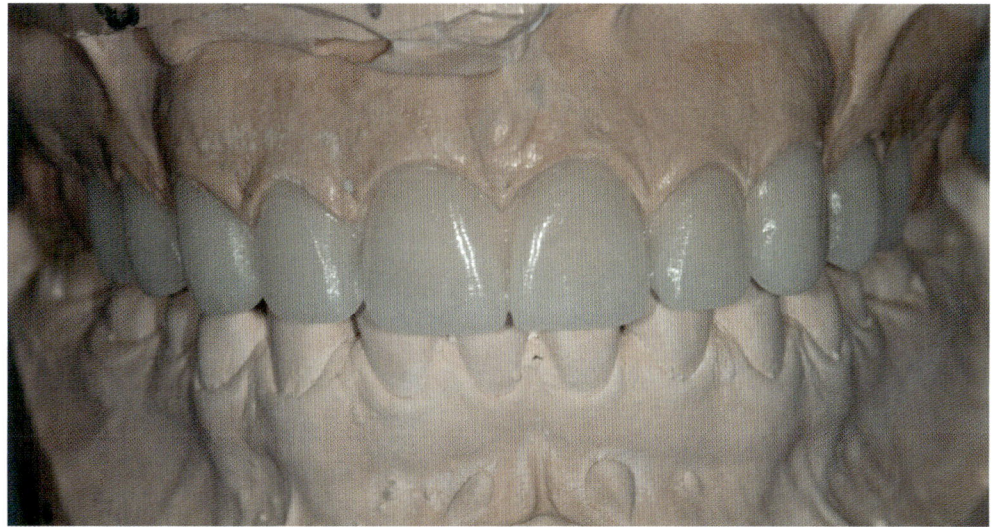

Fig. 1.42 The diagnostic wax-up.

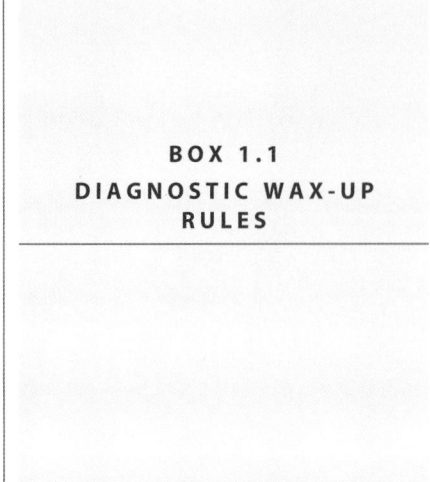

**BOX 1.1
DIAGNOSTIC WAX-UP RULES**

1. Start with the centrals and develop a proper height:width ratio of 80%.
2. Symmetry at the midline: soft tissue height and tooth symmetry (centrals are mirror images of each other). Distalize any imperfections.
3. Establish tooth-to-tooth proportion:

   central–lateral–cuspid

   X   X–2   X–1
4. Axial inclination towards the distal, reflected by proper line angle positions (line angles echo root inclination).
5. Progression of incisal embrasures. Incisal embrasures get larger as we move from centrals to laterals to canines.
6. Create a more interesting display; consider adding slight asymmetries moving away from the midline. Consider cohesive and segregative factors.

can be calculated as 80% of that number (and we know that anywhere in the 75–85% range is acceptable). Based on this width (X mm) Stephen Chu's[11] biometric formula quickly provides the widths of the canines (X–1) and the laterals (X–2). The general guidelines for the wax-up are summarized in Box 1.1.

THE ESTHETIC MOCK-UP

With the wax-up complete, we can now visualize our changes intra-orally by a direct transfer into the patient's mouth. This 'mock-up' technique works well when a case is additive, i.e. expanding the arch or adding length to the teeth. When the case is reductive in nature, as some cases must be, simply presenting the wax-up to the patient and/or utilizing digital imaging are two other ways to convey our vision.

INTRA-ORAL MOCK-UP

A silicone putty or clear injectable silicone (i.e. Memosil, Discus Dental Bite, 3M Express or Heraeus Flexitime) is taken of the diagnostic wax-up (Fig. 1.43). The index is then filled with a provisional material (i.e. 3M Protemp or Dentsply Integrity) and allowed to set on the teeth. If a clear injectable material, such as Memosil, is used then any light-cured provisional material is an option as well.

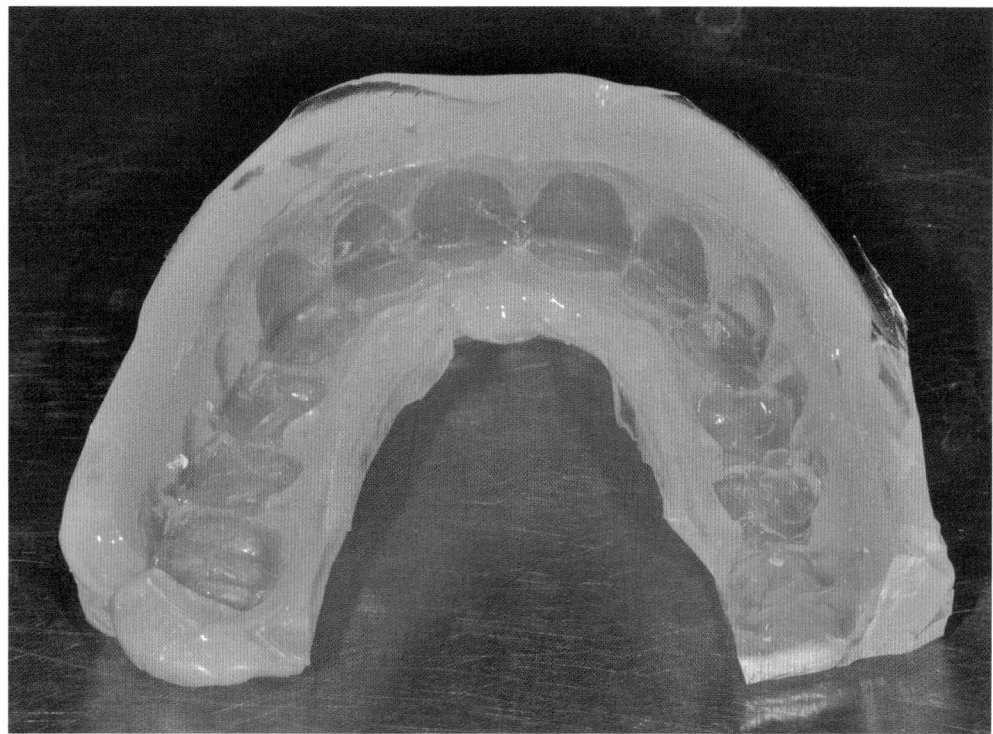

Fig. 1.43 A clear injectable material of the diagnostic wax-up.

In terms of shade, a patient seeking 'straight, white and perfect' would indicate more of a bleached shade for this mock-up, whereas those requesting 'clean, healthy and natural' should be shown a B1 or A1 shaded material.

With the mock-up applied and cleaned up (i.e. any excess is easily removed with a sickle-shaped scalpel) the patient is given a mirror and offered the first glimpse of our 3-dimensional blueprint (Figs 1.44 and 1.45). We can now discuss what the patient likes and does not like esthetically, and make any adjustments directly in the mouth. Once the patient is satisfied with the esthetics of the mock-up, we can check phonetics and occlusion and make any necessary adjustments in those areas as well. Photographs and an alginate impression are then obtained, and it is around this time the patient often asks, 'When do we start?'

CONSIDERATIONS FOR A REDUCTIVE MOCK-UP

When the diagnostic wax-up is not additive (i.e. we are not adding volume and/or length to the teeth and the arch), we need to employ different techniques, alone or in combination, to visualize and discuss the proposed changes.

Computer imaging software (Fig. 1.46A–B) has been available since the late 1980s, and there are a number of highly sophisticated programs available today.

THE ESTHETIC MOCK-UP

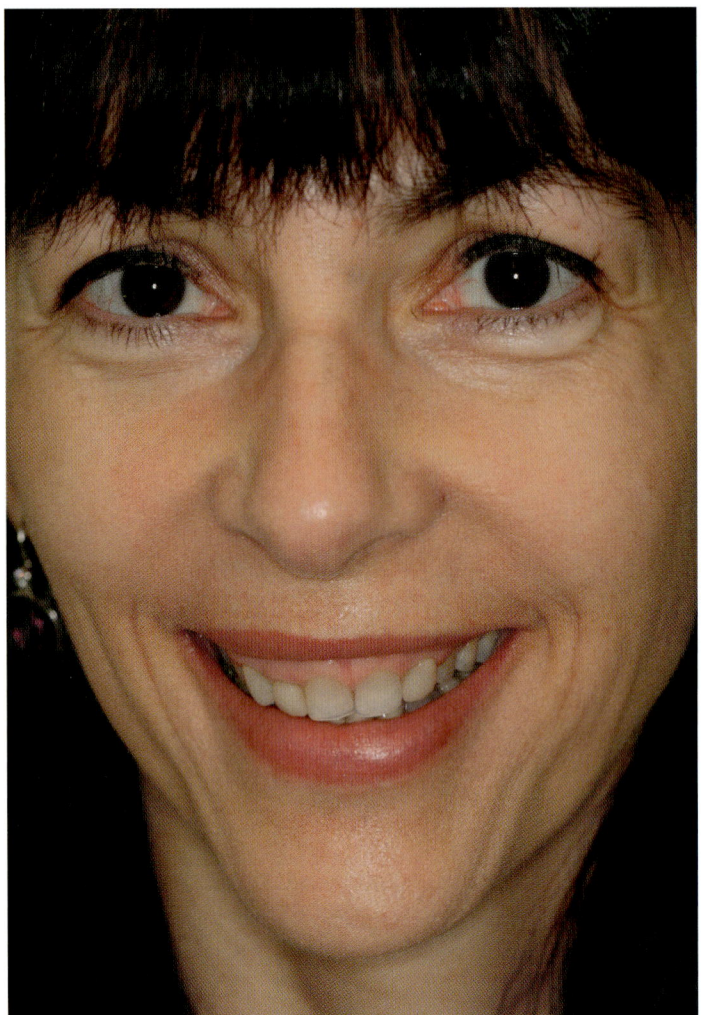

Fig. 1.44 Before the mock up, with a shared vision for the esthetic team of lightening the shade, widening the arch, improving the tooth form and correcting gingival symmetry.

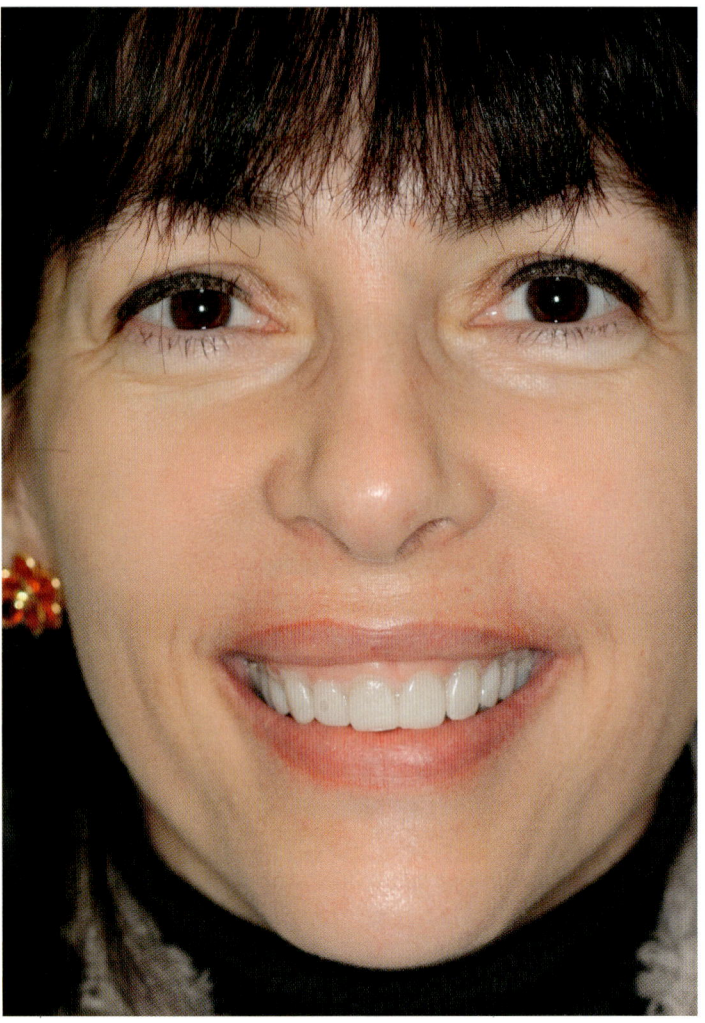

Fig. 1.45 Mock-up. Visualizing the diagnostic wax-up directly in the mouth from the shared vision.

When using imaging software, it is advised that the dentist controls the simulation – versus an assistant or a third party service – as we must be careful not to show anything that may not be achievable.[15] Ideally, this 2-dimensional digital imaging should only reflect changes we have been able to build into the 3-dimensional diagnostic wax-up. Christian Coachman's Digital Smile Design protocol, described in Chapter 9, p. 294, employs calibrated digital rulers that make our digital simulations more precise than traditional digital imaging techniques.

Another technique for visualizing reductive changes is the use of a black marker to shorten the teeth. As the patient opens their mouth the incisal silhouette of the mouth blends in with the black marks at the incisal edges, simulating shortened teeth (Figs 1.47A,B).

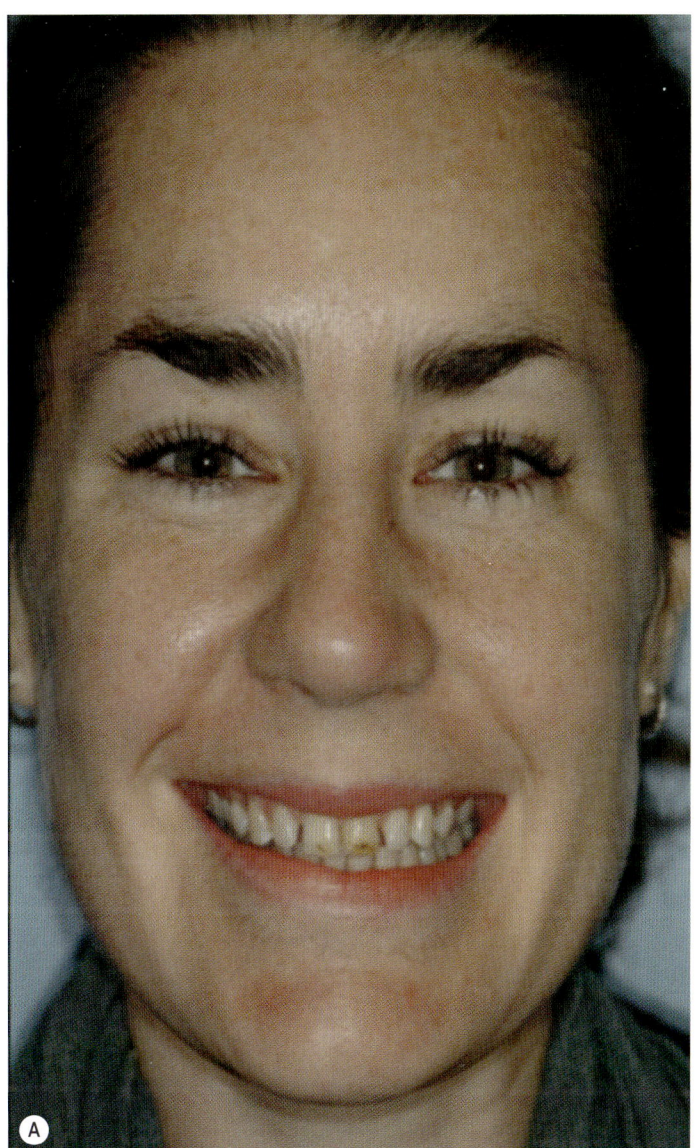
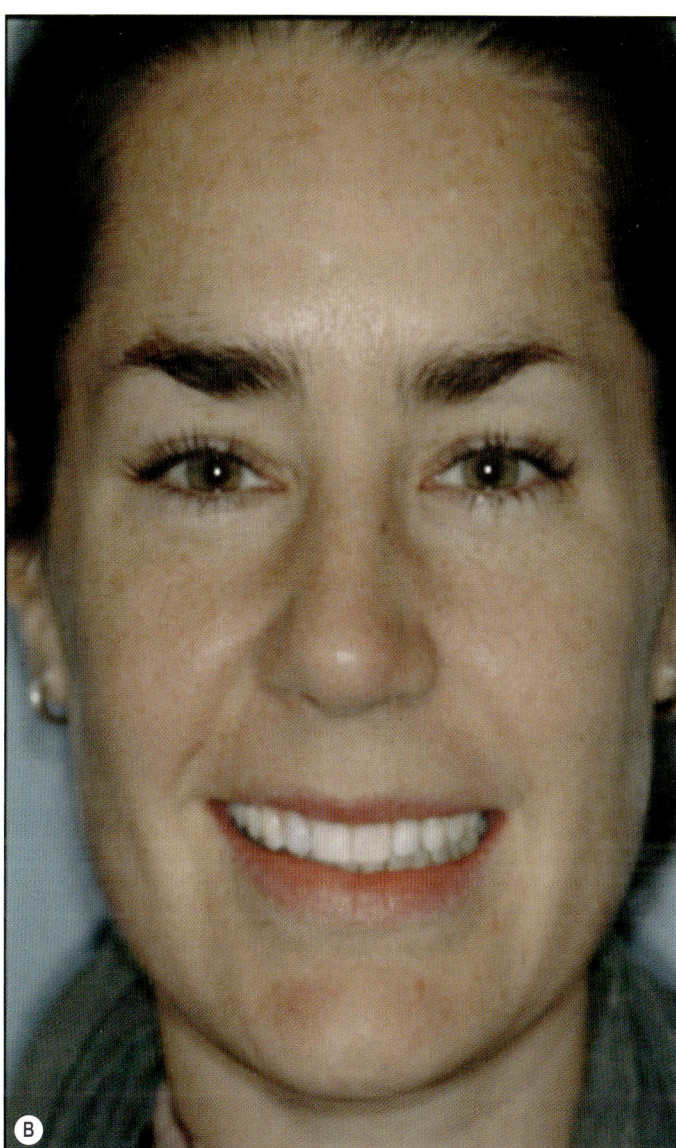

Fig. 1.46A,B Using computer imaging software: (A) before and (B) after.

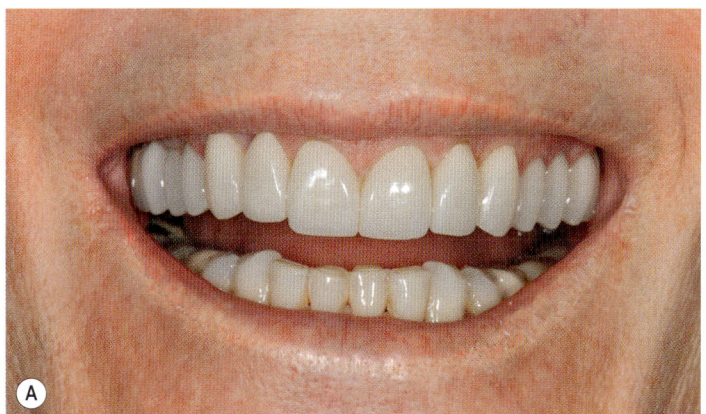
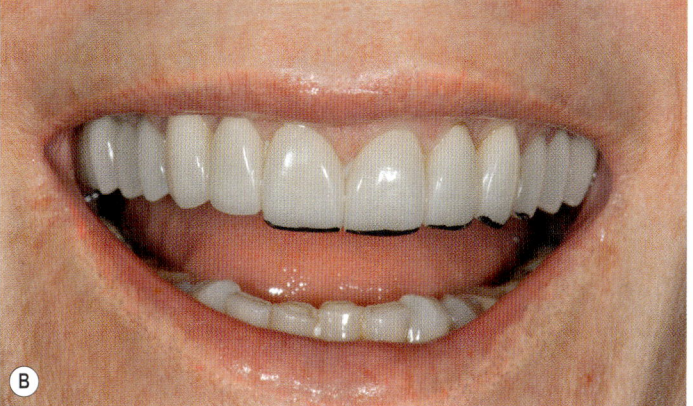

Fig. 1.47A,B The incisal silhouette of the mouth blends in with the black marks at the incisal edges, simulating shortened teeth. (A) Before and (B) after.

Yet another way to visualize reductive changes is to simply present the diagnostic wax-up to the patient, cleanly mounted on an articulator. There are several different colours of wax available for wax-ups, but white wax should be used in this situation. The phonetics and occlusion can be perfected later on when the teeth are temporized.

With our patient's problems identified and the solution visualized, we can now choose the most appropriate course of action and proceed with the case.

SUMMARY

In this chapter we have presented a philosophy for predictable esthetic success. We use an Esthetic Evaluation Form to identify the problems, a diagnostic wax-up on mounted models to visualize the solution, and a direct mock-up or computer imaging to visually discuss the proposal. Once the solution is visualized (and perhaps modified), the most appropriate, conservative technique is chosen.

The esthetic diagnosis starts with open-ended questions to understand the patient's true needs. Maximum communication between the patient, dentist and technician moves us towards a visual proposal of our treatment plan and towards our ultimate goal of esthetic predictability and beautiful, healthy smiles for our patients.

ESSENTIALS

- This chapter described a methodical approach to an esthetics-driven diagnosis: identify the problem, visualize the solution and choose the appropriate technique.
- Identify the problems by utilizing the Esthetic Evaluation Form along with digital photos and mounted study casts. Evaluate macro-esthetics, micro-esthetics and function.
- Visualize the solution through a diagnostic wax-up of the mounted study casts and via intra-oral mock-up.
- Once the solution is visualized, choose the appropriate technique, which means the most conservative option that will achieve our esthetic goals.
- The key objective of the Esthetic Evaluation Form is to establish the incisal edge position and the gingival margin of the maxillary central incisor, two critical landmarks around which the entire case will be designed.

PATIENTS' FAQS

Q. Why are you asking me my opinion? You're supposed to be the expert!

A. Esthetics is subjective, which means that my opinion of beauty might not be the same as yours. It is important to establish, early on, what you consider to be 'beautiful', so we can plan your case accordingly. This whole process will be a team effort among you, the laboratory technician and me.

Q. Why are you taking so many pictures?

A. The more photographs I take, the better I can communicate with our laboratory technician. We want to be able to study your smile in detail and from every angle, and so these photographs are crucial.

Q. How many appointments will this take?

A. Three or four appointments. The next time I see you I will present my treatment plan and give you a preview of your new smile, which is a process we call a 'mock-up'. Depending on how many changes we make, if any, it will take one or two appointments beyond that to finish your case.

Q. How come the mock-up looks so thick?

A. The mock-up is a rough idea of what we are trying to achieve and, because it sits over your existing teeth, it may look and feel slightly more bulky than the final results. A little space will be made to accommodate the porcelain for the actual veneers or crowns, so they will not feel as thick as the mock-up.

Q. How much do you have to shave down my teeth?

A. The materials we use today are incredibly thin. The space required for a typical veneer is 0.3 mm, which is less than the thickness of a fingernail. Often we are adding length or bringing a tucked-in tooth 'out' and we do not need to make any space.

Seminal literature

Matthews T. The anatomy of a smile. J Aesthet Dent 1978;39:1.

Spear FM, Kokich VG, Mathews DP. Interdisciplinary management of anterior dental esthetics. J Am Dent Assoc 2006;137(2):160–9.

Tjan AH, Miller GD. Some esthetic factors in a smile. J Prosthet Dent 1984;51(1):24–8.

REFERENCES

1. Spear FM, Kokich VG, Mathews DP. Interdisciplinary management of anterior dental esthetics. J Am Dent Assoc 2006;137(2):160–9.

2. Vig RG, Brundo GC. The kinetics of anterior tooth display. J Prosthet Dent 1978;39(5):502–4.

3. Arnett GW, Bergman RT. Facial keys to orthodontic diagnosis and treatment planning. Part 1. Am J Orthod Dentofacial Orthop 1993;103(4):299–312.

4. Magne P, Gallucci GO, Belser UC. Anatomic crown width/length ratios of unworn and worn maxillary teeth in white subjects. J Prosthet Dent 2003;89(5):453–61.

5. Chu SJ. Range and mean distribution frequency of individual tooth width of the maxillary anterior dentition. Pract Proced Aesthet Dent 2007;19(4):209–15.

6. Rufenacht CR. Fundamentals of esthetics. Hanover Park, IL: Quintessence; 1990:116–19, 118–19.

7. Kokich VO, Kiyak HA, Shapiro PA. Comparing the perception of dentists and lay people to altered dental esthetics. J Esthet Dent 1999;11(6):311–24.

References

8. Brose M, Tanquist RA. The influence of anterior coupling on mandibular movement. J Prosthet Dent 1987;57(3):345–53.

9. Gurel G. The science and art of porcelain laminate veneers. Hanover Park, IL: Quintessence; 2003:72–3, 75–6.

10. Chu SJ, Tan JH, Stappert CF, Tarnow DP. Gingival zenith positions and levels of the maxillary anterior dentition. J Esthet Restor Dent 2009;21(2):113–20.

11. Chu SJ. A biometric approach to predictable treatment of clinical crown discrepancies. Pract Proced Aesthet Dent 2007;19(7):401–9.

12. Chu SJ, Tarnow DP, Tan JH, Stappert CF. Papilla proportions in the maxillary anterior dentition. Int J Periodontics Restorative Dent 2009;29(4):385–93.

13. Stappert CF, Tarnow DP, Tan JH, Chu SJ. Proximal contact areas of the maxillary anterior dentition. Int J Periodontics Restorative Dent 2010;30(5):471–7.

14. Chiche G, Pinault A. Esthetics of anterior fixed prosthodontics. Hanover Park, IL: Quintessence; 1993:61–2.

15. Levine JB. Photography and smile imaging software, part 2. Aesthetic diagnosis, computer imaging and treatment planning. UK: King's College London.

CHAPTER 2

The Psychological Assessment of the Patient

SYLVIA S. WELSH

Overview of psychological issues pertinent to esthetic dentistry 46

A guideline for evaluating the patient's mental state 47

Summary 49

Consideration of the patient's emotional and psychological suitability and readiness for esthetic dental treatment is an important part of the dentist's initial consultation with the patient. While connected to the esthetic evaluation[1], the psychological assessment of the patient delves deeper into the patient's motivation for treatment and is critical to ensuring a successful outcome. This chapter will provide a brief overview of the relevant psychological issues and disorders that may be contraindications for esthetic treatment and a general guideline for conducting an evaluation of the patient's mental state.

OVERVIEW OF PSYCHOLOGICAL ISSUES PERTINENT TO ESTHETIC DENTISTRY

Patients seeking esthetic dental treatment may suffer from a wide range of emotional and psychological difficulties, but the majority of these difficulties do not pose obstacles to treatment. Nearly everyone experiences times (more or less often) of anxiety, self-doubt, unrealistic thinking, perfectionism, self-loathing and feelings of depression, to name but a few difficult emotional states. These feelings and thoughts are part of the human condition. It is only when such emotional/psychological states occur too frequently or are unremitting and interfere with a person's ability to function that they are considered disorders and may pose risks to treatment.

The most common psychological disorders of concern in esthetic dentistry are anorexia nervosa, bulimia nervosa, and body dysmorphic disorder. All three of these disorders are detailed in the DSM-V (*Diagnostic and Statistical Manual of Mental Disorders*, fifth edition).

Anorexia nervosa (DSM-V 307.1) is characterized by an obsession with body weight, an intense fear of gaining weight, a distorted perception of body weight and a dangerous restriction in calorie intake (i.e. eating) resulting in extreme weight loss. Efforts to control weight often entail excessive physical exercise and may include vomiting after eating, the use of laxatives, diet aids and diuretics. Severe cases of anorexia nervosa can result in death.

Bulimia nervosa (DSM-V 307.51) refers to an eating disorder characterized by episodes of secretive overeating, commonly known as binge eating. Binges are followed by compensatory behaviours such as vomiting or 'purging', abuse of laxatives and diuretics, and excessive exercise. Unlike anorexia, patients with bulimia can fall within the normal range for weight and age. However, they share an intense fear of and preoccupation with gaining weight and distortions in body image.

It is well known that both of these eating disorders can cause gum disease and enamel erosion. If a patient's oral health seems particularly poor in these regards and the classic signs of bulimia are observed (islands of amalgam, demineralization of the palatial aspect of the maxillary anteriors), the dentist should include in his psychological evaluation (detailed below) questions about the patient's diet, smoking habits, exercise routine, sleep patterns, etc. If there is a question as to whether a patient is currently anorexic or bulimic, a psychological consultation is in order. On the other hand, a patient's oral clinical picture may be the result of a past eating disorder, one the patient no longer suffers from. In this case, esthetic treatment may still be appropriate. It is unwise to provide esthetic treatment to a patient who currently suffers from an eating disorder, as their oral health will continue to be affected by it.

Body dysmorphic disorder (DSM-V 300.7): Many people are dissatisfied with one or more of their body parts. The nose may be too large or too small, ankles too skinny or too thick, cheekbones too sharp or too flat, breasts too full or too small, etc. *Any* part of the human body, including teeth or the entire body itself, may become the focus of a patient's unhappiness. Body dysmorphic disorder (BDD) is an emotional disorder involving persistent and intrusive thoughts about one's perceived physical flaws. The irrational idea or fantasy underlying such obsessions in BDD is that the patient's 'bad' part of themselves is the reason for their unhappiness or misfortune. Hence, it would stand to reason that 'correcting' it, getting it *just* so, would lead to happiness.

To some extent, we all have it. But the degree of obsession and distortion is what distinguishes BDD from more ordinary displeasure with one's appearance. In the extreme, an obsession with real or imagined physical imperfections may lead to many unneeded cosmetic surgeries, ultimately resulting in disfigurement. Michael Jackson's well-known obsession with his nose and the colour of his skin is an extreme example of body dysmorphic disorder.

Most patients presenting for esthetic dentistry, however, do not suffer from severe psychological disorders such as these. The guideline below is intended for that majority of patients.

A GUIDELINE FOR EVALUATING THE PATIENT'S MENTAL STATE

An assessment of the patient's emotional and psychological state is interwoven with the esthetic evaluation. The key here is to establish a rapport with the patient. Patients seeking esthetic enhancement often experience shame, both about the 'defects' for which they are consulting you and the desire for cosmetic change itself. Shame about perceived physical defects, particularly if those defects are the result of the patient's negligence, such as poor dental hygiene, may be a powerful deterrent to seeking an esthetic consultation in the first place. Shame may also pose a significant obstacle to the patient revealing thoughts and ideas they fear would evoke disapproval in the dentist. The dentist must strive to create a safe environment, one in which the patient's fears of self-expression are minimized. A non-judgmental and empathic stance, conveyed through tone and posture, is critical to the dentist gaining a clear understanding of the patient's motivation for esthetic treatment and their expectations of outcome.

The most important tool the dentist has in conducting an effective consultation is the dentist herself. Interpersonal skill is as important as technical expertise in putting a patient at ease and gaining their trust. Two of the open-ended questions in the esthetic evaluation section are also useful in evaluating the patient's psychological readiness and appropriateness for treatment. They are:

1. A. If there was anything you could change about your smile, what would that be?

    C. History of esthetic change

These two questions are connected and are at the heart of the psychological assessment of the patient, particularly the patient's history of esthetic change.

Obtaining a detailed history of the patient's esthetic change will aid the dentist in his determination of whether the patient's current request for esthetic dentistry is more or less rational. In addition to the question 'If there was anything you could change about your smile, what would that be', follow-up questions such as these may be useful:

1. How long have you wanted to make this change?
2. Have you had any previous esthetic dental work? Here, it is important to ascertain the number of previous treatments, dates performed, the details of each procedure and whether the same dentist was used.

    In regard to each previous dental procedure, ask the patient:

3. Were you happy with the results at the time?
4. What pleased you?
5. If you were not satisfied with the results, what specifically still bothered you?
6. Were you able to speak with your dentist about it?

In general, if a patient has had multiple esthetic dental procedures and is still unhappy with the results, it is likely that additional treatment will lead to a negative outcome. It is best, under these circumstances, for the dentist to convey her concern about the patient's motivation for treatment and to ask the patient whether he or she would like a referral to a mental health professional.

There are instances, however, when a patient has had several past esthetic procedures and still has reasonable cause for dissatisfaction with the results.[2] In such instances, the dentist must use his professional judgment, based on his own esthetic evaluation and his evaluation of the patient's mental state, to decide whether or not to recommend further esthetic treatment.[3,4] If the dentist decides to treat the patient, the dentist must very clearly communicate to the patient what he intends to and, ideally, show the patient, through digital imaging, a close approximation of the results.

SUMMARY

Understanding the emotional state of our patients is critical to determining whether or not a psychological consult is necessary prior to performing esthetic dental work. Under certain psychological conditions, esthetic treatment may not be appropriate. The use of a 3-step analysis allows us to maximize communication and gain a clear understanding of the patient's esthetic desires and determine the best treatment plan.

Additionally, an effective consultation for esthetic change must include an assessment of the patient's mental and emotional readiness and appropriateness for treatment. This is best accomplished by creating a non-judgmental, safe environment in which a good rapport with the patient is established.

Seminal literature

American Psychiatric Association. Diagnostic and statistical manual of mental disorders. 5th ed. Washington, DC: American Psychiatric Press Inc; 2013.

ANAD. Bulimia nervosa. Retrieved from: <http://www.anad.org/get-information/bulimia-nervosa/>; 2015.

Anxiety and Depression Association of America (ADAA). Body dysmorphic disorder. Retrieved from: <http://www.adaa.org/understanding-anxiety/related-illnesses/other-related-conditions/body-dysmorphic-disorder-bdd>; 2014.

Mayo Foundation for Medical Education and Research. Diseases and conditions: anorexia nervosa. Retrieved from: <http://www.mayoclinic.org/diseases-conditions/anorexia/basics/definition/con-20033002>; 2015.

REFERENCES

1. Goldstein C, Goldstein RE, Garber D. Imaging in esthetic dentistry. In: Levine JB, editor. Esthetic diagnosis. Curr Opin Cosmet Dent 1995;9–17.

2. Kokich V, Kiyak HA, Shapiro PA. Comparing the perception of the dentist and lay people to altered dental esthetics. J Esthet Dent 1999;11:311–24.

3. Rosentiel SF, Rashid RG. Public preferences for anterior tooth variations: a web-based study. J Esthet Restor Dent 2002;14:97–106.

4. Kokich VO, Kiyak HA. Perceptions of dental professionals and laypersons to altered dental aesthetics: asymmetric and symmetric situations. Am J Orthod Dentofacial Orthop 2006;130:141–51.

CHAPTER 3

Integration of Function and Esthetics

JEFFREY McCLENDON, JONATHAN B. LEVINE

The biologic model	**55**
The neutral zone	**62**
Soft tissue profile analysis	**63**
Clinical occlusal analysis	**66**
Introduction of seven line FEE analysis	**69**
The 'FEE appliance' for diagnosis, stabilization and visualization	**72**
Clinical case 3.1	**76**
Clinical case 3.2	**79**
Clinical case 3.3	**81**
Clinical case 3.4	**82**

Optimal smile design should integrate facial balance and harmony with natural form, fit and function of the teeth and jaws. A proper treatment plan should address not only the esthetic needs of our patient, but also improve or sustain the health of the entire orofacial complex. The smile reflects the quality, quantity and functioning of the component parts of this entire system. Achieving the 'right stuff' requires the right teeth, in the right place and with the right timing. Ultimately, the quintessential test of this system is the smile, and the key to evaluating the smile is the 3-dimensional position of the maxillary central incisors. Simply stated, the maxillary central's incisal edge links dental, dental–facial and facial esthetics with mandibular movement and jaw function (Fig. 3.1).

A beautiful smile reflects proper function, healthy teeth, a healthy neuromusculature and healthy temporomandibular joints (TMJs). Each tooth has its natural position and form for a reason: to play a very specific role as our

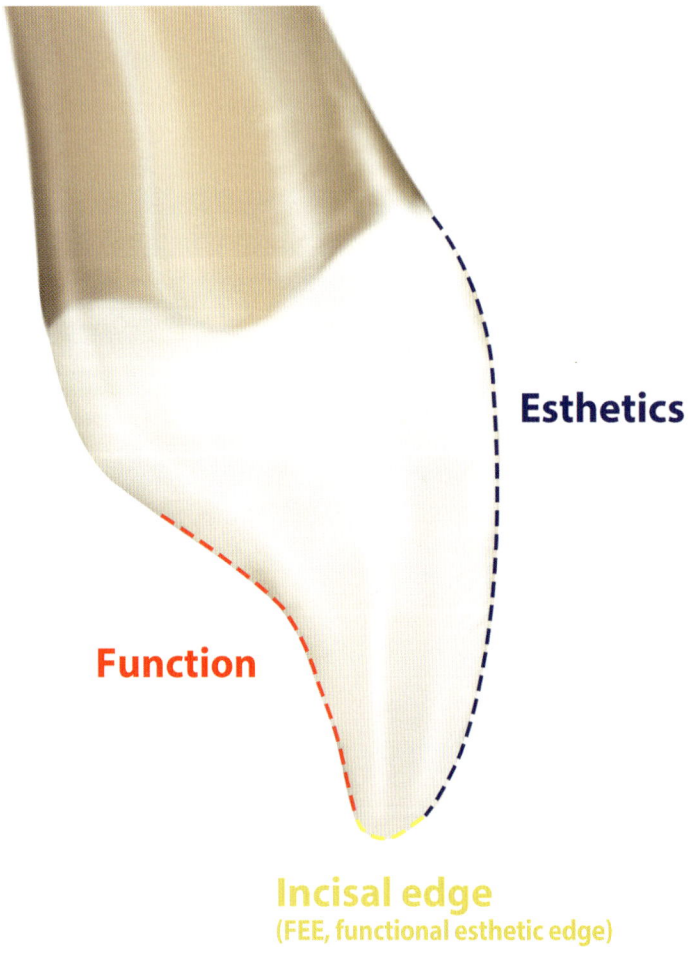

Fig. 3.1 The maxillary central's incisal edge links dental, dental–facial and facial esthetics with mandibular movement and jaw function.

mandible moves through chewing, speaking and swallowing. When the tooth form or position is not ideal, the system adapts functionally and structurally and does not function as designed; pathology develops over time (i.e. wear facets, mobility and pain on function). The fundamentals of occlusion play out over the teeth, muscles and joints, and ultimately our facial expression and smile. A properly designed smile will be coincidentally beautiful. When the hard tissues provide the optimal scaffolding for the facial soft tissues, we see a 'beautiful' smile, one that all appreciate and few can forget.

When planning comprehensive treatment, the clinician must initially determine whether the patient's dentition is in a state of health or adaptation/pathology. If there are signs of pathology present (hypermobility, abfractions, wear facets or pain on function), then the aetiology must be diagnosed and addressed if we want our patients to be comfortable and our restorations to last.

THE BIOLOGIC MODEL

The biologic model, first introduced by Dr Bob Lee,[1] describes the following basic requirements of a stable occlusion and optimal mandibular function. These four positions (Fig. 3.2) are evaluated during the occlusal analysis, as part of the Aesthetic Evaluation Form, and test the adequacy of the patient's overbite and overjet in the context of their occlusal plane, curve of Spee, and condylar inclination. If the mandible cannot move into and out of these positions without interference, pathology will be present in the mouth in the form of wear facets, hypermobility, abfractions or pain. As discussed in the diagnosis chapter (see Chapter 1), once that pathology has been noted, the 'habitual' mandibular position can no longer be trusted and a centric relation bite must be recorded. The models will be mounted, studied and waxed-up just before the first point of contact, rather than in the maximum intercuspation position. Centric relation gives us a reproducible mandibular position, from diagnostics all the way to the final restorations.

Maximum intercuspation or centric occlusion is the position the mandible assumes while swallowing. What we are seeking here are small point contacts (0.2 mm) of equal timing and intensity throughout the mouth (Fig. 3.3 A–C) with vertical, axially directed forces at closure. When the mandible moves into and out of complete occlusion (Fig. 3.4), there should be no deviation or deflecting contacts on tooth inclines. Any such interferences are noted on the Aesthetic Evaluation Form. Optimal jaw posture has minimal stress when the difference between centric occlusion and centric relation is minimal.

THE BIOLOGIC MODEL

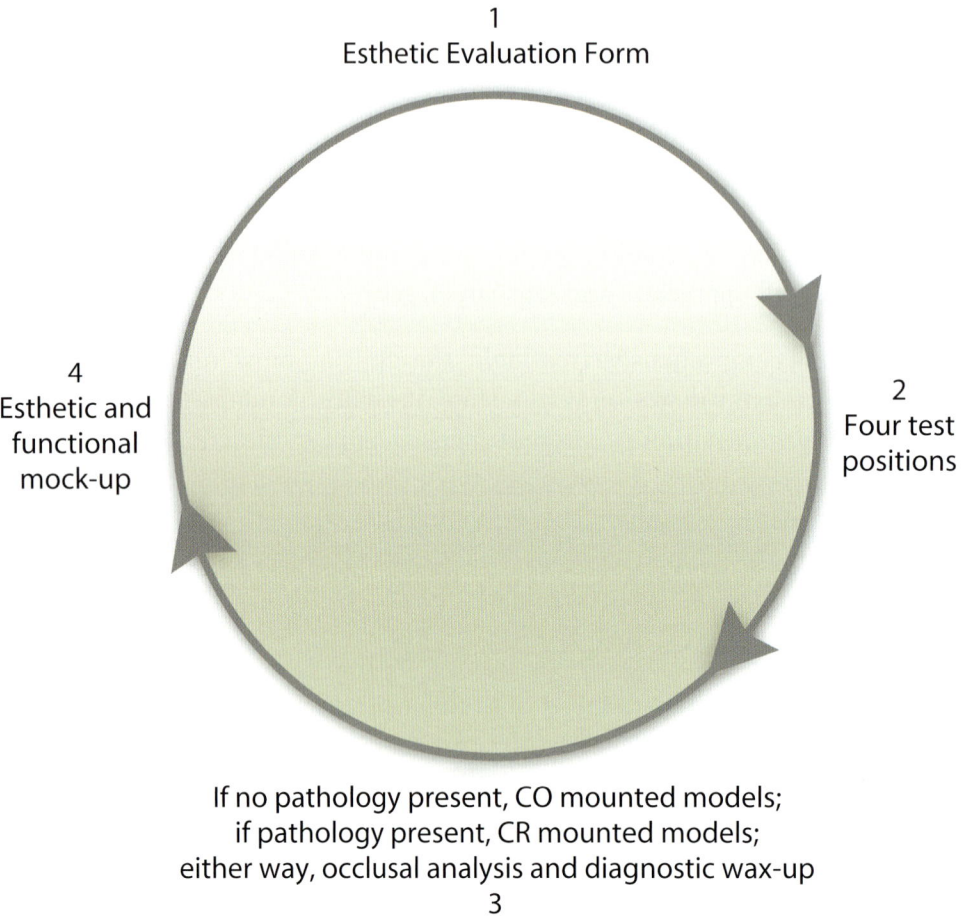

Fig. 3.2 Occlusal analysis. CO: complete occlusion; CR: centric relation.

KEY POINT SUMMARY

Biologic model

- Concept of natural tooth form, fit and mandibular function observed and reported by Dr Bob Lee.[1]
- Provides for Class I dental fit and skeletal pattern, and a relatively flat plane of occlusion.
- Provides for an interference-free, canine-guided lateral chew and central incisor guidance for speaking, swallowing and smiling.
- Provides for mandibular movement 3 mm left, right or forward from complete occlusion so that the posterior second molars separate 2–3 mm due to the anterior tooth contact. This pattern of movement provides for optimal space to swallow, chew, bite, speak and smile.

POSITION 1: COMPLETE OCCLUSION (TEETH TOGETHER) (Fig. 3.4)

The biologic model requires the following relationship of the occluded anterior teeth: the central incisors overlap vertically ('overbite') 3–5 mm and horizontally ('overjet') 2–4 mm, and the cuspids overlap vertically 4–6 mm and horizontally

CHAPTER 3
INTEGRATION OF FUNCTION AND ESTHETICS

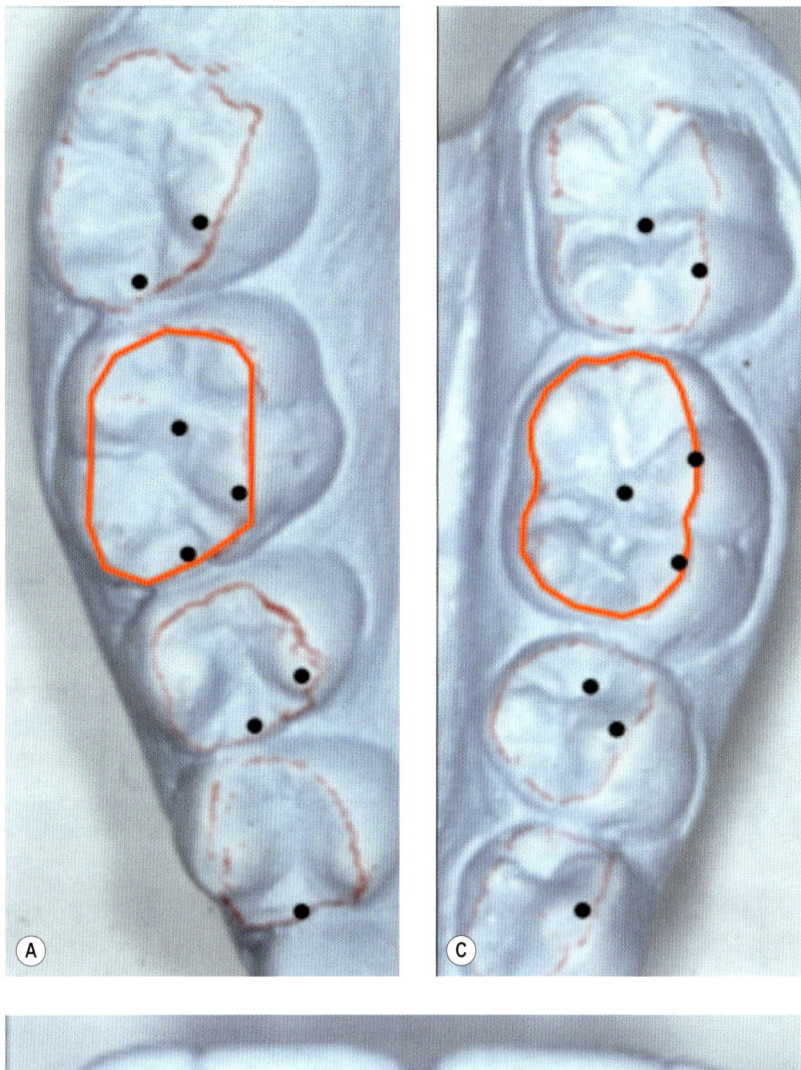

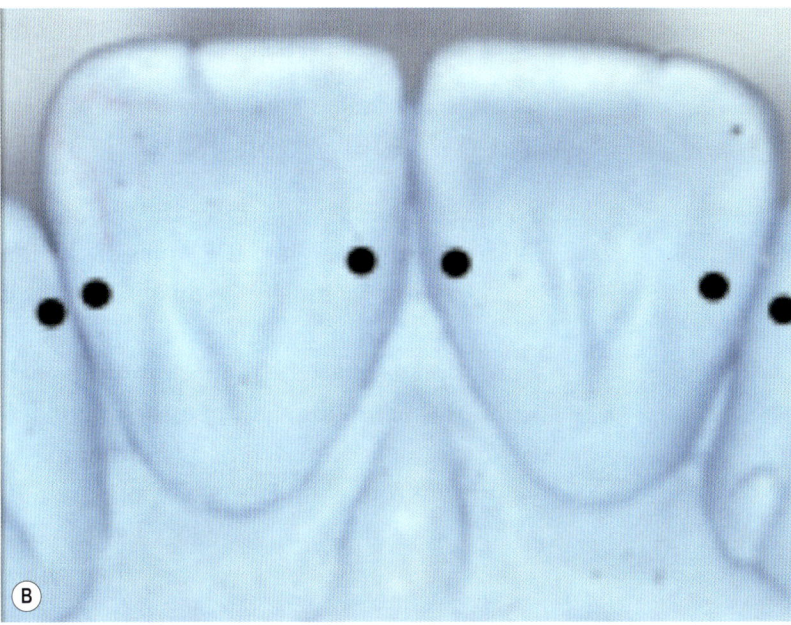

Fig. 3.3A–C Ideal tooth contacts illustrated on a model. The contacts should be small, i.e. 0.2–0.3 mm areas. Red pencil outlines the occlusal table to show buccal–lingual tooth width relationship and tooth contacts relative to the occlusal outline.

THE BIOLOGIC MODEL

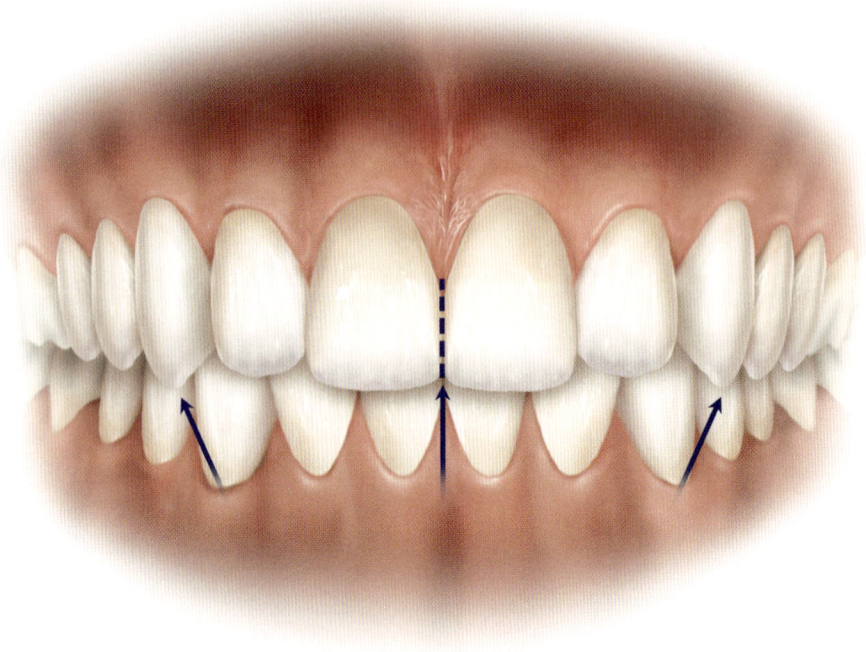

Fig. 3.4 Position 1: complete occlusion (teeth together).

0.5–1 mm. This anterior overbite and overjet relationship (Fig. 3.5) allows contact-free movement of the posterior teeth until closure, when all teeth, including the anterior teeth, contact. Having sufficient overbite and overjet allows lateral canine guidance and chewing without anterior incisal edge contact or wear (Fig. 3.6).

POSITION 2: INCISIVE POSITION (Fig. 3.7)

This position demonstrates the patient's ability (or inability) to separate all posterior teeth when just the edges of the incisors are in contact. As the mandible moves from complete occlusion into this 'edge-to-edge' position, the palatal contours of the maxillary anteriors and the facial surfaces of the mandibular anteriors 'guide' the motion and the posterior teeth separate. This is known as anterior 'coupling' between the maxillary and mandibular incisors. Any posterior contacts ('interferences'), either at the incisive position or on the way to this position from complete occlusion, are noted on the Aesthetic Evaluation Form. Once incisal wear has caused the maxillary centrals to no longer separate the posterior teeth (Fig. 3.8), then the wear accelerates both anteriorly and posteriorly.

CHAPTER 3
INTEGRATION OF FUNCTION AND ESTHETICS

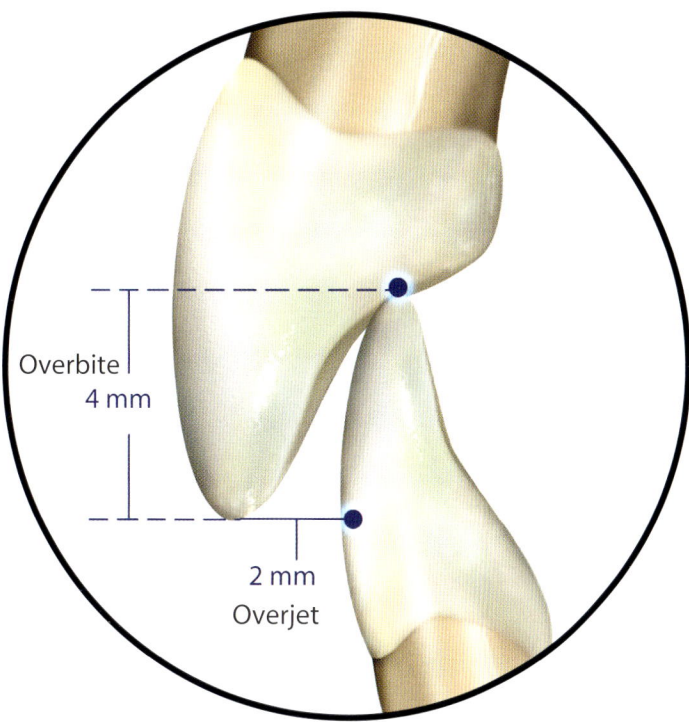

Fig. 3.5 The biologic model showing appropriate overbite and overjet between the central incisors. This relationship is key.

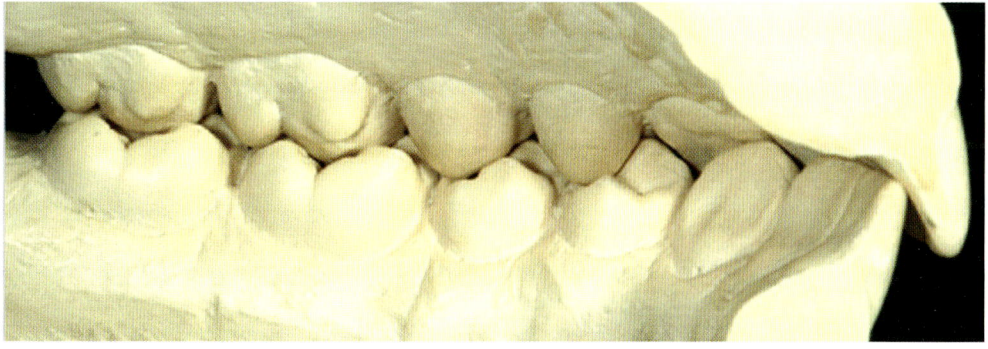

Fig. 3.6 View from tongue laterally and showing lingual relationships. Verticalizing posterior contacts that support the anterior teeth. This provides a stabilizing effect on the condylar position at closure and swallowing. Note the sluiceways and interproximal relationships of occluded dentition, and the relationships at embrasures and mesial slopes of uppers and distal slopes of lowers.

POSITIONS 3 AND 4: RIGHT AND LEFT CHEW POSITIONS (Fig. 3.9A,B)

The patient is instructed to move the mandible left and right, from complete occlusion, while keeping the teeth together. There should be no contact across any incisal edges and there must be complete separation of all posterior

THE BIOLOGIC MODEL

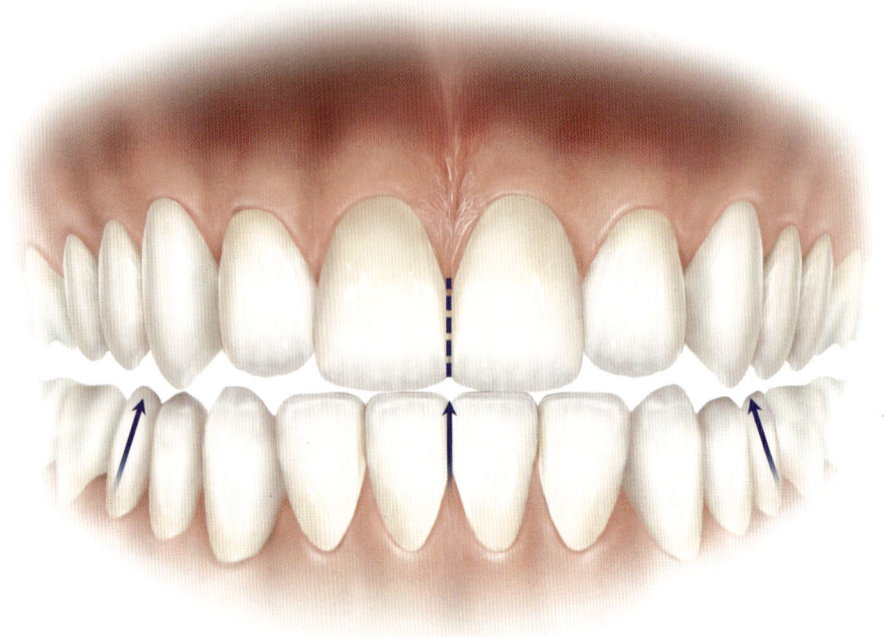

Fig. 3.7 Incisive position.

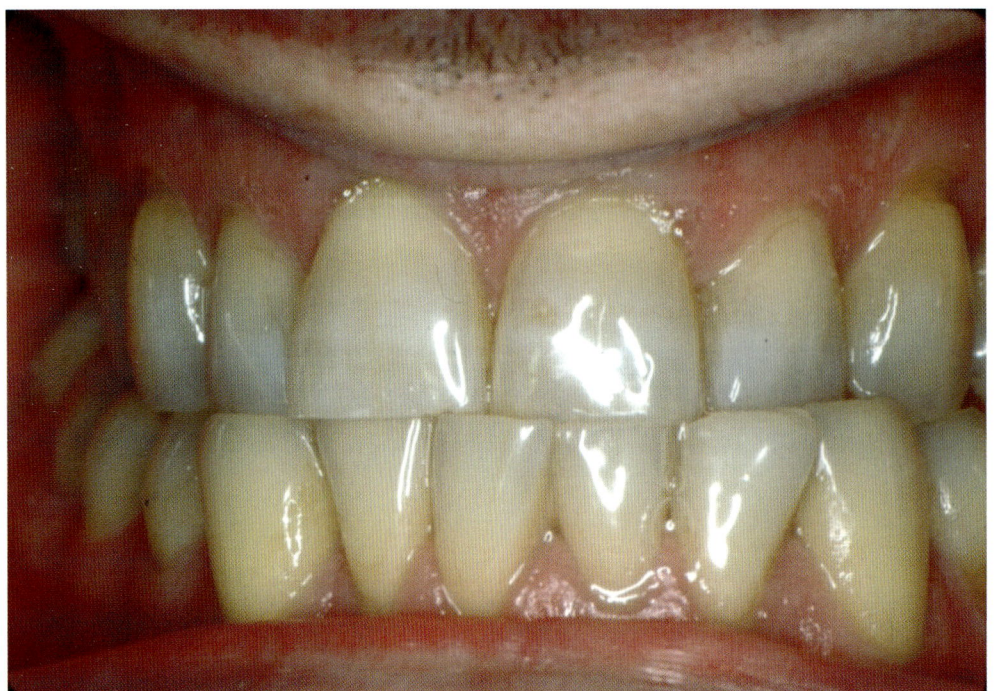

Fig. 3.8 A lack of posterior separation when in the incisive position. This will cause accelerated wear. A deficient overbite/overjet relationship causes this lack of posterior disclusion.

CHAPTER 3
INTEGRATION OF FUNCTION AND ESTHETICS

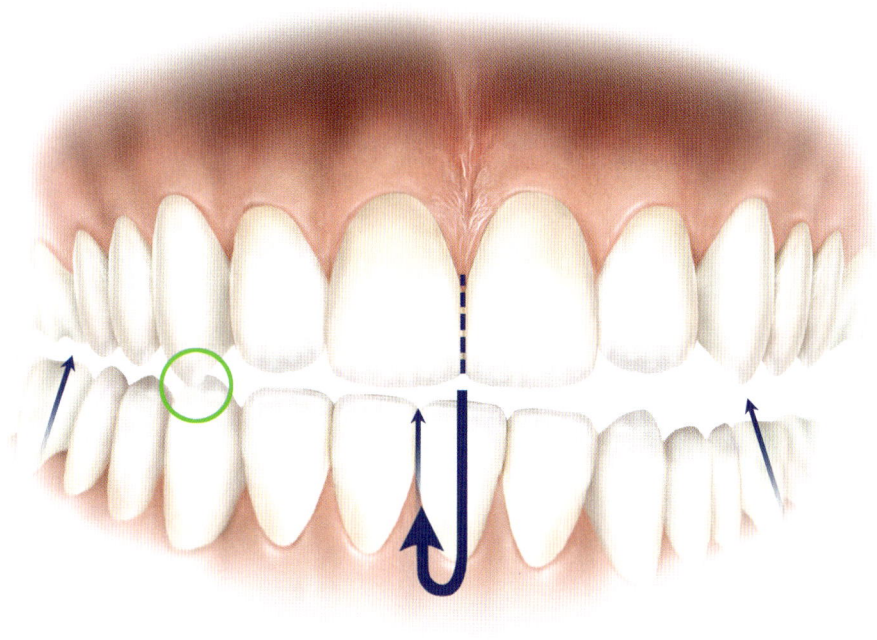

(A)

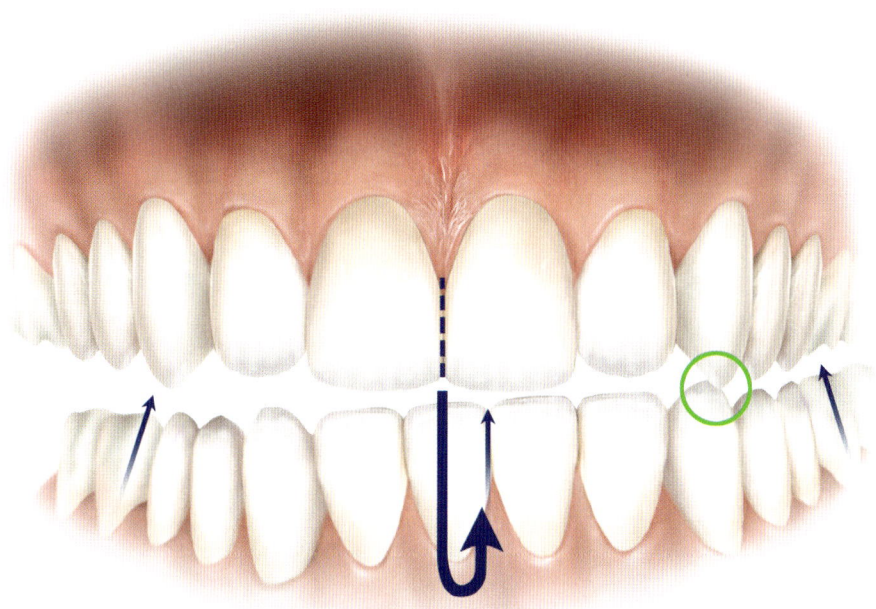

(B)

Fig. 3.9A,B The right (A) and left (B) chew positions. When the canine is tip-to-tip on the chewing side (the furthest lateral point of the cycle), the second molars on that side should be separated by 1–2 mm and the opposite (non-chewing) second molars should be separated by 2–3 mm.

teeth on the 'non-chewing' side (i.e. the side from which the mandible moves away, also known as the 'non-working' side). On the 'chewing' side, the canines provide posterior separation, termed 'canine rise'. When the excursive motion is performed in reverse (as is done while chewing), it is the contours of the guiding canine teeth that lead the mandible back into complete occlusion. When the lateral chewing guidance is not present, the anterior incisal edges will quickly wear, followed by the premolars. Once the jaw begins to chew across these wear facets, the research indicates, the patient may parafunction in the same pattern. Note that, usually, wear on a cuspid coincides with interferences on the contralateral, non-working side molar(s).

'Occlusion' is the movement of the mandibular teeth into the fit of the maxillary teeth; however, clinically, we assess these positions in reverse. The patient slides to the right, left and forward, whereas actual function sees the mandible moving into these positions.

The biologic model provides guidelines for natural tooth form, fit and function and provides for comfortable condyles and atraumatic mandibular function. However, the occluded tooth mass must be considered in the context of the soft tissues as well. When creating a facially directed treatment plan, assessing only the dental view is not enough. We need to consider the 'neutral zone' and soft tissue profile analysis to connect the teeth to the face.

THE NEUTRAL ZONE

KEY POINTS

Neutral zone

- The neutral zone is the concept described by Dawson where the teeth are maintained in balance by the lip and tongue pressure.
- Teeth erupt 'into' the neutral zone and are maintained there by the lips and tongue.
- Anteriorly, the neutral zone is the perioral musculature described by orbicularis oris. The neutral zone extends posteriorly as the buccinator and anterolaterally to the buccinator raphe, which shares the superior constrictor of the pharynx, thus having a direct connection to the airway. The tongue inserts posteriorly as the anterior wall of the pharynx and plays a role in the airway.
- The neutral zone, first noted by Earl Pound[2] and further described by Dawson,[3] provides for balance and harmony of the teeth between the lips and the tongue. The teeth erupt into the neutral zone and are maintained in balance between the opposing forces of the tongue pushing outward and the lips pulling inward (Fig. 3.10).

CHAPTER 3
INTEGRATION OF FUNCTION AND ESTHETICS

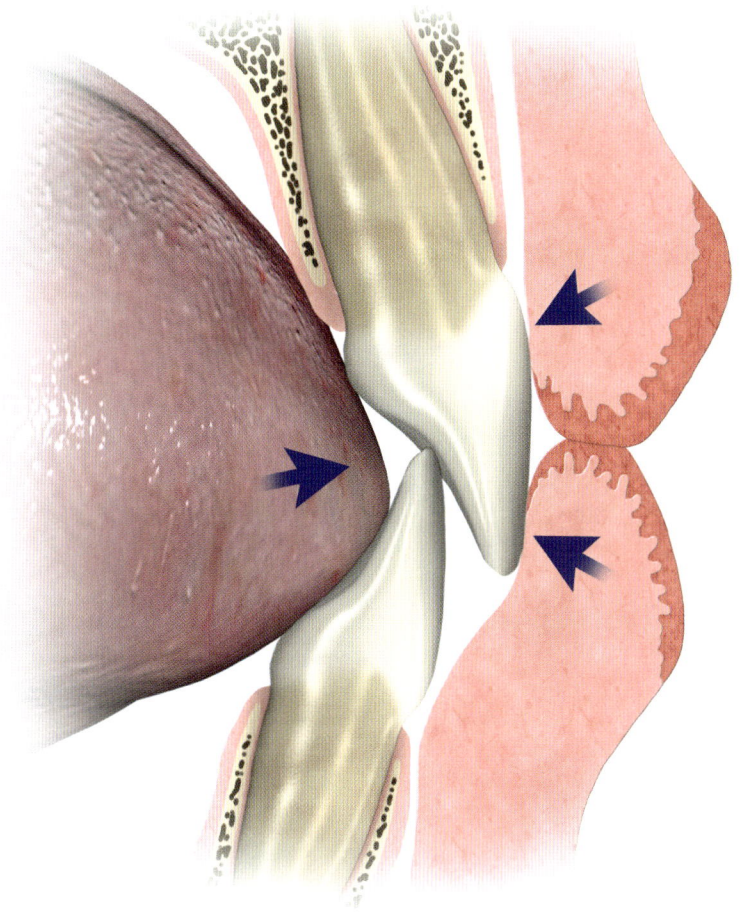

Fig. 3.10 The teeth erupt into the 'neutral zone', where they are held in balance between the opposing forces of the tongue and the lips.

An unworn maxillary central incisor supports both the upper and lower lips (Fig. 3.11). When the tooth wears and loses its edge, however, the lips become 'inverted' rather than 'everted', thinning out and flattening the patient's facial profile (Fig. 3.12).

Lengthening a worn incisal edge will not only rejuvenate by increasing display at rest ('Emma'), it will give back the supported, fuller lips seen in youthful, less stressed faces. For this reason, the face can be thought of as an extension of the neutral zone (Fig. 3.13).

SOFT TISSUE PROFILE ANALYSIS

A soft tissue analysis of a profile-view photograph can be used to compare the positions of subnasale, upper and lower lip projection and soft tissue pogonion

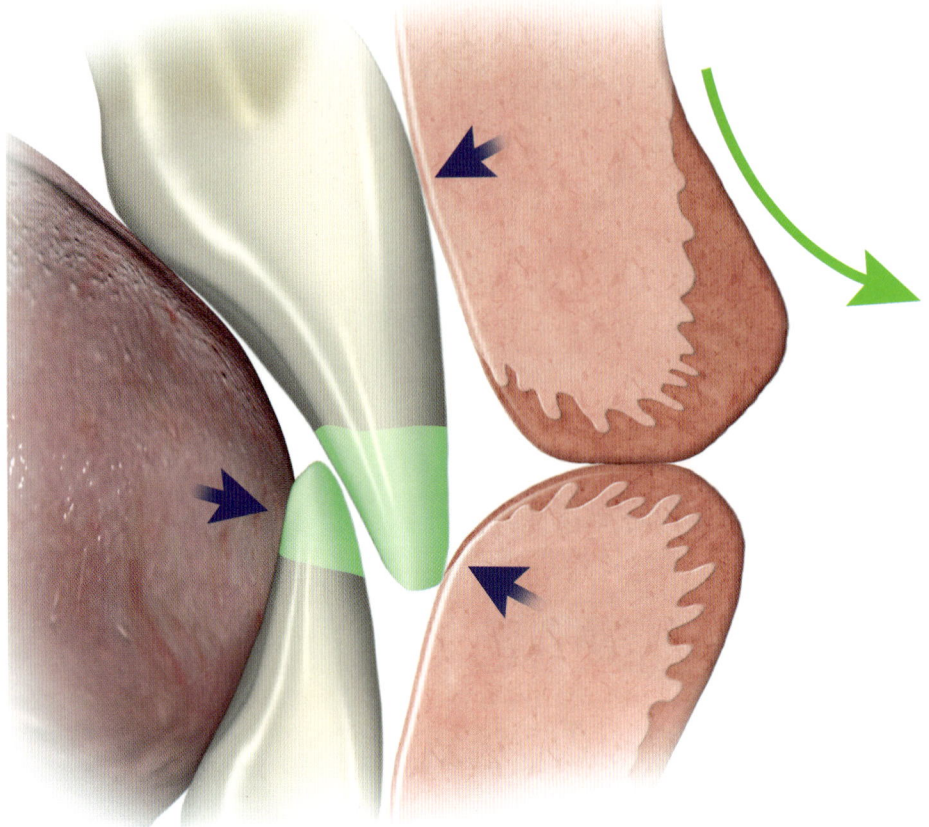

Fig. 3.11 The unworn maxillary central incisor's edge supports both the upper and lower lips.

(Fig. 3.9B). The 'true vertical' line, drawn from subnasale with the patient in natural head position, is used to assess upper and lower lip projection (Fig. 3.14). The acceptable range for the upper lip is 2–5 mm anterior to the line and 0–3 mm for the lower lip. The soft tissue pogonion (anterior-most aspect of the chin) is ideally situated 0–3 mm posterior to this line.

The Ricketts' E-plane and the nasolabial angle are two other important guidelines, described previously in the esthetic diagnosis chapter (see Chapter 1), that provide evaluation of the facial profile. These measurements relate to smile design in that the relative convexity or concavity of a profile guides our anterior tooth form and position, known as facially directed treatment planning. Recall that a concave profile indicates restorations on the larger end of the 10–12 mm central incisor range, while for a convex profile the teeth would be downsized and the central incisor's length would be closer to 10 mm.

Facially directed treatment planning synergizes three concepts: the neutral zone (tongue, lips and teeth), the biologic model (optimal tooth form, fit and function,

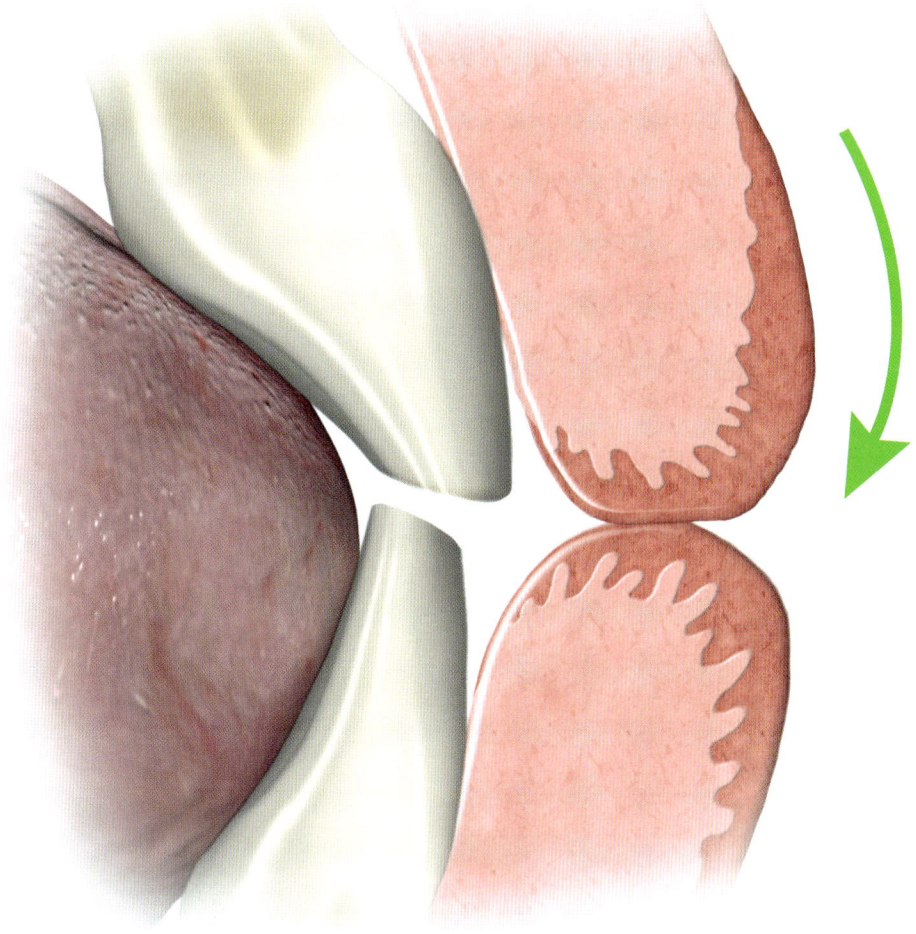

Fig. 3.12 Loss of the incisal edges results in inverted, flattened lips.

and relatively flat occlusal plane to the horizontal) and soft tissue facial analysis (optimal projection of lips relative to subnasale and soft tissue pogonion). Consideration paid to these areas will ensure improved dental–facial harmony, patient comfort, predictability and the longevity of our treatment and restorations.

KEY POINTS

Occlusal plane

- The key to smile design (after placement of the central incisors) for health, wellness and symbiotic function and esthetics is optimal placement of the occlusal plane within the context of the face.

- The integration of the vertical dimension of the occluded tooth mass, its horizontal plane of orientation and its balanced relationship within the neutral zone, provides individual functional and esthetic smile integrity.

CLINICAL OCCLUSAL ANALYSIS

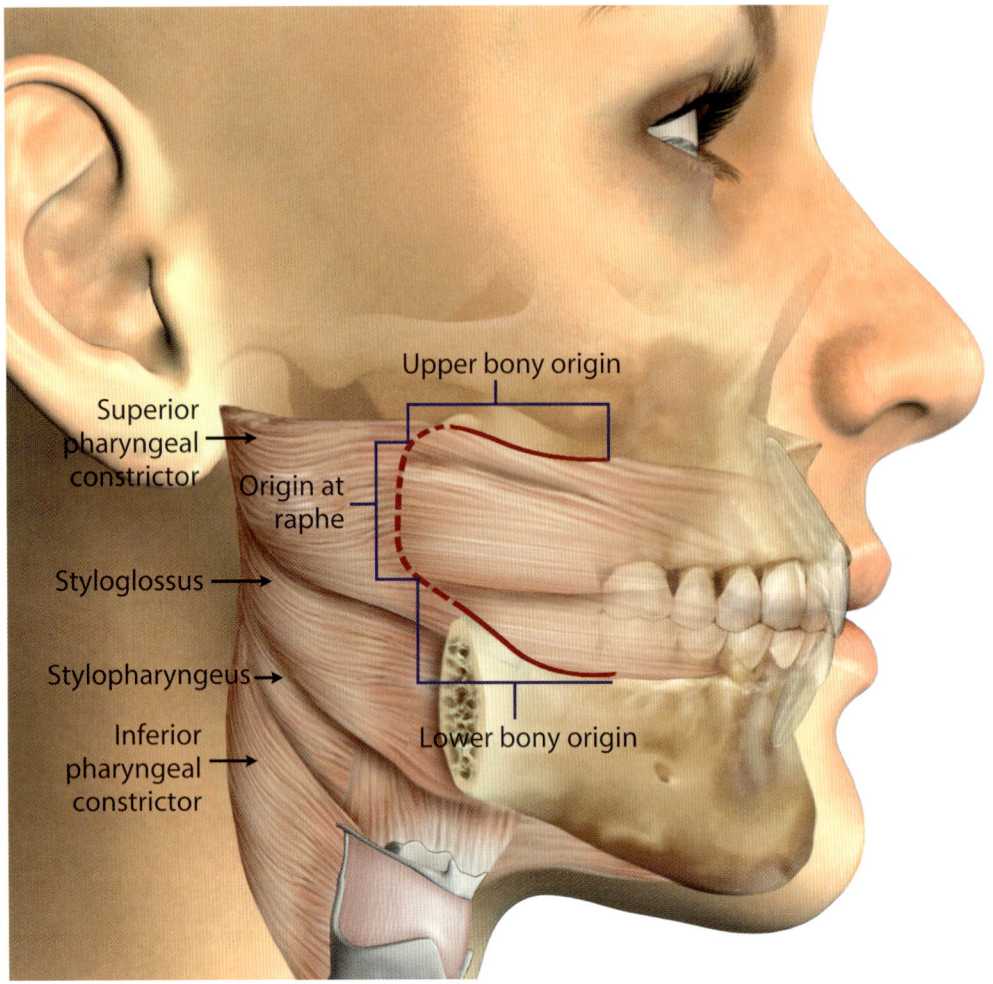

Fig. 3.13 The face can be thought of as an extension of the neutral zone.

CLINICAL OCCLUSAL ANALYSIS

In addition to assessing the four test positions (complete occlusion, incisive, right chew, left chew), the following must be checked before comprehensive dentistry is performed:

1. Painless palpation of the muscles of mastication (masseter and temporalis, Fig. 3.15) and intra-oral palpation of the temporalis insertion gives a sense of neuromuscular harmony.

2. Range of motion and opening, looking for symmetry or deviation, and movement to the left and right are performed.

3. The ability of the TMJ to rotate and translate smoothly may be assessed by lateral palpation anterior to the ear canal and within the ear canal, or via use of a stethoscope.

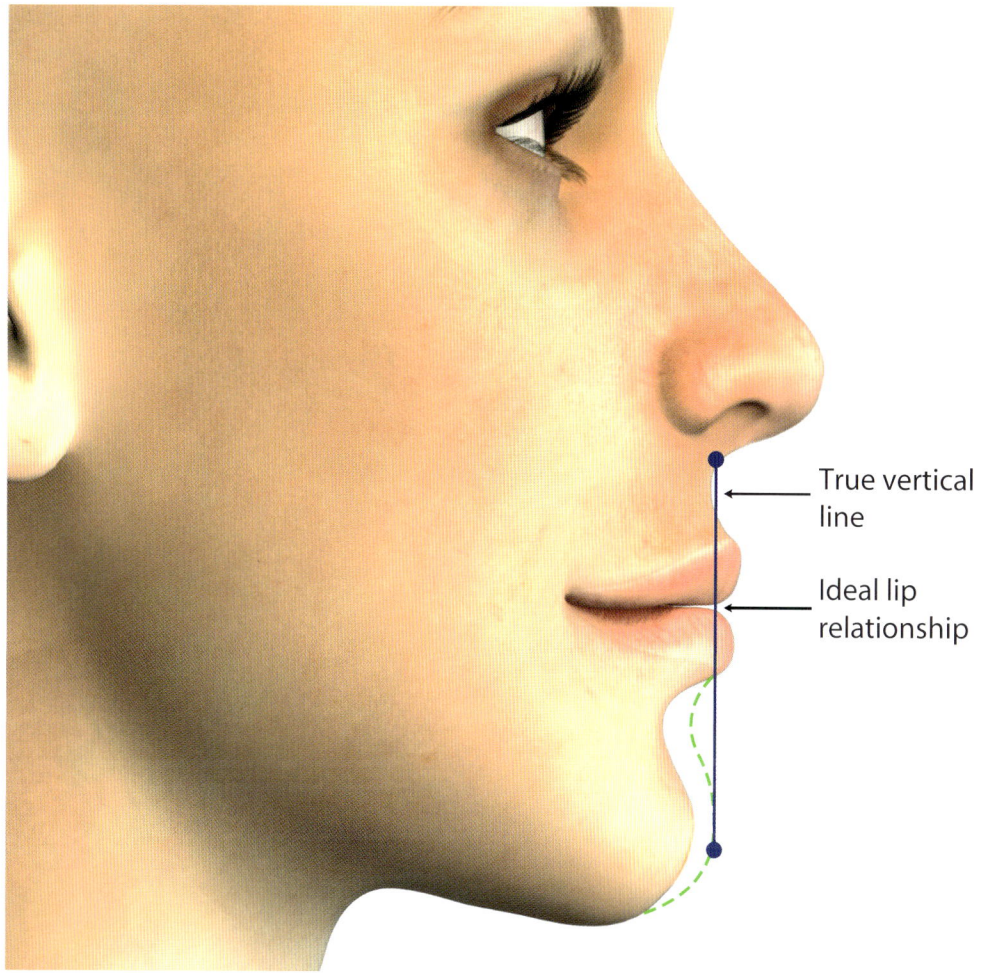

Fig. 3.14 A 'true vertical' line helps assess protrusion of the lips. Ideally, the upper lip lies 2–5 mm anterior to this line, the lower lip projects just 0–3 mm beyond, and the soft tissue pogonion is situated 0–3 mm posterior to the line.

4. Opening, closing and right and left lateral jaw movement against resistance also provide information of the condyle–disc functional status.

5. Load testing the joint by closing firmly on a cotton roll anteriorly across the anterior teeth. Pain indicates disc displacement and pressure on retrodiscal tissue.

Any popping, clicking or pain needs further evaluation before comprehensive dental treatment starts. MRI evaluation for disc position and CBCT evaluation for eminence and condyle form may provide additional information.

Due to the protective nature of the neuromusculature, the fit of the teeth represents an adapted mandibular posture that is anterior and inferior to its optimal position. To realize the intra-arch relationship purely from the basis of joint

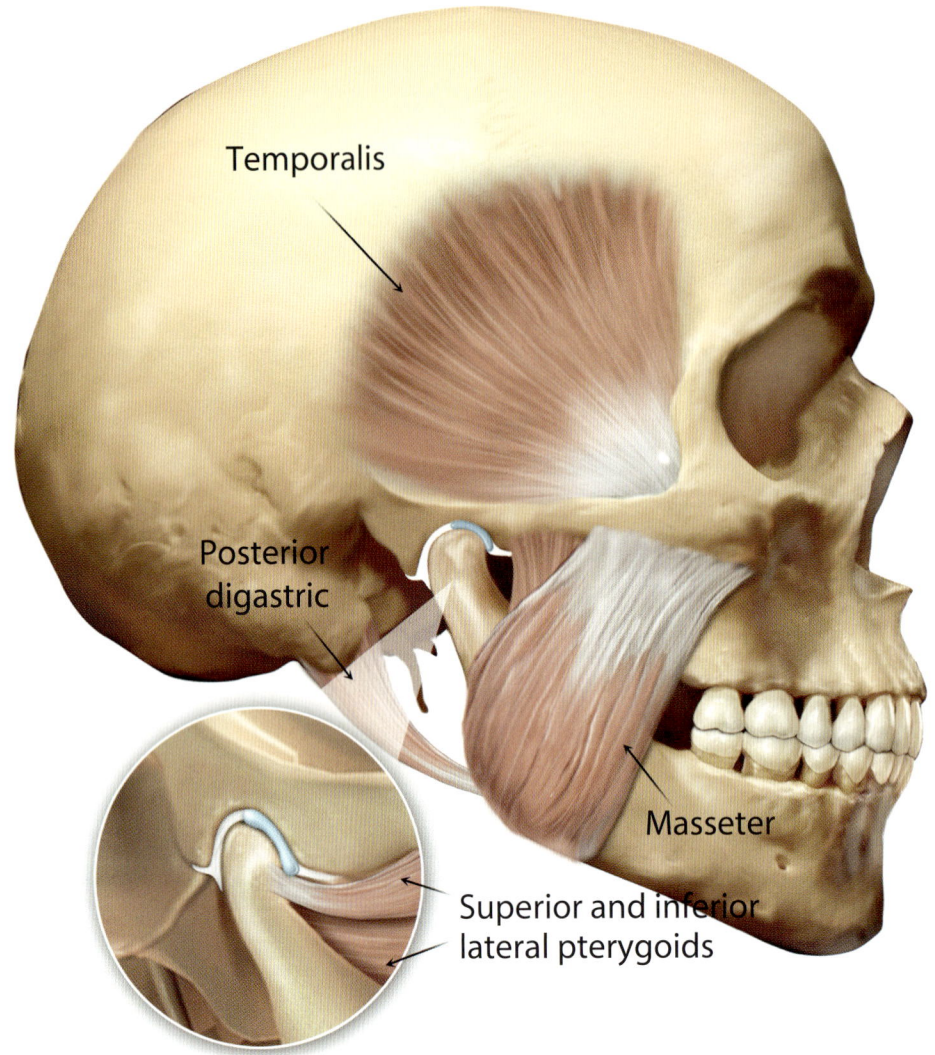

Fig. 3.15 The muscles of mastication: superior and inferior lateral pterygoids. The medial pterygoid is not shown.

orthopaedics, a seated, rotation-only recording of the maxilla to mandible is made. A recording material such as heated soft wax or polyvinyl siloxane records a minimal posterior opening provided by an anterior stop. Mounted models referenced to the patient's TMJ rotation are evaluated in the same four test positions as the clinical examination. Inspection of dental models improves evaluation of tooth form, fit and jaw function and augments the clinical examination findings.

Articulated models do not have a neuromusculature and show the primary condylar determinant of jaw movement. Clinically, the patient's neuromusculature integrates tooth form into fit by muscular force, which may alter the mandibular pathway. When the patient has signs or symptoms of dysfunction, the use of an occlusal splint to improve condylar function and relax the neuromusculature may be considered. Appliances may be used therapeutically, diagnostically or protectively. Design and adjustment should provide fit to the arch and to the teeth. Contacts and jaw movement should mimic occlusion treatment goals.

Figures 3.16A–C and 3.17 are instructive when considering conformative versus reformative treatment.

INTRODUCTION OF SEVEN LINE FEE ANALYSIS

Seven horizontal lines (Fig. 3.18) may be appreciated within the biologic model's 'complete occlusion' diagram, and can be utilized as our functional esthetic evaluation (FEE) which then serves as a guideline for the diagnostic wax-up. The first five lines establish esthetic parameters for the gingiva.

1. The first horizontal line is that of the incisal edge of the maxillary central incisors, which is of course the link between function and esthetics, and thus the most important. The edge, midline and inclination of the central incisors relative to the upper lip at rest provide evaluation of tooth display, symmetry to the lips and face, and support of the upper lip beneath the nose and subnasale. Extension of this line laterally to the tips of the canines, and parallel to the horizon, allows further evaluation of the esthetic plane. We call this the 'FEE' line, known as the functional esthetic evaluation, and it is best evaluated when the patient smiles broadly, or with retracted lips and head in natural head position.

2. The second line, aiding in evaluation of the maxillary plane, is one passing through the gingival zeniths of the maxillary central and canines.

3. The third line corresponds to the gingival margin of the maxillary lateral incisors, and is parallel and slightly coronal to the centrals/canine gingival line.

4. Line 4 passes through the mandibular incisor's gingival margin will provide evaluation of relative eruption, to each other and to the canines at the corner of the arch.

5. The fifth line, again parallel to all the others, connects the gingival zeniths of the mandibular canines. This line should be about 1 mm apical to that of the four mandibular incisors.

6. The sixth line passes through the incisal edges of the four lower incisors. This line corresponds to the proper amount of incisor overbite when compared to line 1.

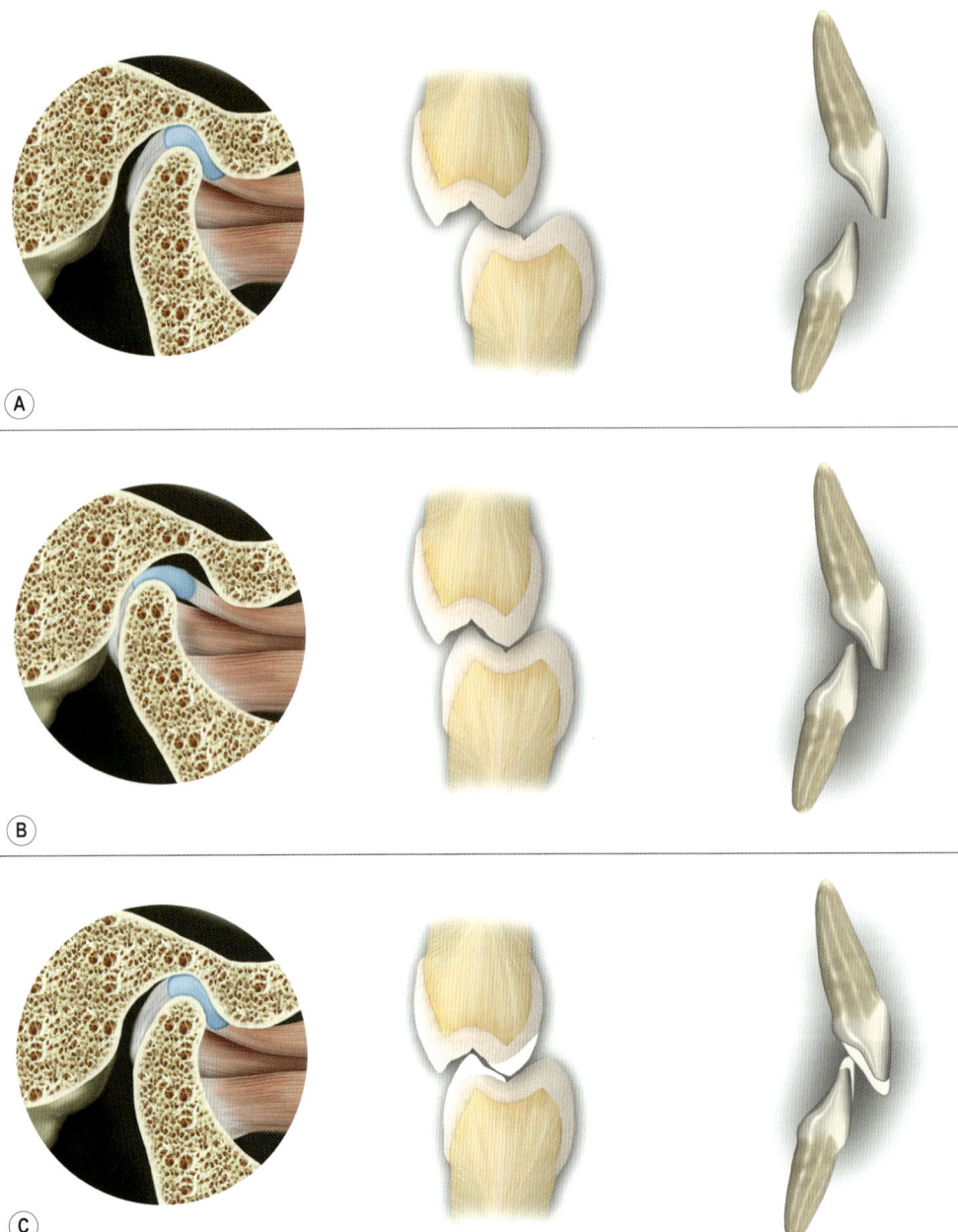

Fig. 3.16A–C   (A) This shows the joint and tooth relationships as the mandible rotates to first contact (maintaining superior, anterior condyle/disc relationship). (B) The neuromusculature postures the mandible to maximize contacts at the end of each chewing cycle and to swallow. When this neuromusculature adaptation exceeds the structural or functional tolerances within the gnathic system, there is breakdown. (C) The reformative choices are shown and the additive form is depicted in white. The goal of system balance and harmony must be provided across the tops of the teeth, the condyle/disc/eminence and tongue and lips.

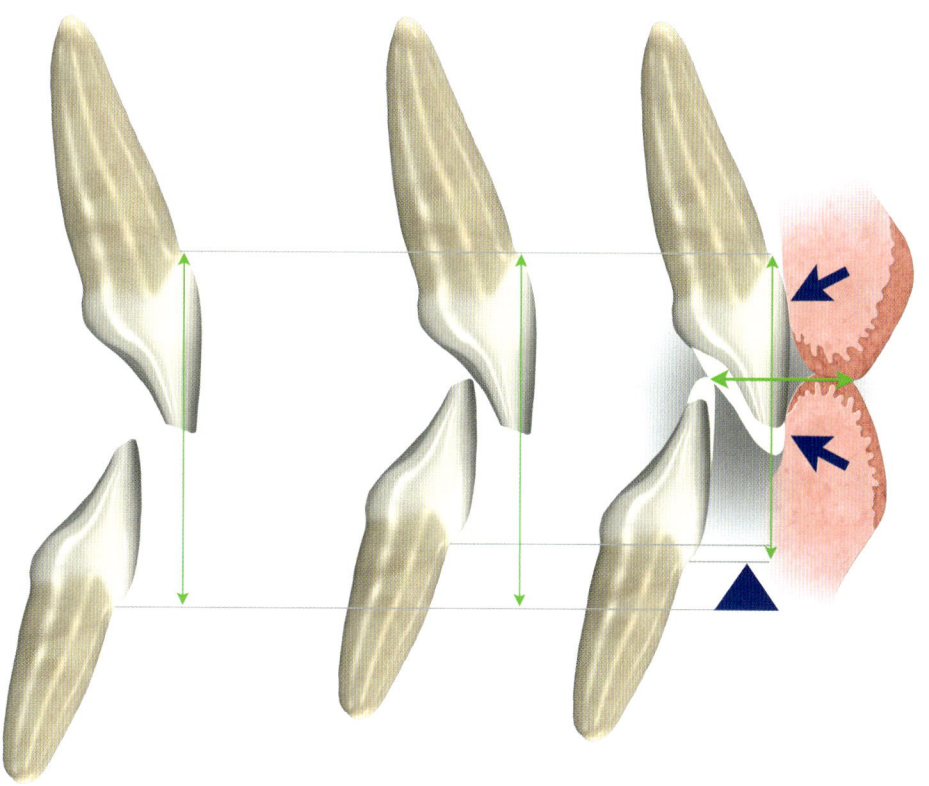

Fig. 3.17 An illustration of the dynamic interplay between the anterior teeth. The process for optimal incisor position and orientation of the occluded teeth (occlusal plane) is started by identifying the maxillary central incisal edge relative to the stomion with lips together and unstrained, and the display with lips in repose (say 'Emma') and in full smile (say 'eeee').

The blue triangle depicts the parameter for vertical anterior tooth mass change to provide an optimal amount of overbite and overjet, creating comfortable jaw posture and smile dynamics. The final tooth form positions can be achieved by restorative or orthodontic means, and in rare cases require orthognathic surgery.

7. The seventh line passes through the tips of the mandibular canines. This line should be parallel to the mandibular incisor line, but slightly coronal (1–1.5 mm). This reflects the increased overbite between the canines relative to the incisors.

As we connect the FEE line (Box 3.1) from the centrals' edges straight across to the canines' tips, designing the four teeth to be of equal length, we restore a pleasing esthetic with improved lateral chewing motion. The amount of clearance on the non-chew side is directly related to the canine-guiding relationship. Additionally, the difference in tooth length provides for more upper lip support and fullness, lower lip support and eversion, and a more verticalized chewing envelope, providing for more axially directed forces. Beauty, indeed, is in the 'eyetooth of the beholder'. Natural forms in function seem to provide the most 'biological' smile system.

THE 'FEE APPLIANCE' FOR DIAGNOSIS, STABILIZATION AND VISUALIZATION

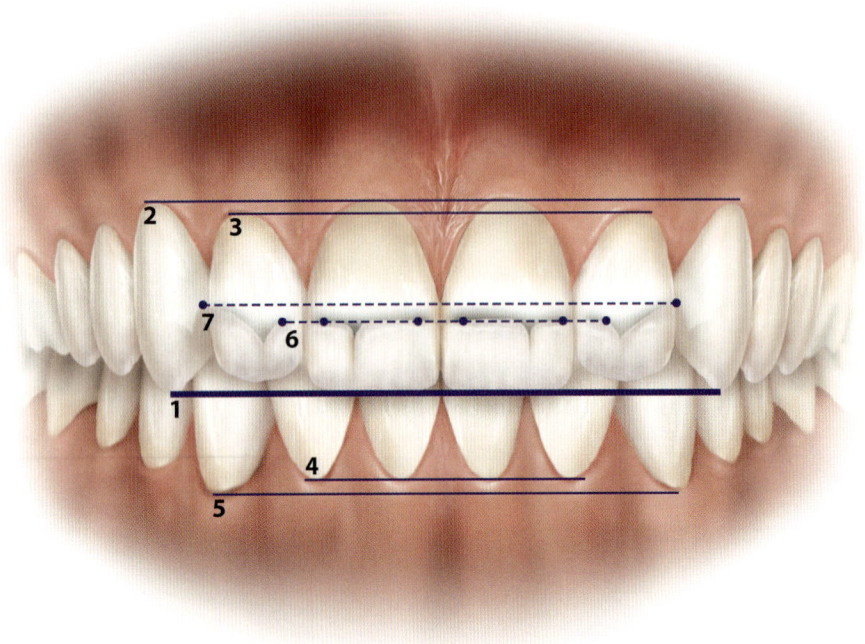

Fig. 3.18 The seven 'FEE' lines used to evaluate symmetry, balance and harmony. Additionally, the concepts of golden proportion, gingival height symmetry, axial inclination and gradation effect can be appreciated in this frontal view of the occluded dentition.

THE 'FEE APPLIANCE' FOR DIAGNOSIS, STABILIZATION AND VISUALIZATION

As described in the esthetic diagnosis chapter (see Chapter 1), a crucial part of our 3-step analysis is the visualization of our proposed treatment. In addition to the visualization methods of computer imaging and an intra-oral mockup, a technique utilizing an appliance named a 'FEE appliance' allows us to test the patient's neuromuscular response to the new incisal edge position, the esthetics and any change in vertical dimension. Similar to our provisionals, but without preparing any teeth, this appliance is an occlusal splint fabricated from the diagnostic wax-up that the patient wears, which provides a functional, esthetic and phonetic dress rehearsal.

Clinically, we determine the FEE by first establishing the length of the maxillary central incisors relative to the upper lip in repose. With the patient in natural head position and looking straight forward, flowable composite is added directly to the centrals, using the pronunciation of 'emma' and 'F' sounds to guide the vertical position of the incisor edge. The canine tips should then be made on a

BOX 3.1
FUNCTIONAL ESTHETIC EVALUATION (FEE) LINE

- Horizontal reference line in the frontal plane that passes through the maxillary central incisor edges and cuspid tips. Ideally, is perpendicular to the long axis of the face, passing through the midline of the maxillary central incisors.

- The FEE line reveals the functional movement of the mandible. Loss of tooth mass at the incisal edge indicates a system that is functionally adapted and may continue to diminish if structural or functional issues are not identified and treated.

- When the incisal edge or cusp tip is lost then form diminishes and tooth proportion decreases. Structure, function and biology have their own 'esthetic'. When form is diminished, then so is function and the 'esthetic' of the system will be decreased.

- Dental, dental–facial and facial esthetics synergize with optimal function when the FEE line provides 4 mm of upper central display with the lips in repose, and the guidelines of the biologic model and neutral zone are met.

- The FEE line evaluates a horizontal line passing through the maxillary central incisors' incisal edges and cusp tips of the maxillary canines in the frontal plane.

- The esthetic line of the maxillary esthetic plane represents the integration of the envelope of mandibular function with the function of lip closure.

- The maxillary central incisors are the keystone to the esthetic plane. This represents the maxillary dental arch through the buccal cusp and incisal edges when viewed in the frontal plane.

- Ideally, a horizontal line from the tip of maxillary canines and central incisors.

- FEE line is a measure of the vertical components of the maxilla.

- The FEE line quantitates the quality of the incisal edges from maxillary canine to canine.

- Optimal function, and dental, dental–facial and facial esthetics synergize when the FEE line is in the relationship indicated by the biologic model and the neutral zone.

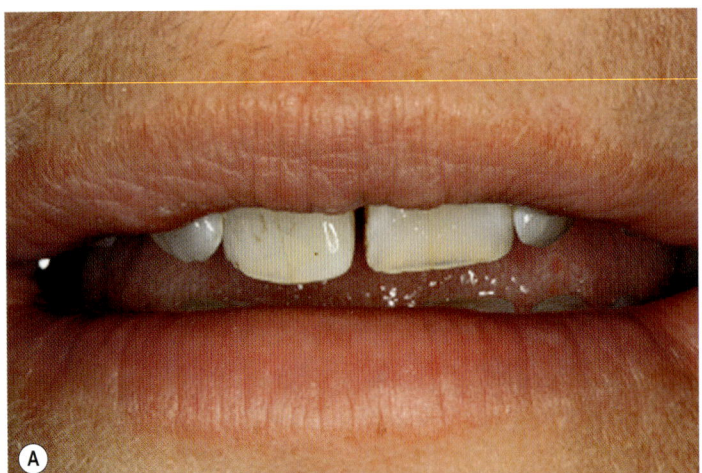 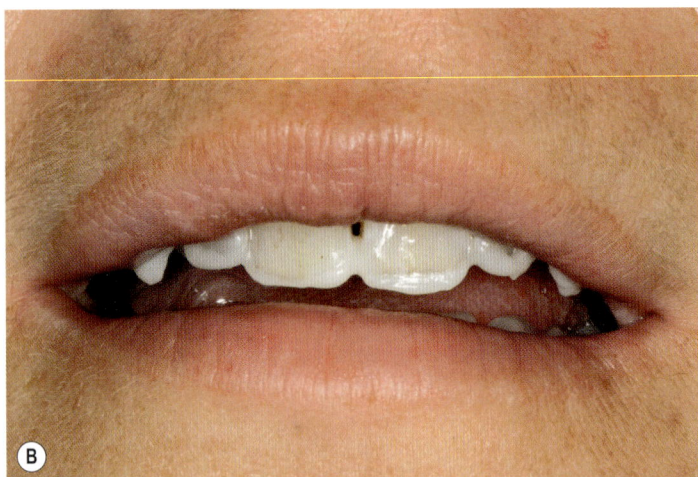

Fig. 3.19A,B (A) 'Emma'. Uneven incisal edges and exposure with lips in repose. (B) FEE line from maxillary canine to canine through central incisor edges established with flowable composite on lubricated teeth. Incisal display is re-evaluated. When optimal tooth length is achieved, an impression is taken and sent to the technician to guide wax-up fabrication.

parallel line to the centrals (Fig. 3.19A,B). Once the cuspid tips are of equal length and parallel to the centrals, composite is added to the laterals following the embrasure guidelines from Rufenacht[4] and Chu[5].

The upper six anterior teeth establish the esthetic plane, or 'FEE line', and the information is transferred to the lab by photography, direct measurement or incisal edge indexing (polyvinyl siloxane). This assists visualization for laboratory waxing for integration of incisal edge function and esthetics.

Once the position of the FEE line is established, the information can also be utilized to make a removable esthetic visualization and stabilization appliance ('FEE appliance') for use in more complex treatment requiring alteration of vertical dimension or joint stabilization. Once optimal display and symmetry are achieved across the maxillary anterior teeth, a model is fabricated and 0.04 inch Essix A+ material is vacu-formed over it. The intaglio of the aligner is primed with bonding agent, flowable composite is placed in the additive areas, the aligner is seated on lubricated teeth, and the composite is cured.

PATIENTS' FAQS

Q. What is the connection between my smile and my face?

A. The face is comprised of the overlying soft tissue and the hard tissue scaffolding beneath, and, most importantly for the smile, the dental arches and teeth. For it is when we smile we reveal our teeth!

Q. Can you really 'design a smile'?

A. Each smile is a unique physical facial pattern that has many social, psychological and emotional cues. Though we can't control when someone smiles, we can ensure that they have the right stuff for that right time.

Q. What is a healthy smile?

A. Health exists in the realm of absence of disease, and movement is the test of form in function. Symmetry is always a sign of health in nature. When the optimal proportions of teeth and gums are revealed from behind well-shaped lips, within the context of a rather symmetrical face, beauty is in the 'eye of the beholder'.

Q. Is a healthy smile a measure of overall health?

A. A healthy smile is effortless and reveals the harmony of forms in function. The quality and quantity of parts from tooth proportion, supporting bone and gum tissue, to facial skeletal type are interrelated to each other through a feedback system of contacts and mechanosensory flow. Within the context of our metabolism, everything we do metabolically is processed through our face and airway. One cannot be truly healthy if the tooth form, fit and function are not in harmony with the form and function of the jaws and facial structure.

The smile may be the ultimate simple measure of overall wellness, for it is a measure of how well all the parts are integrated and functioning.

FAQS

Q. Where do you start?

A. Display of the upper incisors relative to the upper lip, with the lips relaxed and teeth slightly apart. With the lips in repose, say the word 'Emma' and you should see 2–4 mm of tooth depending on age and sex. A measurement of 3–5 mm is considered youthful, and 1–3 mm is normal or with minimal adaptation. Lack of display is usually a sign of being aged and worn and indicates stress across the system.

Q. What are the special guidelines when starting with the upper central incisors?

A. With the lips in repose, relative to the upper lip, the incisal edges should have 2–4 mm of display, midline centered to the philtrum, and be inclined to support the upper lip and provide for lip competence and unstrained lip seal on lip closure.

Q. What is a healthy smile?

A. Within the context of the face a healthy smile refers to natural forms that fit and function in harmony (with little or no adaptation) with the jaw joints, neuromusculature and airway. The quality and quantity of parts, tooth proportions, supporting bone and gum tissue provide for ideal tooth proportions (white) framed by gum (pink). When the pink:white mass is arranged most favourably between the tongue and lips, the neutral zone of balance and harmony has been achieved.

Q. What is natural head posture and how is this used?

A. This is a reproducible manner to orientate the head for esthetic evaluation of the face, e.g. as if the patient was looking in a mirror or at the horizon.

Q. What is the true vertical line?

A. The vertical line is from the subnasale (base of the nose) when the head is in natural head position. This is used to evaluate upper and lower lip projection and the chin relative to the base of the nose. It is also used as a 'soft tissue cephalometric analysis'.

CLINICAL CASE 3.1

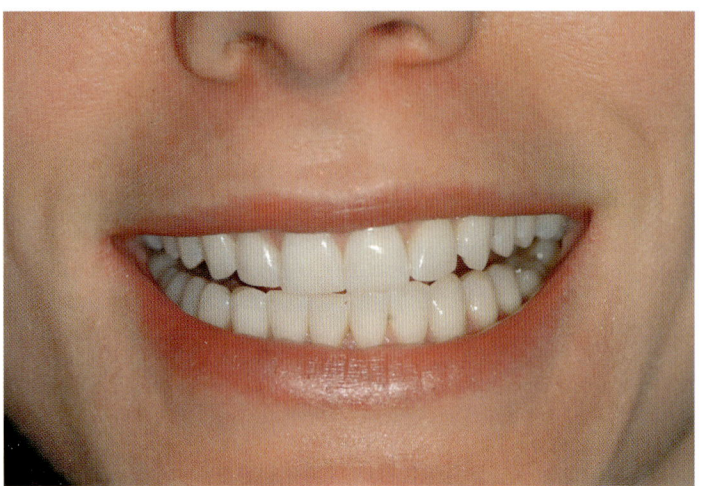

Fig. C3.1.1 Patient presents with a parafunctional habit that has caused wear of the maxillary centrals' incisal edges. The consequence is a lack of posterior disclusion when in the edge-to-edge position, which in turn causes accelerated wear of both anterior and posterior teeth.

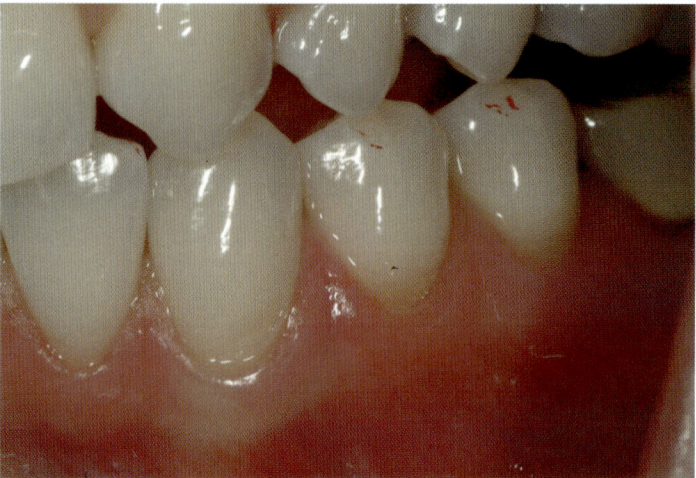

Fig. C3.1.2 The tooth contacts on teeth #20 and #21 with resulting wear and gingival recession.

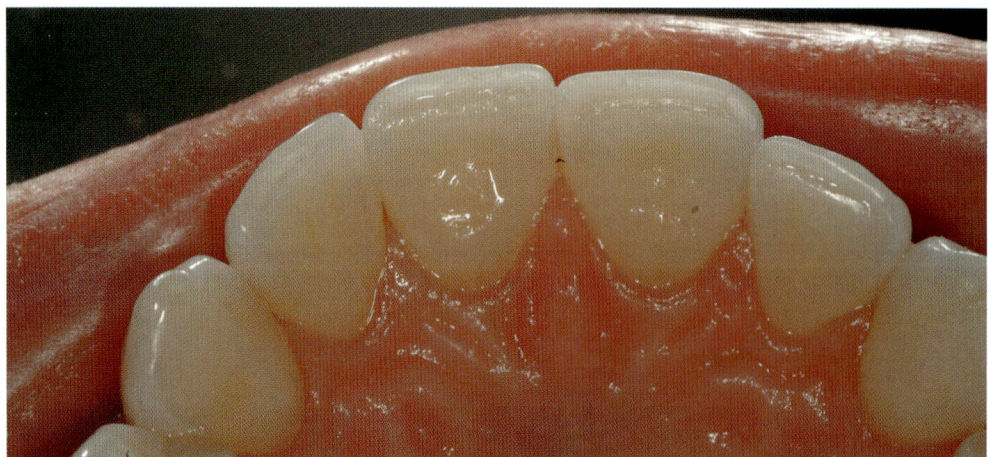

Fig. C3.1.3 Occlusal view showing worn incisal edges of maxillary anterior teeth.

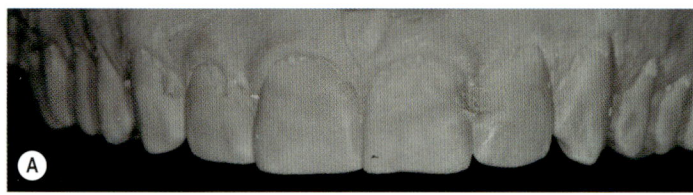
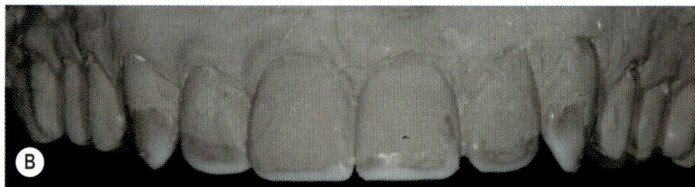

Fig. C3.1.4A,B Wax is added to the model to restore lost tooth structure.

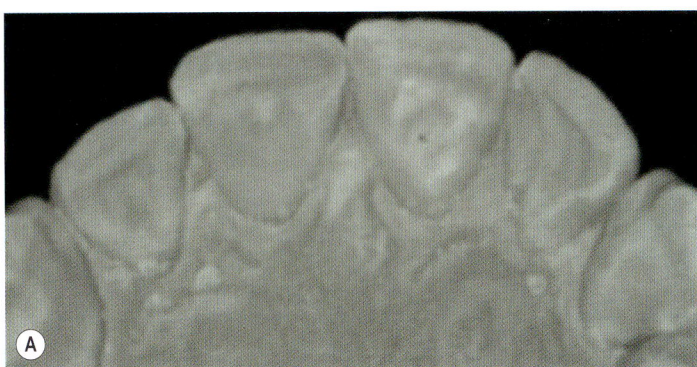 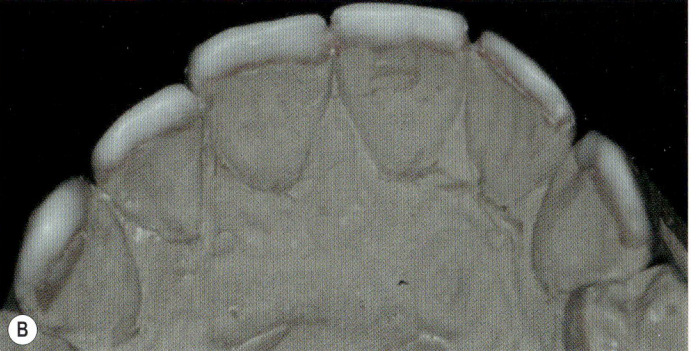

Fig. C3.1.5A,B Occlusal view of the diagnostic wax-up. Lengthening the incisal edges will provide steeper anterior guidance and an improved overbite/overjet relationship.

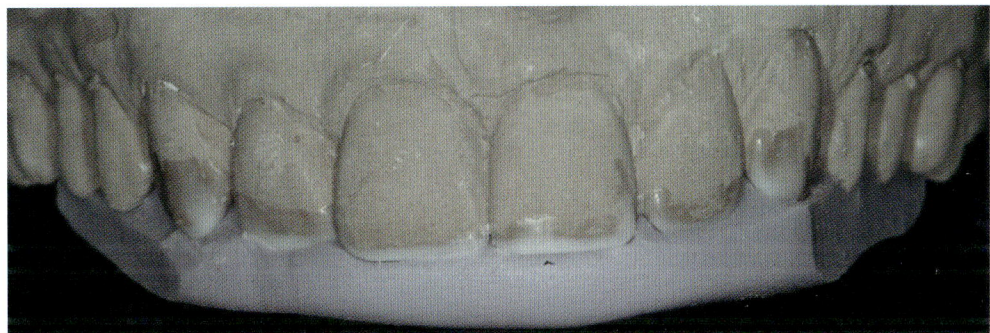

Fig. C3.1.6 A polyvinyl siloxane impression material index is fabricated on the diagnostic wax-up.

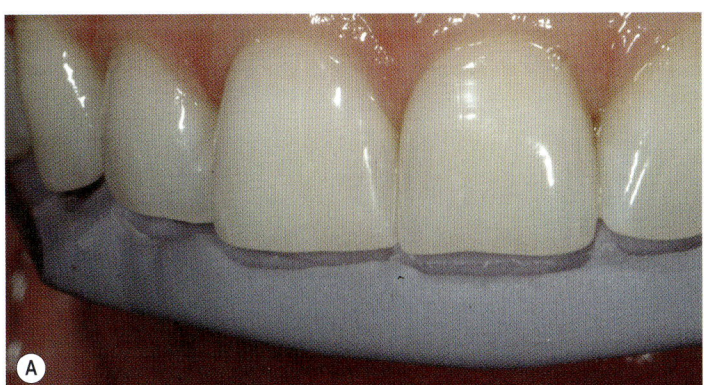 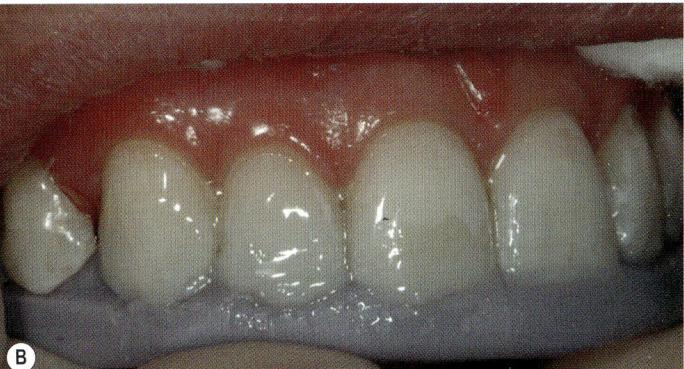

Fig. C3.1.7A,B The incisal edges are etched, bonding agent is applied (A), and highly loaded resin is indexed into place (B).

CLINICAL CASE 3.1

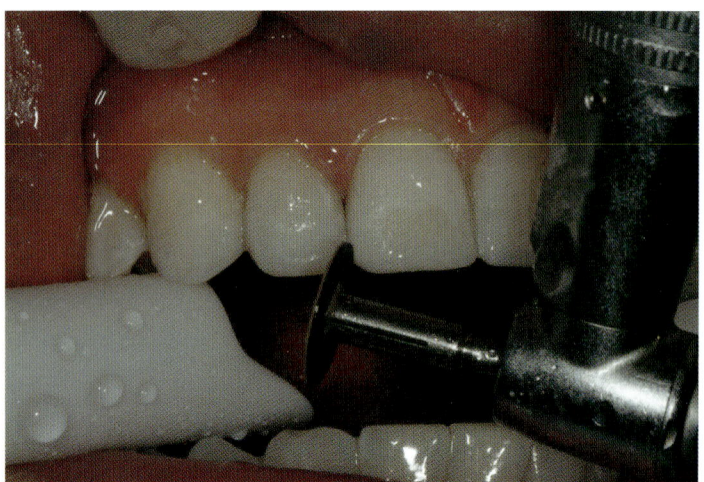

Fig. C3.1.8 Embrasures are refined and occlusion is finalized.

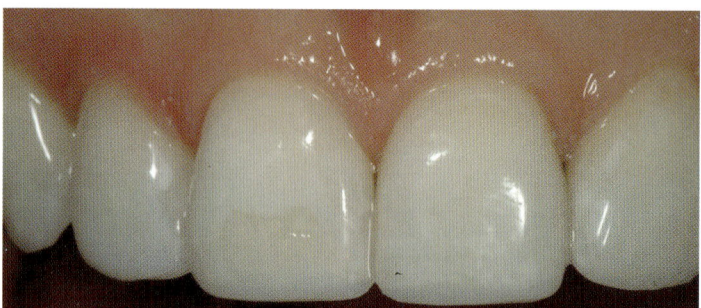

Fig. C3.1.9 The completed composite bonding.

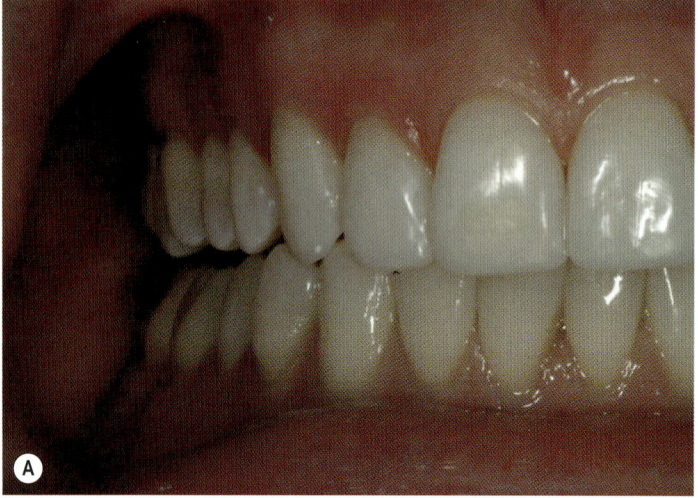

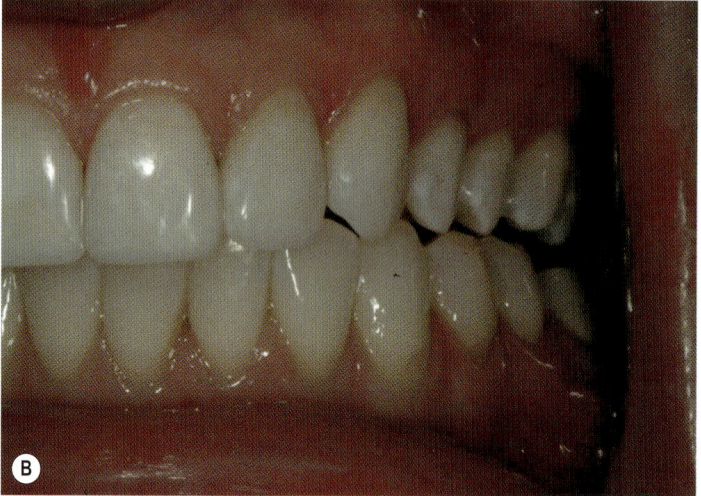

Fig. C3.1.10A,B Working positions now exhibit steeper canine rise, which eliminates interferences on the inner inclines of the posterior teeth.

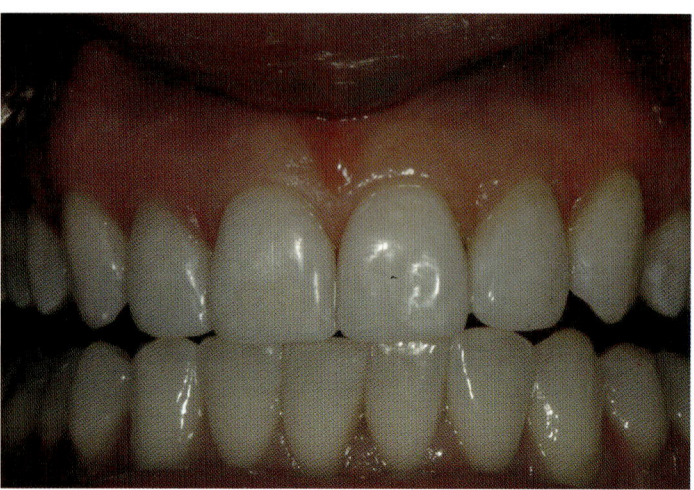

Fig. C3.1.11 The incisive position now demonstrates improved anterior coupling, with greater posterior separation. Improved function and esthetics have been achieved.

CLINICAL CASE 3.2

The following series shows a patient before and after orthodontic treatment, followed by FEE appliance, then bonding from #3–#14 and #21–#28, and final tooth contacts.

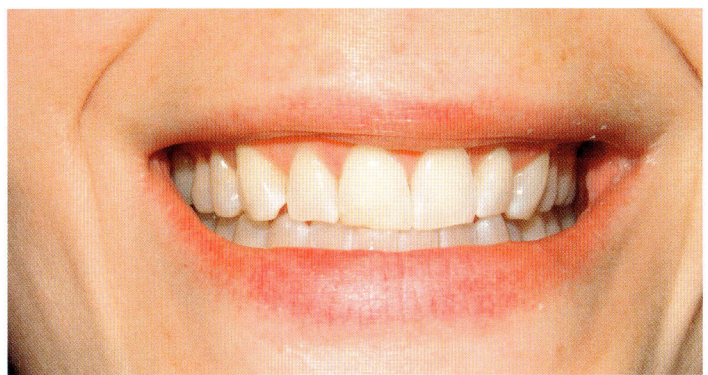

Fig. C3.2.1   Pre-orthodontics.

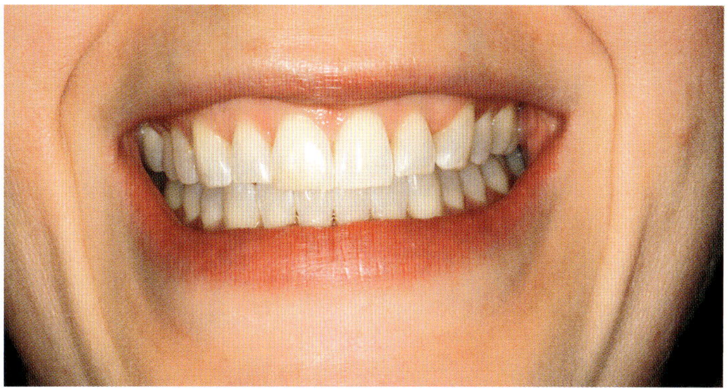

Fig. C3.2.2   Post-orthodontics.

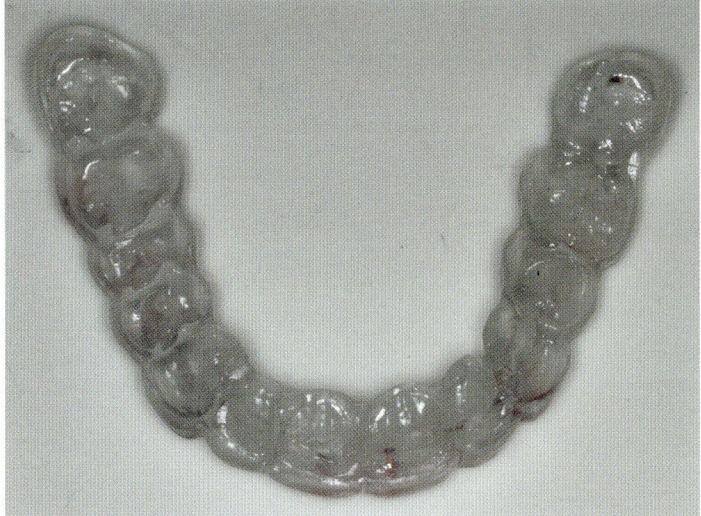

Fig. C3.2.3   The FEE appliance, fabricated on a cast of the diagnostic wax-up (or, alternatively, upon a model of direct composite bonding).

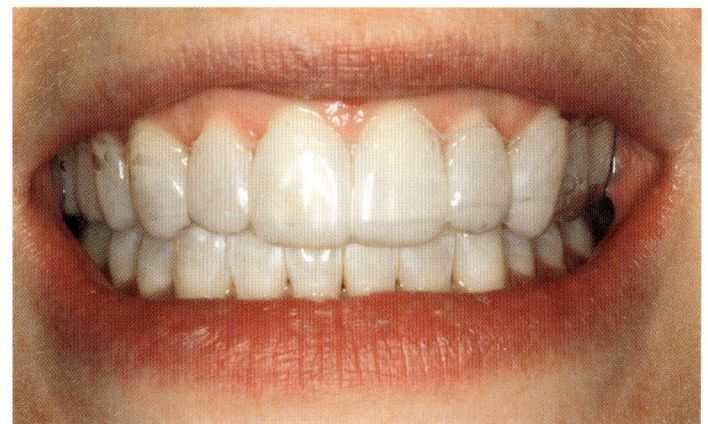

Fig. C3.2.4   The FEE appliance in place. This provides more verticalized movement that gives more anterior and posterior clearance.

CLINICAL CASE 3.2

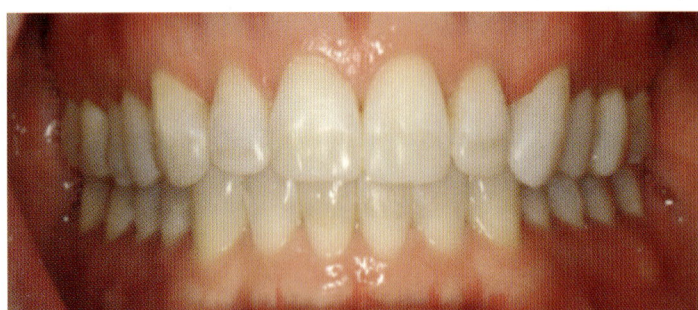

Fig. C3.2.5 Final composite restorations following the same tooth form as the wax-up and FEE appliance.

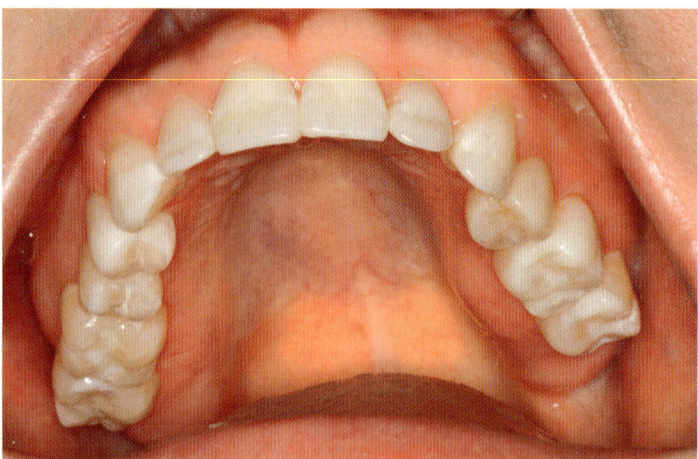

Fig. C3.2.6 Composite bonding #3–#14.

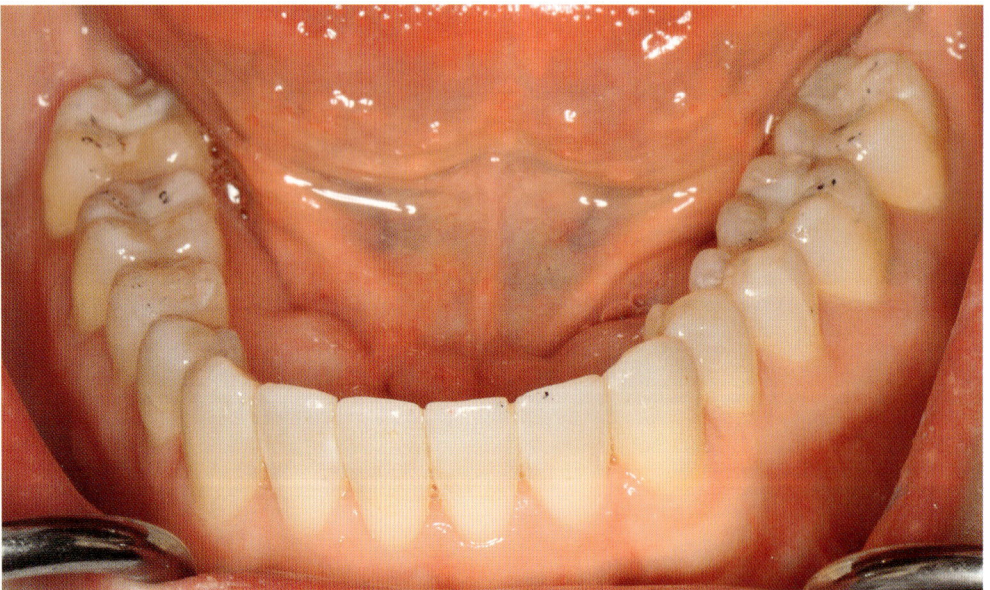

Fig. C3.2.7 Composite bonding #21–#28.

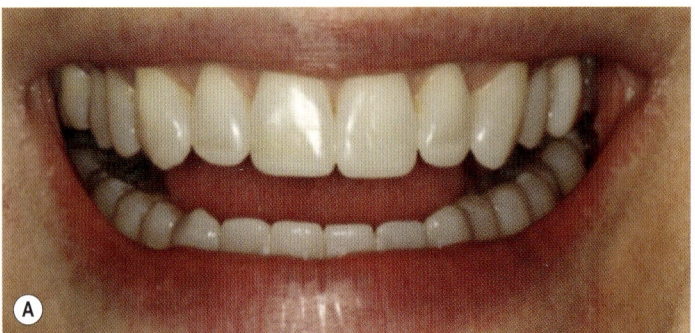
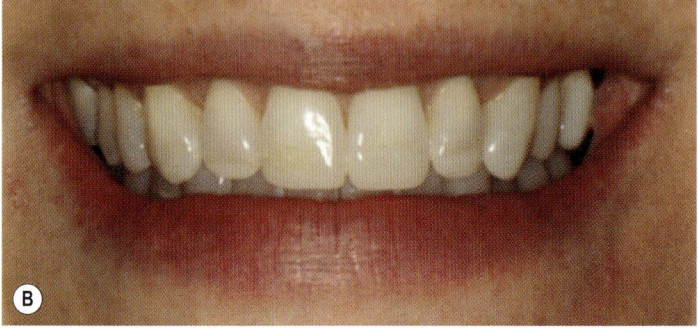

Fig. C3.2.8A,B The post-treatment smile, displaying improved esthetics and function.

CLINICAL CASE 3.3

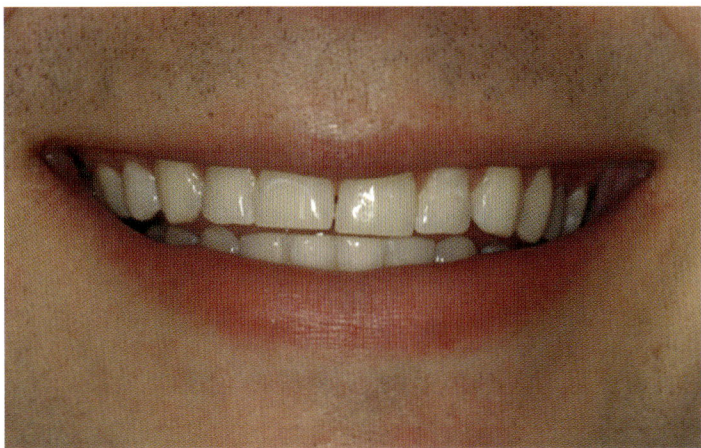

Fig. C3.3.1 A 27-year-old male presents with upper and lower incisal edge wear.

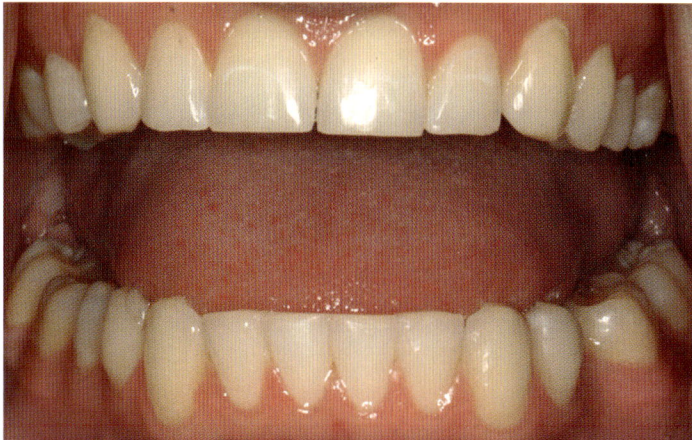

Fig. C3.3.2 The retracted pre-treatment view reveals lower second molars with steepened curves of Spee and Wilson compared to the rest of the arch.

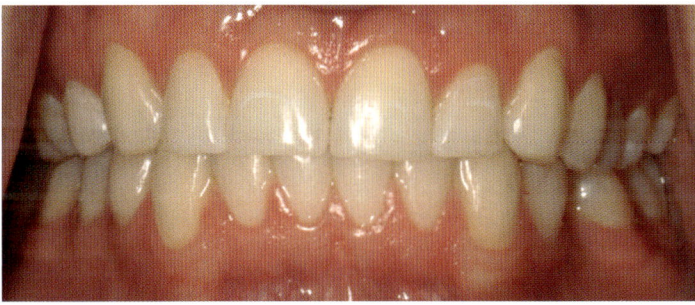

Fig. C3.3.3 When occluded, the arches are coordinated (history of orthodontics) but the forms are not functioning well, and there is esthetic decline occurring. The anterior overbite is not sufficient to provide separation at the second molars in right chew, left chew and incisive positions.

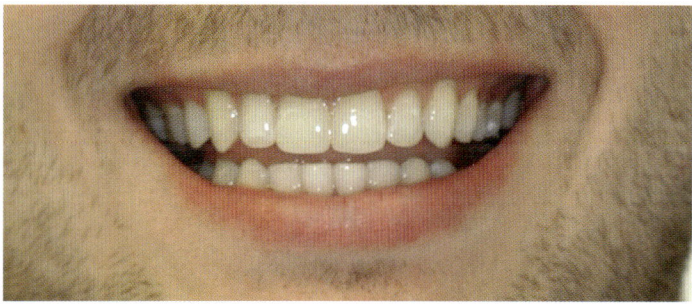

Fig. C3.3.4 Post-treatment. Composite bonding was used to restore teeth #3–#12 to natural lengths and proportions after the posterior bite was adjusted.

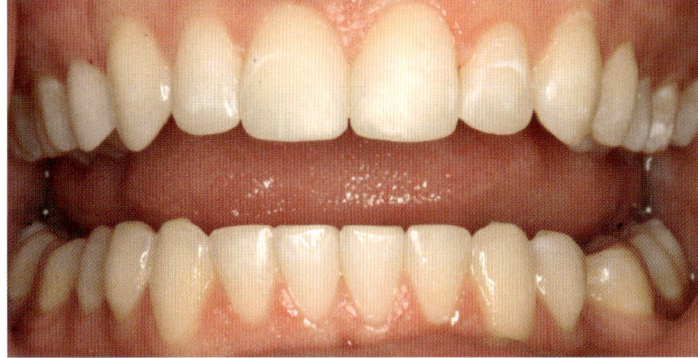

Fig. C3.3.5 Post-treatment retracted view. The incisal embrasures of the lower anteriors have been reshaped to create a less worn appearance (recall that worn teeth lose their rounded incisal embrasures). Additionally, negative coronoplasty was performed on the premolars and molars to equilibrate the occlusion.

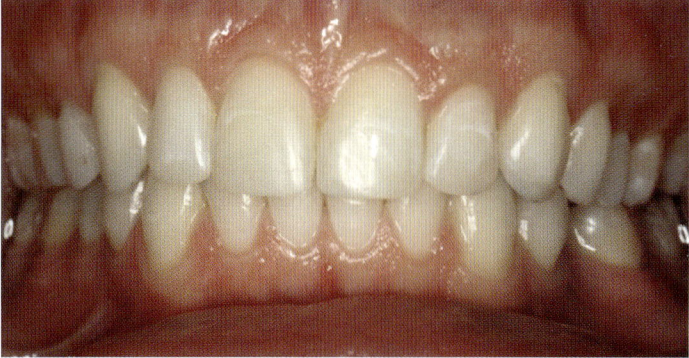

Fig. C3.3.6 Improved overbite and overjet. Composite on lingual marginal ridges of upper incisors provides anterior contacts to the lower incisors.

CLINICAL CASE 3.4

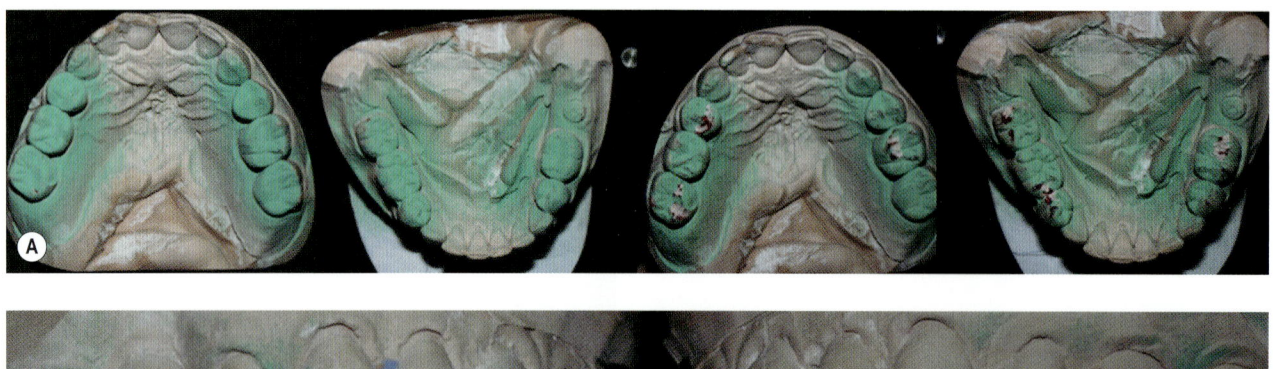

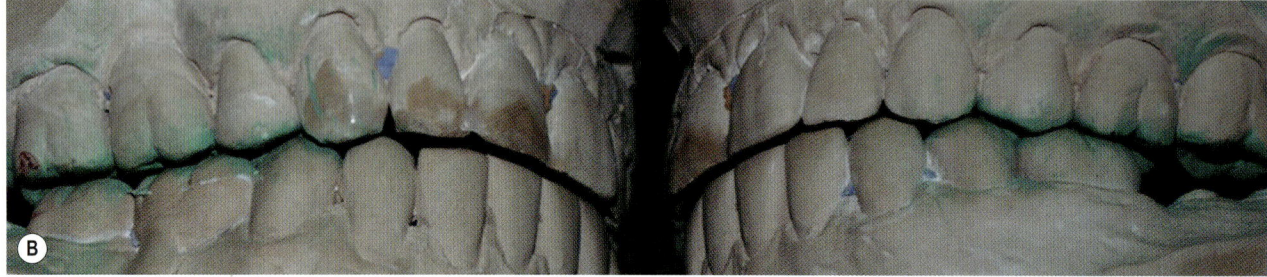

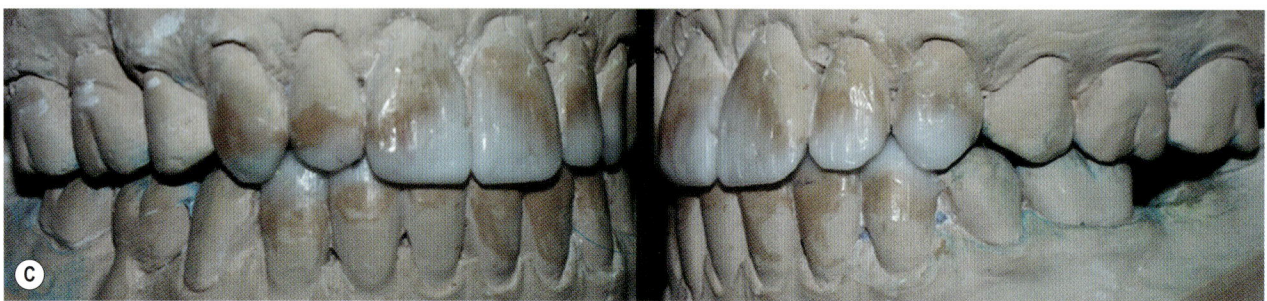

Fig. C3.4.1A–C (A) The diagnostic casts are mounted and sprayed with Occlude before occlusal adjustment. Posterior teeth are adjusted until the first premolars contact. (B) Model equilibration showing lack of anterior tooth contact and minimal overbite and overjet. (C) Form is added in wax to #6–#11 and #22–#27 for contact, esthetic proportion and function. A polyvinyl siloxane index is used to translate these new forms into hybrid composite restorations. Eventually, the same form was followed for porcelain restorations.

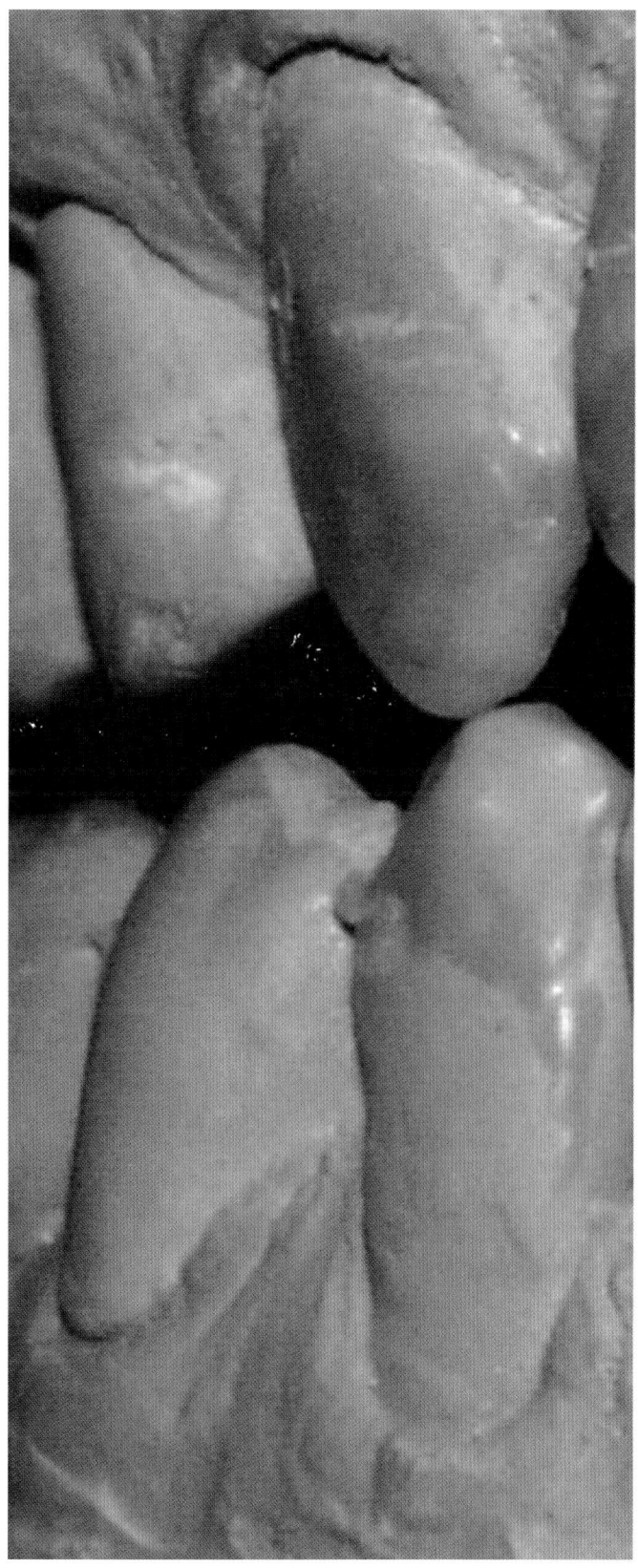

Fig. C3.4.2 A detail of the diagnostic wax-up displaying more verticalized right jaw chewing movement.

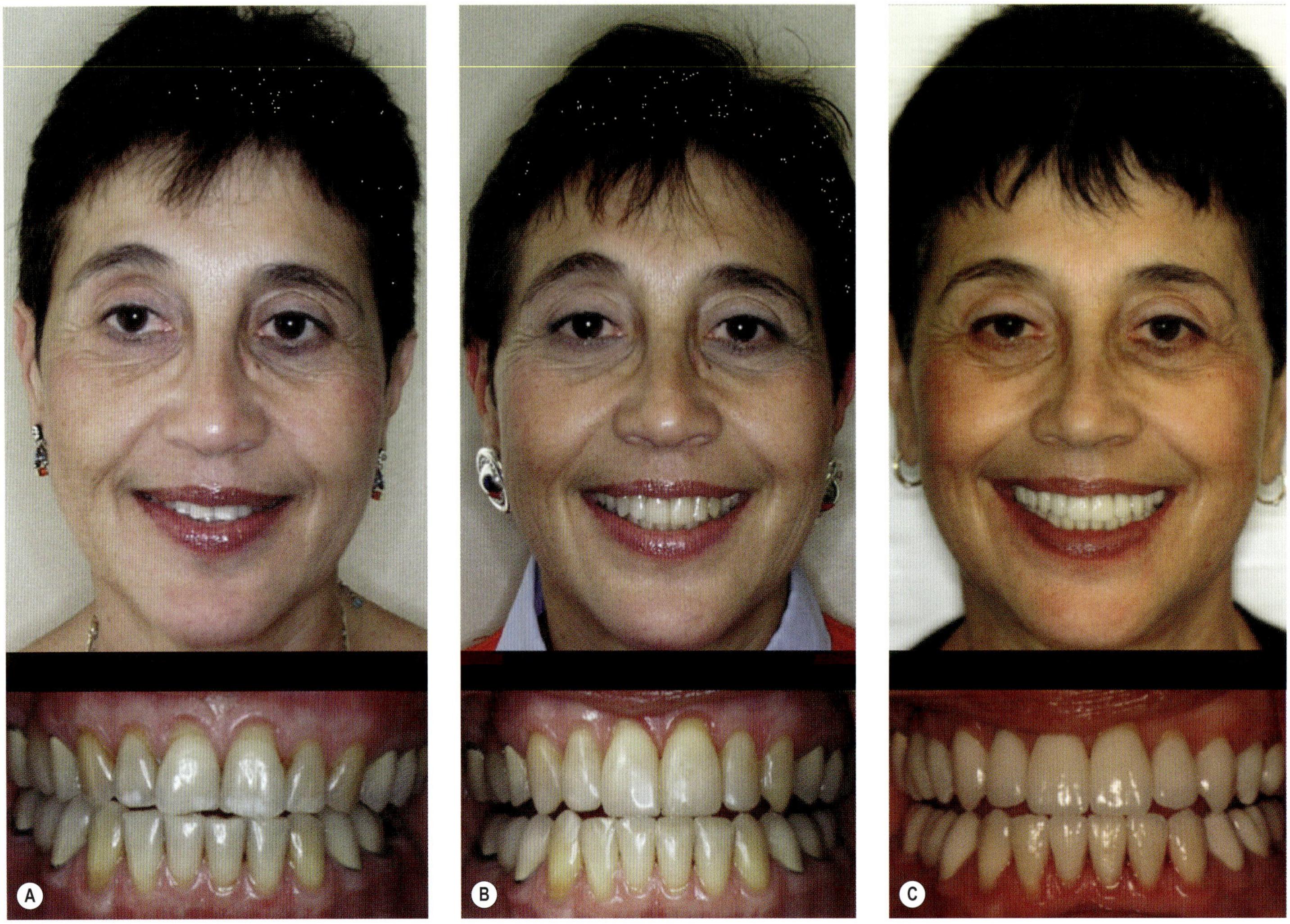

CLINICAL CASE 3.4

Fig. C3.4.3A–C Pre-treatment view of incisive position (A), followed by composite restorations to restore proper occlusion (B), and eventual porcelain restorations following the same form (C).

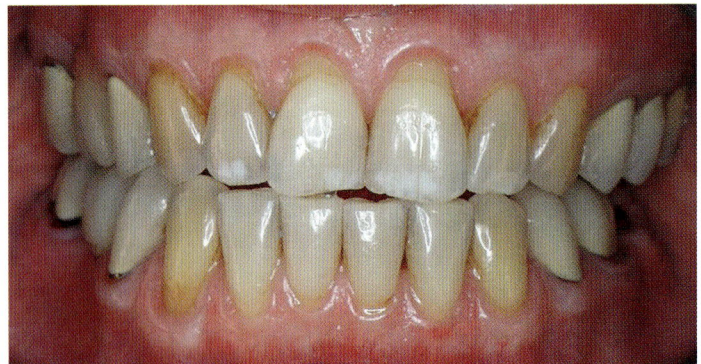

Fig. C3.4.4 Pre-treatment right chew position demonstrating multiple interferences, anterior tooth contact, and a lack of posterior separation.

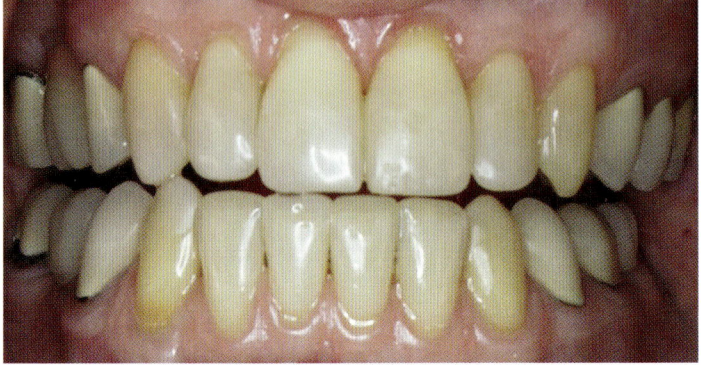

Fig. C3.4.5 Restored form (at the composite stage) in right chew test position. Note the increased posterior separation and no anterior tooth contact.

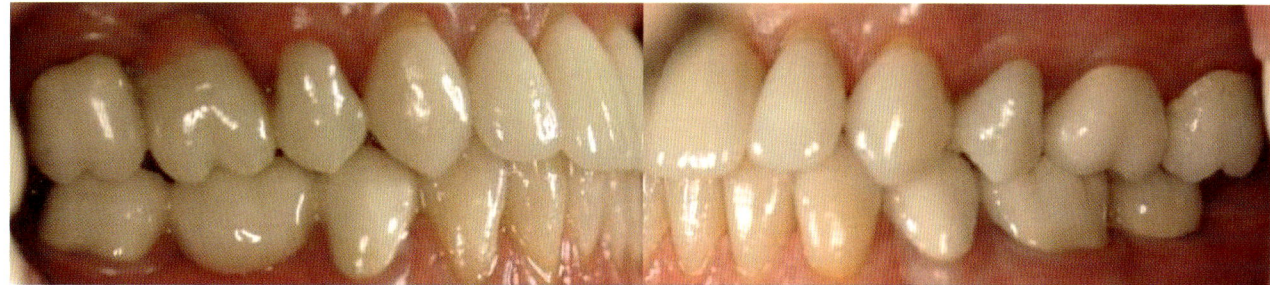

Fig. C3.4.6   Final porcelain restorations. Note maxillary right first molar implant crown with gingival porcelain.

Seminal literature

Arnett GW, Bergman RT. Facial keys to orthodontic diagnosis and treatment planning. Part 1. Am J Orthod Dentofacial Orthop 1993;103(4):299–312.

Nineteen facial traits are presented with the face in frontal and profile views in order to better evaluate the face before treatment. The authors argue that tooth movement to correct the bite may result in facial decline. Isolated dental model analysis or cephalometric analysis without consideration of the face may not provide the best result. Patients are examined in natural head position, centric relation and relaxed lip posture.

Magne P, Gallucci GO, Belser UC. Anatomic crown/length ratios of unworn and worn maxillary teeth in white subjects. J Prosthet Dent 2003;89(5):453–61.

This study provides maxillary tooth dimensions and proportions that may be useful guidelines for diagnosis and treatment planning and make a clear distinction between unworn and worn centrals, laterals and cuspids. These guidelines are useful for restorative dentistry and periodontal surgery.

Spear FM, Kokich VG, Mathews DP. Interdisciplinary management of anterior dental esthetics. J Am Dent Assoc 2006;137(2):160–9.

The authors present their time-tested process for working as an interdisciplinary team. Starting with esthetics, the first step is to identify the edge, midline and inclination of the upper incisors. Gingival levels followed by arrangement, contour and shade precede evaluating lower incisal edges relative to the face. Following esthetics, function, structure and biology should then be considered.

Further reading

Andrews LF. The six keys to normal occlusion. Am J Orthod 1972;62(3):296–309.

Arnett G, McLaughlin W, Richard P. Facial and dental planning for orthodontists and oral surgeons. New York: CV Mosby; 2004.

Arnett GW, Bergman RT. Facial keys to orthodontic diagnosis and treatment planning, part 1. Am J Orthod Dentofacial Orthop 1993;103(4):299–312.

Kraus BE, Jordan RE, Abrams L. Dental anatomy and occlusion. Baltimore: Williams and Wilkins Co.; 1969.

Levy JN. Teeth as sensory organs. Vistas 2009;2(3):14–19.

Lundeen HC, Gibbs CH. The function of teeth. USA: L & G Pub; 2005.

Okeson JP. Management of temporomandibular disorders and occlusion. 4th ed. St Louis: CV Mosby; 1999.

Renner RP. An introduction to dental anatomy and esthetics. Chicago: Quintessence; 1985.

Spear FM, Kokich VG, Mathews DP. Interdisciplinary management of anterior dental esthetics. J Am Dent Assoc 2006;137(2):160–9.

REFERENCES

1. Lee RL. Esthetics and its relationship to function. In: Rufenacht CR, editor. Fundamentals of esthetics. Chicago: Quintessence; 1990. p. 137–209.

2. Pound E. Lost fine art in the fallacy of ridges. J Prosthet Dent 1954;4:6–16.

3. Dawson PE. Evaluation, diagnosis and treatment of occlusal problems. 2nd ed. St Louis: CV Mosby; 1989.

4. Rufenacht CR. Esthetics and its relationship to function. Fundamentals of esthetics. Chicago: Quintessence; 1990. p. 140.

5. Chu SJ. A biometric approach to predictable treatment of clinical crown discrepancies. Pract Proced Aesthet Dent 2007;19(7):401–9.

CHAPTER 4

Clinical Photography in Esthetic Dentistry

NICHOLAS A. HODSON

Uses of dental photography in esthetic dentistry . . . 90
Consent and other medico-legal aspects 92
Photographic equipment 92
Basic principles of dental photography 93
General photographic technique 104
Standard photographic views 106
File types and digital workflow 107
Clinical cases 108

Clinical photography is a critical skill to develop for successful esthetic dentistry. The digital revolution has allowed increased efficiency in our field, improving communication between the dental profession and our patients. Proper photographs, combined with thorough diagnostics, allow us to document, plan and execute our cases predictably.

USES OF DENTAL PHOTOGRAPHY IN ESTHETIC DENTISTRY

TREATMENT PLANNING

Esthetic treatment planning of smile design requires an understanding of the relationship between the patient's smile line and lip rest position in relation to the size and position of the front teeth, as well as relating this to the face as a whole.[1] Standard dental photographs allow these to be considered when planning cases in the absence of the patient and enable the presentation of the proposed treatment plan to the patient. This planning can consider the gingival contour and tooth proportions and can be used in planning crown lengthening, with annotated digital images used to show the patient what is intended (Fig. 4.1),[2,3] or to facilitate communication between restorative and surgical dentists.[4] Some practitioners have advocated the use of digital simulations to increase patient acceptance of a treatment plan such as crown lengthening[4] and diastema closure.[5] However, simulation software needs to be used carefully; if you overpromise and under deliver, you can create unfulfilled expectations and an unhappy patient. We strive, instead, for under promising and over delivering for our patients.

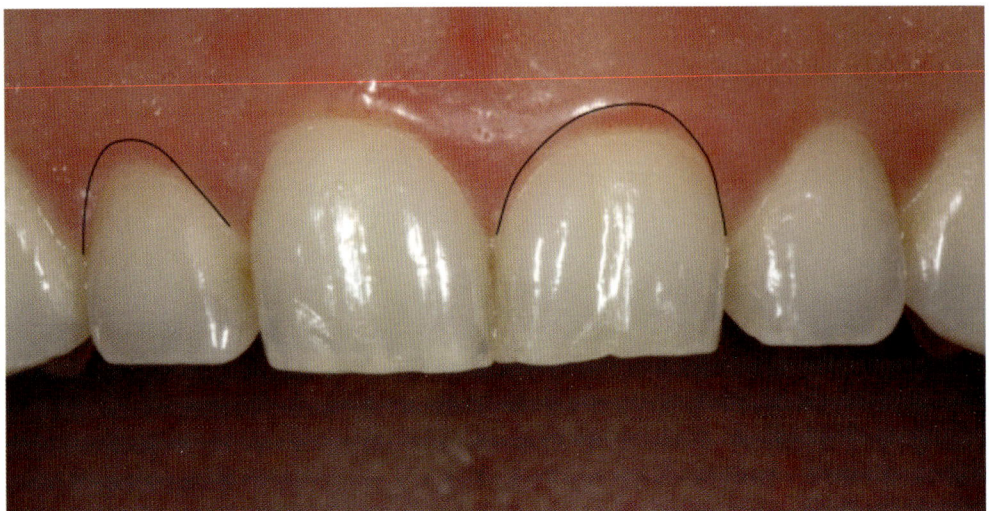

Fig. 4.1   Planning crown lengthening on a digital photograph.

COMMUNICATION WITH THE DENTAL TECHNICIAN

Photographs allow a quick and effective way to communicate esthetic characteristics, such as translucency, opalescence, opacity, maverick colours and size and shape of incisal mamelons, of a tooth to be seen by the technician.[6-9] At present it is not possible, due to the lack of colour accuracy, to use digital photographs taken with a single-lens reflex (SLR) camera alone to accurately determine shade; however, inclusion of shade tabs in the photograph is considered to be the best way of communicating colour.[10]

BLEACHING

Monitoring the progress of bleaching by recording photographs of shade tabs against the teeth is possible and gives a record of pre-bleaching tooth colour. Alternatively, if you want a more precise approach then you could use a standard neutral reference and Adobe Photoshop (Adobe Systems Incorporated) to more accurately measure the change in shade.[11]

MARKETING

Marketing is communication. We have an enhanced tool to visually represent our abilities and how we create beautiful smiles. There is an increasing need to promote practices in order to increase business. A series of cases displayed in a 'coffee table book' style in the waiting room or on practice websites can give patients an idea of what sort of treatments are offered in your practice and acts as a good marketing tool to demonstrate your clinical skills.[12] If you are intending to use photographs in this way then you need to be careful about your consent procedures for photographs (Box 4.1).

OTHER USES

Photographs are also useful for other general areas of dentistry, such as lectures and training for colleagues. Documentation before, during and after the work is

---

BOX 4.1 CONSENT

Consent is required from patients for all dental photography, irrespective of whether they can be identified, and for the subsequent use of the images. Specific consent should be obtained if an image will be used in electronic publishing.

Hood CA, Hope T, Dove P. Videos, photographs, and patient consent. BMJ 1998;316(7136):1009–1011.

done helps the dental team understand the challenges, and how these challenges were managed. This fosters the mindset of 'constant improvement' for the dental team and can be used for personal reference and for educational purposes within our profession. This is critical for the clinician to achieve the goal of predictable esthetic results and for considering how this can be better accomplished.

CONSENT AND OTHER MEDICO-LEGAL ASPECTS

As with all aspects of dental treatment, demonstrating consent (Box 4.1) is important and this should ideally be in a written form. The consent should cover permission for photographs being taken and how they are going to be used. Is the photograph for clinical records, publication in practice literature or articles, educational use or other possible use? In general, three levels of consent are used:[13,14]

1. For use in medical/dental records only
2. For use in teaching healthcare staff and students
3. For publication.

It is important to remember that any clinical photographs you take are part of the patient's clinical record. Medico-legally, these should be stored with the other clinical records for the patient, either as hard copies or digitally on a computer. This storage should be secure (i.e. password protected) in order to comply with data protection legislation and the confidentiality of patients. The other medico-legal use of the photographs is a record of the pre-treatment appearance of the teeth when esthetic treatment plans are considered.[6,15]

PHOTOGRAPHIC EQUIPMENT

The most appropriate camera for good quality clinical photography is a digital SLR camera with a high quality macro lens and ring flash (Fig. 4.2) or dual flash.[9,11,16] These will allow appropriate and necessary control over the aperture, shutter speed of the camera and illumination of the teeth. Some compact cameras allow limited control over these aspects; however, they are a compromise and lack predictability for high quality images.[11,17]

Most SLR cameras offer through-the-lens (TTL) viewing of the teeth to allow you to frame your photograph, although the latest digital SLRs also allow the option of viewing the output on a liquid crystal display (LCD). You should select either manual or aperture (Av) settings on the camera so that you can choose an appropriate aperture for the clinical situation.

Most digital SLRs have a sensor that is smaller than standard 35 mm film. This is important as it means that the image captured will appear magnified compared to the same image captured with a 35 mm SLR camera. The degree of magnification depends on the size of the sensor. For example, the Nikon D7000 sensor is 23.6 mm × 15.6 mm giving a 1.5 × magnification; and the Canon 450D has a 22.2 × 14.8 mm CMOS sensor giving a 1.6 × magnification. This has to be kept in mind when selecting the appropriate reproduction ratio on your lens. More recent digital SLRs have a sensor the same size as a 35 mm film and so no correction is required, e.g. Canon EOS 5D.

The resolution of the digital camera that you need depends upon how you wish to display the photograph. If you are planning to show patients pictures as photographs or on a laptop or an iPad then you need to consider the 'pixels per inch' (ppi) and the size of the screen.[18] For photographs, a resolution of 300 ppi is recommended, which would allow you a print of 6 × 8 inches (4 megapixels), 8 × 10 inches (6 megapixels) or 11 × 14 inches (12 megapixels) dependant on your camera. An iPad 2 has a screen resolution of 1024 by 768 pixels at 132 ppi and can only show an image of 0.8 megapixels, and even the retina display of an iPad 3, with a resolution of 2048 by 1536 pixel at 264 ppi, can only show an image of 3.1 megapixels. On this basis, for most practitioners, 6 megapixels would be more than sufficient unless you are planning to move into poster prints of your work!

A macro lens of between 90 and 105 mm is ideal for dental photography (Fig. 4.3). This will allow the range of reproduction ratios required and enable a comfortable working distance from the mouth. This lens can also be used for portrait photography without the distortion that can occur with a smaller focal length.

BASIC PRINCIPLES OF DENTAL PHOTOGRAPHY

Intra-oral photography is essentially macrophotography, which is a photographic technique that allows you to take magnified images of the teeth. Classically, macrophotography is where the image on the sensor or film is the same size as the object itself, i.e. a reproduction ratio of 1:1. For intra-oral photography it is not just a question of being able to focus really close to your patient's teeth, as this can be uncomfortable or even claustrophobic for the patient, but of being able to choose an appropriate working distance. Your

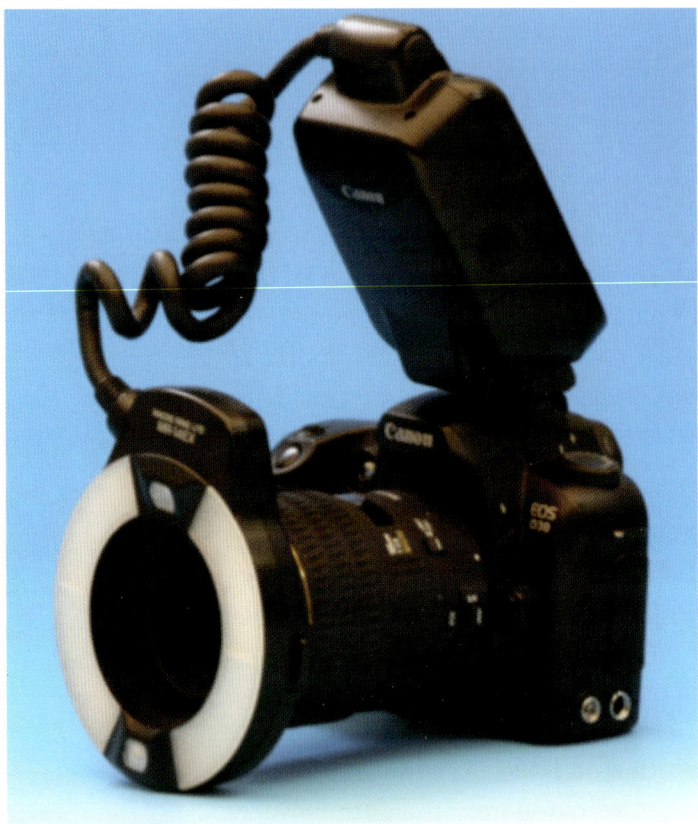

Fig. 4.2 A digital single-lens reflex (SLR) camera with a high quality macro lens and ring flash.

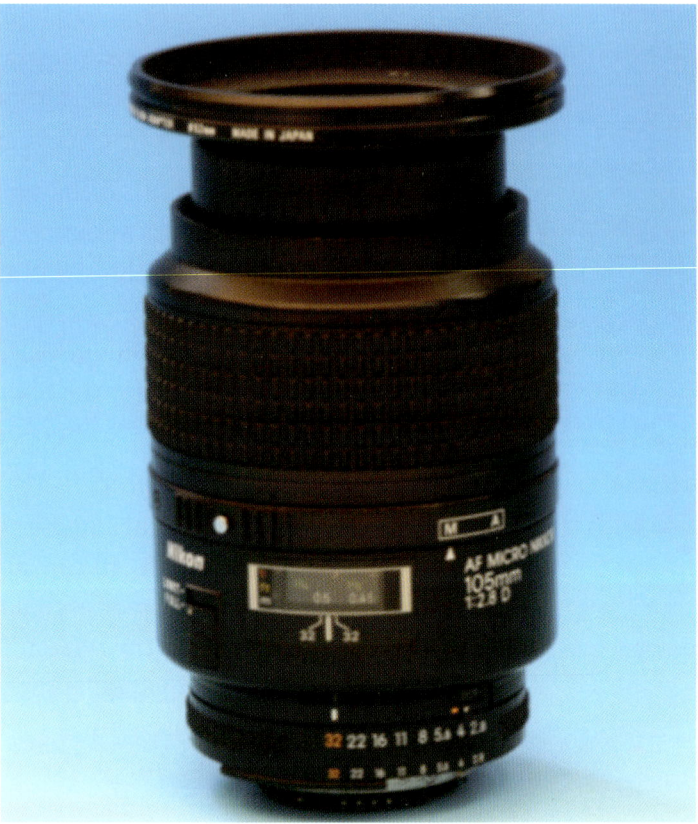

Fig. 4.3 A 105 mm Nikon macro lens.

working distance must also allow sufficient light from your flash to get to the teeth that you are photographing without the patient's cheek getting in the way. The importance of this is most obvious if you want to take a photograph of a single tooth towards the back of the mouth. The main challenges of macrophotography in dentistry are that it tends to limit the depth of the photographic field and makes it difficult to illuminate objects to get the correct exposure.

REPRODUCTION RATIO

Different reproduction ratios are used in dental photography; however, intra-oral photography needs somewhere between 1:1 and 1:3 (Fig. 4.4). Lenses capable of producing these reproduction ratios are known as macro lenses. The different ratios for different intra-oral photographs will be discussed later; however, it is important to be consistent with the ratio that is used for the

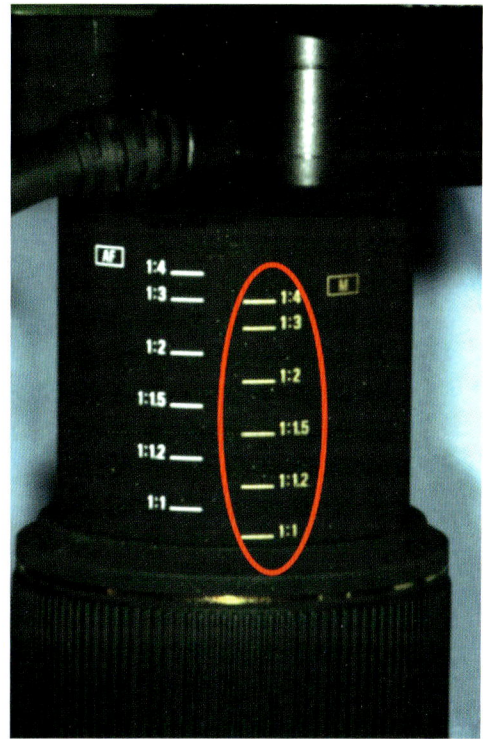

Fig. 4.4 Reproduction ratios used in intra-oral photography on a 105 mm macro lens.

different views that you take. When you take a photograph it is sensible to make a note of the reproduction ratio as part of the information that you record about the photographs, as this will enable you to use the same settings for any subsequent photographs. This consistency allows 'before' and 'after' photographs to be comparable without adding to your workflow by requiring resizing or cropping of the images.

DEPTH OF FIELD

The depth of field of a photograph is the distance in front and behind an object that the camera has been focused on (focal plane) that appears to be in focus. In general, approximately 50% of the depth of field is in front of the focal plane and 50% behind the focal plane. The depth of field is dependent upon the size of the aperture or metal diaphragm inside the lens, which is usually referred to as an f-stop (Fig. 4.5A–D). A good depth of field is determined by a large f-stop (Fig. 4.6A,B). The problem with a small aperture, however, is that this limits the amount of light getting to the film or sensor in your camera and therefore affects the exposure of the object.

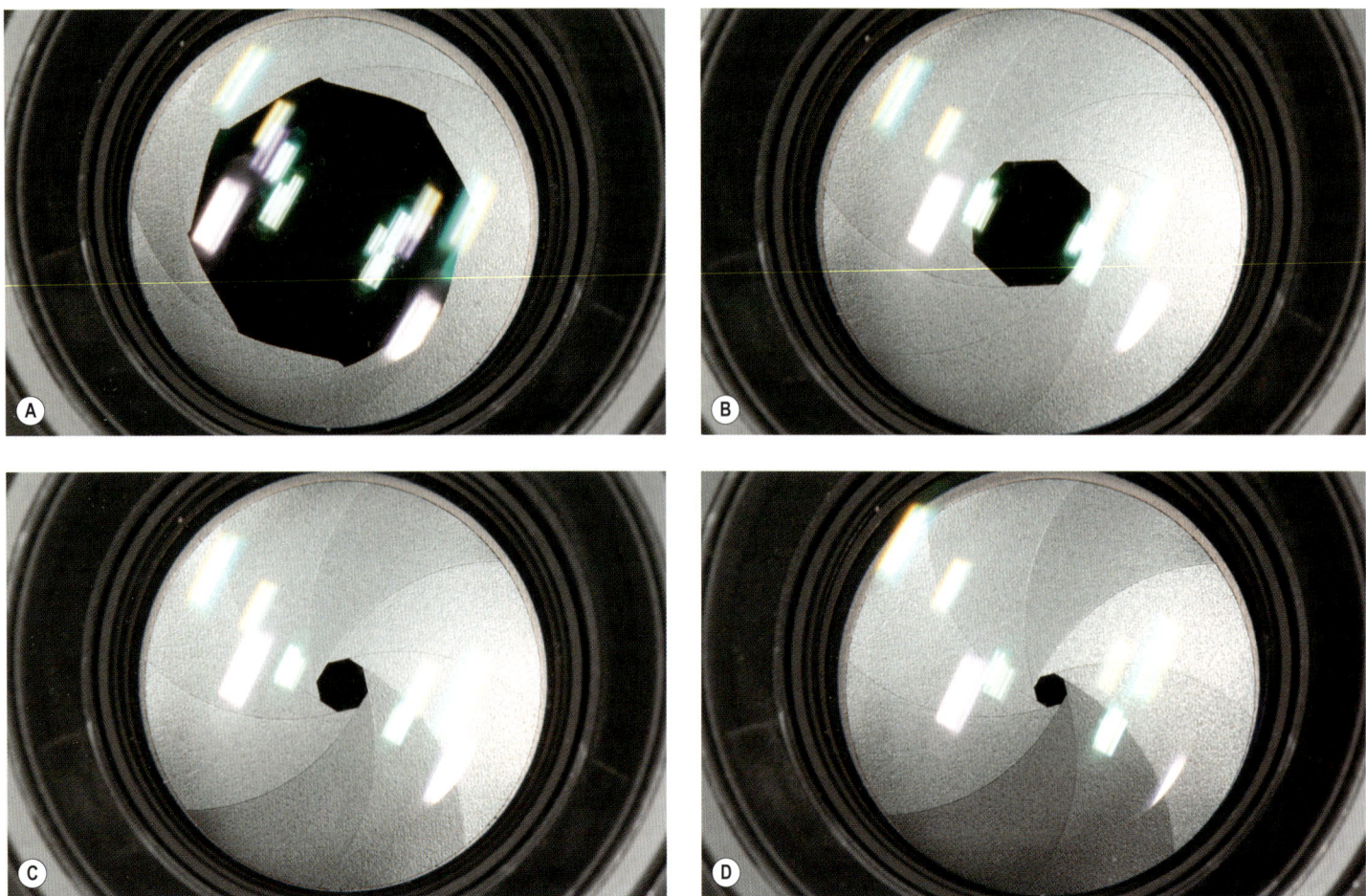

Fig. 4.5A–D The relationship between f-number and aperture opening.

PATIENTS' FAQS

Q. What are you going to use the photograph for?

A. You might explain that photographs before treatment commences are important to help show the patient those areas you think need addressing and as a pre-treatment record of their mouth. If you want to use them for other areas such as teaching or for publication then your consent process must cover this, although patients are often happy to oblige.

Q. What if I decide that I don't want photographs to be used for teaching or publication after consent?

A. You should reassure the patient that they can view images at any time and withdraw consent for use. It is important, however, to discuss clearly with the patient if you are planning to use the pictures on a website as they must understand the irretrievability of photographs put online.

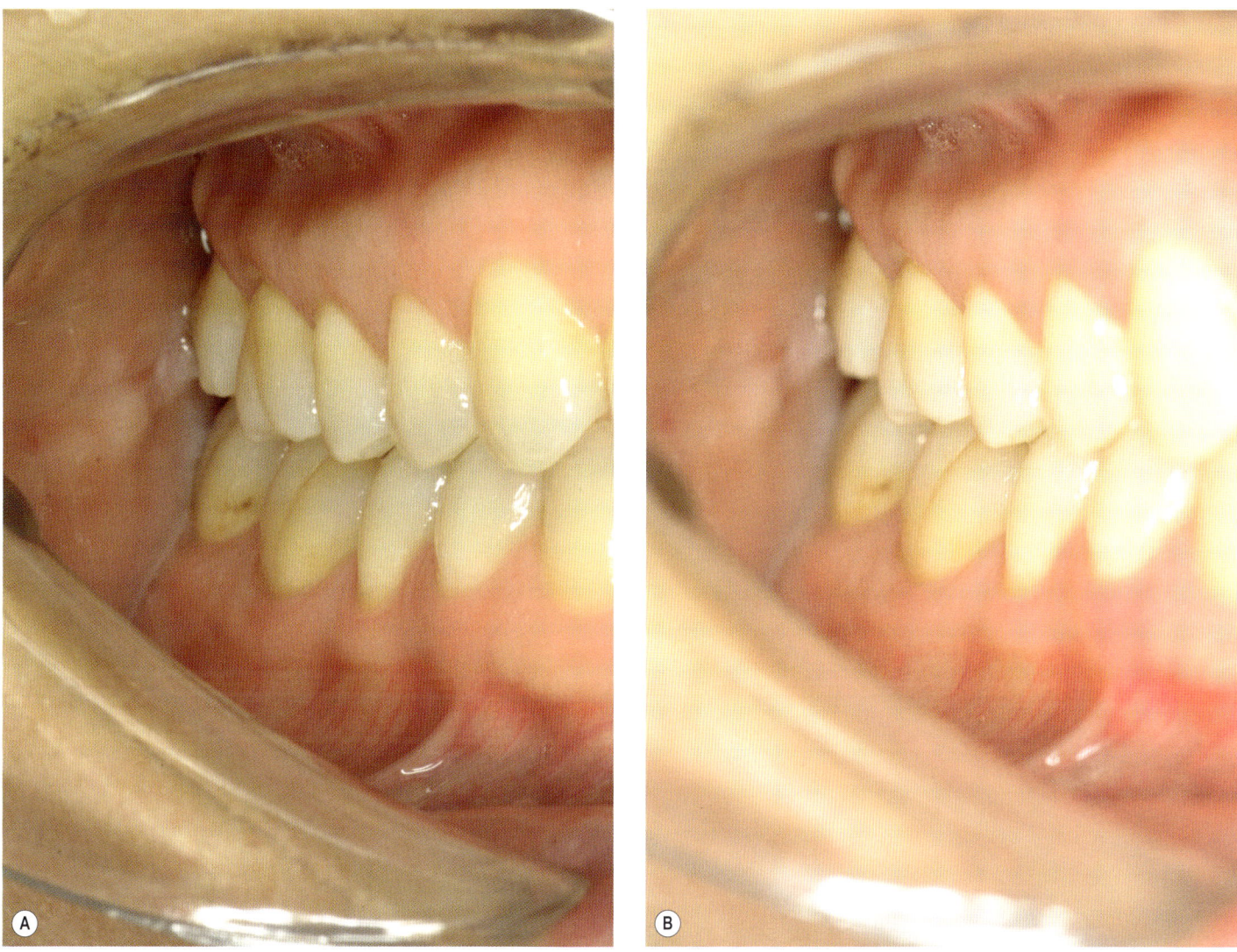

Fig. 4.6A,B The differences in depth of field between large and small f-numbers can be seen with all the teeth looking in focus in (A) but only the second premolar in focus in (B).

EXPOSURE

Exposure relates to whether the image is too light (overexposed, Fig. 4.7) or too dark (underexposed, Fig. 4.8). If a tooth is overexposed then you will lose highlight details and the teeth will look 'washed-out' or all white. In general, exposure can be controlled by the aperture or shutter speed of the camera and the output of the flash. For dental photography, the aperture is determined by the depth of field that we want, and the shutter speed has to be synchronized with the flash unit (usually between a shutter speed of 1/60 and 1/250 seconds). This means we need to have a camera which either allows aperture priority

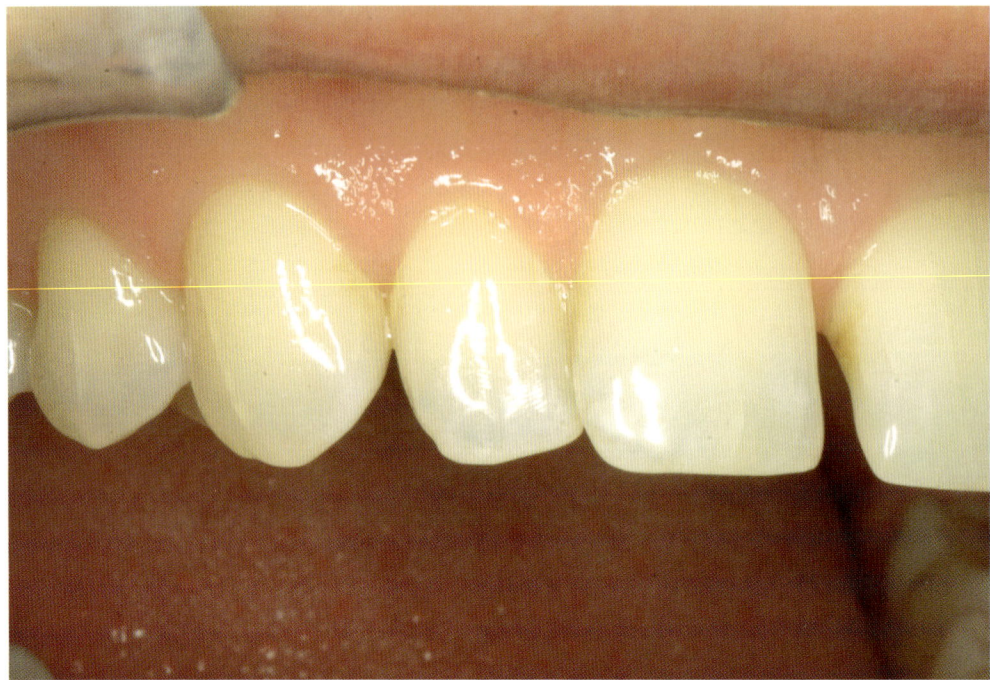

Fig. 4.7 Overexposed teeth showing a lack of details and 'washed-out' appearance.

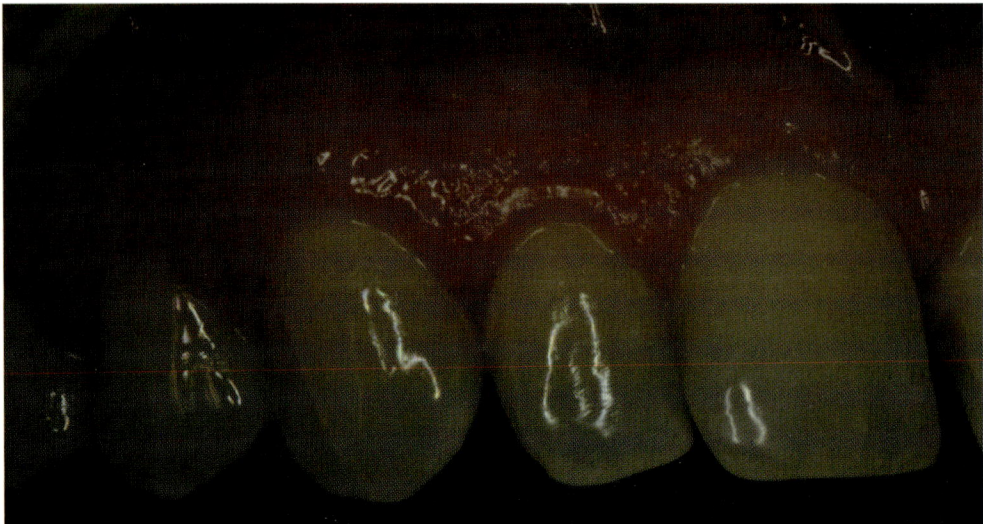

Fig. 4.8 Underexposed photograph of the upper right anterior teeth.

(control of the aperture) or a manual mode (control over both aperture and shutter speed).

The exposure of teeth in the mouth can be altered by several different methods. In addition to adjusting f-stop, as described above, the exposure can be controlled by the flash unit using TTL exposure metering. The TTL exposure metering works by averaging the amount of light from the object, equating it to a midgrey and choosing the correct settings to get this mid-grey in the picture.

Alternatively, if the object is still underexposed because the maximum light output of the flash is insufficient to illuminate the object then it is possible to make the sensor more sensitive. This involves changing the ISO value from 100 to 200. It is also possible to reduce the f-number as a means of increasing the light entering the camera but this has to be balanced against the loss of depth of field.

Finally, it is possible to modify the TTL exposure metering using exposure compensation (+/− EV) settings (Fig. 4.9). You may need to do this when you are taking very close-up pictures of teeth that will be brighter than mid-grey and so TTL exposure results in the teeth being underexposed. This will require a positive exposure compensation. Experimentation will show how much this positive compensation needs to be, e.g. +1 EV. You might also need to increase the exposure compensation by +1 to +2 EV when taking a mirror shot for an occlusal photograph. This will compensate for the lack of illumination provided by the flash (as a result of loss of light through reflection and increased distance between flash and object).

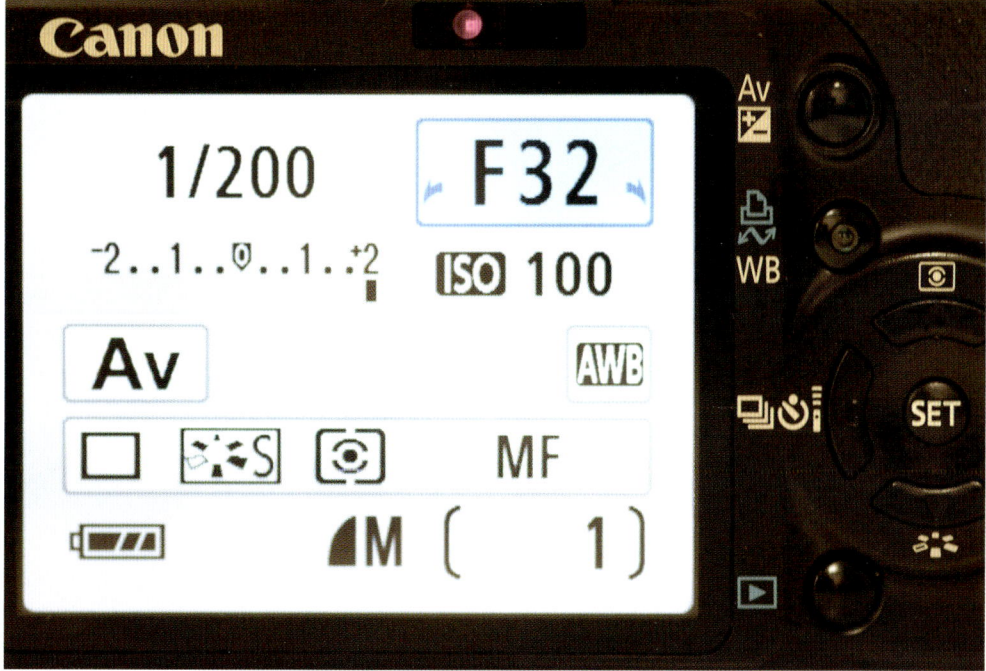

Fig. 4.9 An example of the exposure compensation setting button and scale.

ILLUMINATION

Intra-oral photographs should be carried out using a ring flash (Fig. 4.10) or twin flash that gives an even illumination of the teeth. The unit should allow modification of its output by TTL metering. The main reported disadvantage with ring flashes is that they can produce multiple reflections from the surface of the tooth with a flattening effect as they eliminate shadow (Fig. 4.11A,B).[17,19]

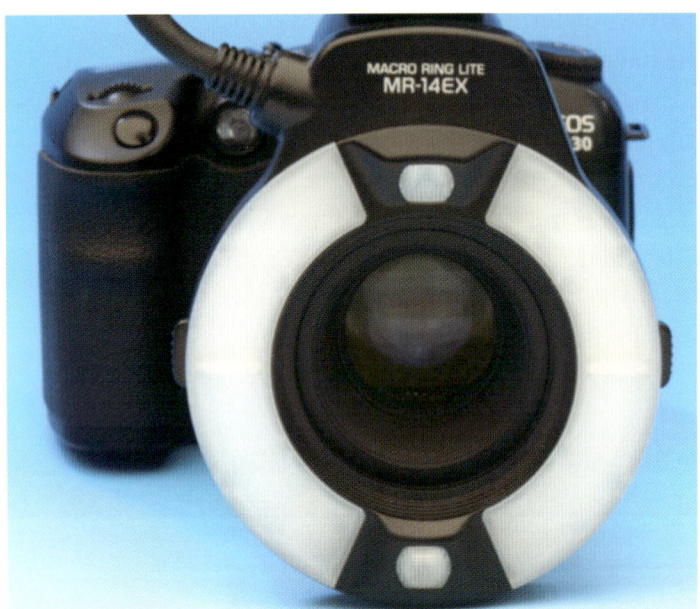

Fig. 4.10   A Canon Macro Ring Flash MR-14EX showing a two-tube arrangement that allows some variation in the balance of illumination from the left or the right side.

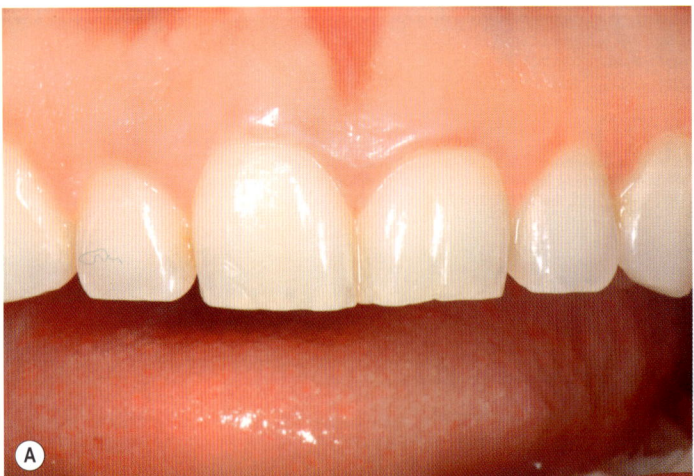 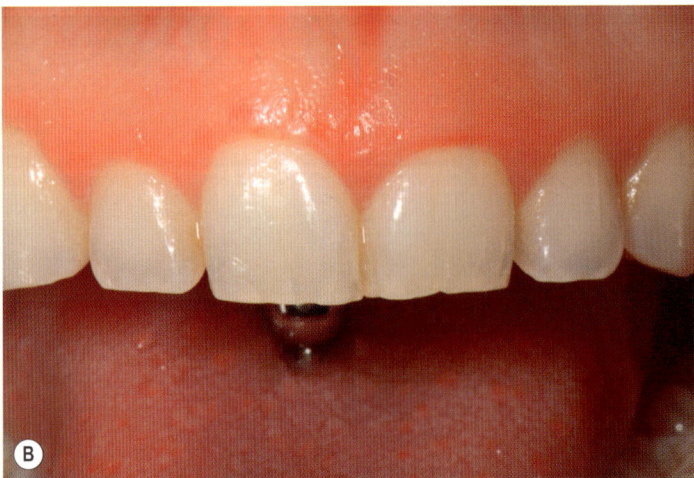

Fig. 4.11A,B   A comparison of the illumination from a ring flash showing a flattened surface (A) compared to illumination from a two-tube ring flash with illumination predominantly from the right side (B).

If light can be directed from the side, then some slight shadowing can be produced in order to give texture and depth to the teeth.[16,19] Some ring flashes contain two tubes which allow the light to come predominantly from one side to produce an image with more apparent contours (Fig. 4.11A,B).

KEY CLINICAL TECHNIQUES

Before you begin

- Ensure that the teeth are clean of plaque, lipstick and any other debris and suction excessive saliva.
- Warm up occlusal mirrors in a hot water bath to avoid fogging.
- Moisten cheek retractors before use.

Taking a photograph

- Set the reproduction ratio on the lens.
- Position the patient in a reclined position and move their head to make taking the view as easy as possible.
- Move in and out towards the subject to focus.
- Try to keep the centre line of the face in the midline of the photograph.
- Compose the photograph and think about the balance and symmetry and then take the photograph.

A dual flash system is an alternative to a ring flash that provides less flattened images, with better visualization of translucency and line angles. The dual flashes can be adjusted and thus the direction of our illumination can be controlled. Figure 4.12 shows the characteristics of photos taken with a dual flash system using direct frontal light, direct lateral light and indirect lateral light. As Figure 4.13A–D shows, photos taken with direct lighting appear much more flat and static, versus the volume and dimensionality seen with indirect lighting. Note that a diffuser, or 'bouncer', can be attached to each dual flash to provide softer, indirect light.

OTHER PHOTOGRAPHIC EQUIPMENT

Cheek retractors

Cheek retractors are important for keeping the soft tissues away from the teeth and allowing easy camera viewing of the dentition. Generally, these come in plastic or stainless steel, although plastic retractors are more comfortable for patients (Fig. 4.14). It is important to ensure that these are autoclavable.

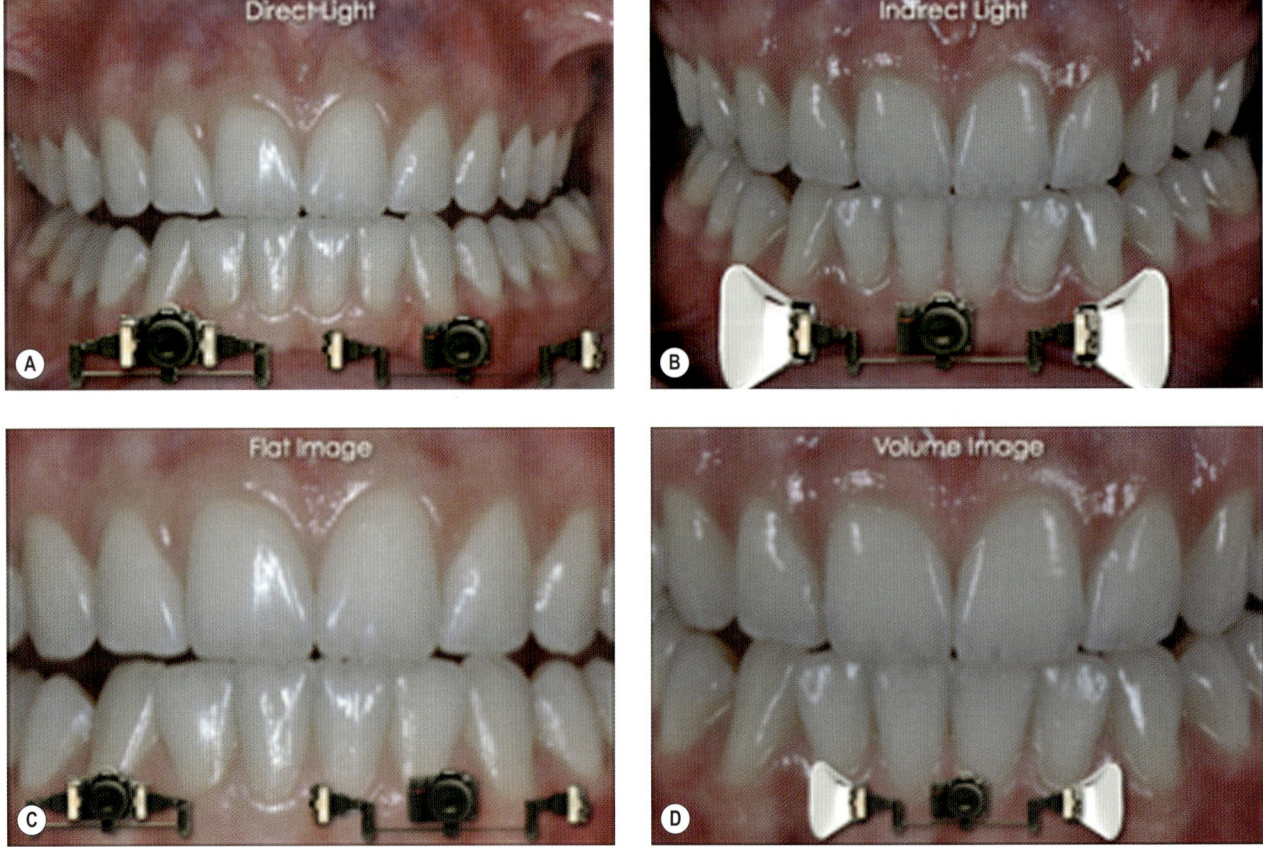

Fig. 4.12 The characteristics of photographs taken with a dual flash system used with direct frontal light, direct lateral light and indirect lateral light.

Fig. 4.13A–D Photographs taken with direct lighting versus indirect lighting.

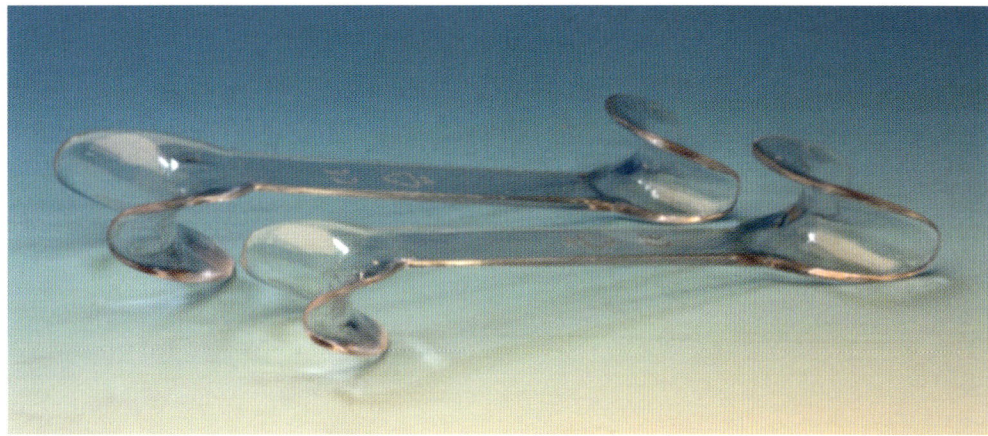

Fig. 4.14 Autoclavable plastic cheek retractors.

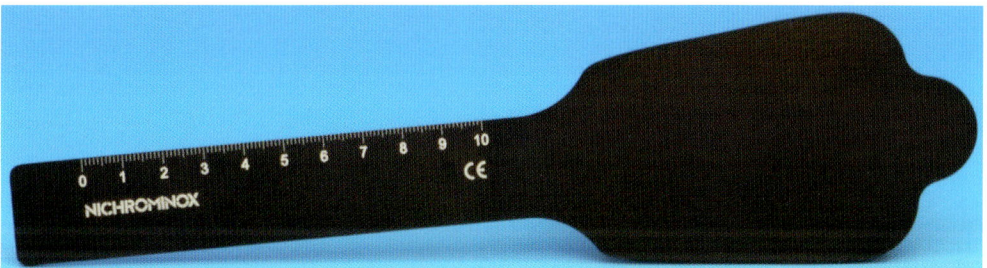

Fig. 4.15 Contrasters used to give a 'blacked out' background to anterior teeth.

Contrasters

These are used to give a 'blacked out' background to the anterior teeth and remove the distraction of the tongue or other soft tissues (Fig. 4.15). The reason for their use is to provide a contrast to the lightness of the teeth and improve the exposure of the front teeth. They also help improve the visualization of the translucency and colour of the front teeth. Check all such photographic aids can be autoclaved.

Photographic mirrors

Two main types of mirrors are needed: occlusal mirrors or lateral mirrors. They can be either metal or glass and have their individual advantages and disadvantages. It is essential that the mirrors are autoclavable. Metal mirrors are usually highly polished stainless steel and therefore virtually indestructible. Glass mirrors produce a much higher surface reflectance than metal mirrors, which produces sharper images, but they are more breakable and easily scratched (Fig. 4.16). When choosing mirrors, ensure that they are top-silvered and not bottom-silvered. This is essential in order to avoid possible double images created by reflection from the surface of the glass as well as the mirrored surface.

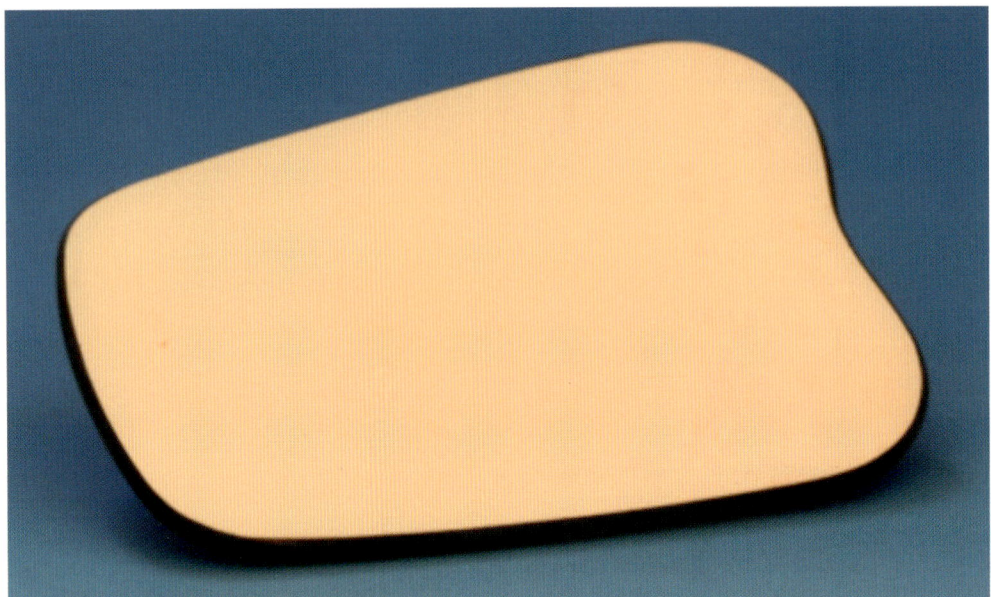

Fig. 4.16 A glass top-silvered photographic mirror.

It is important to ensure that the surface of the mirror is not scratched and has no smears or saliva from contact with oral tissues, which might affect the image quality.

The general technique for use of mirrors is to warm them up prior to use. This is most easily done by placing them into a warm water bath and then drying the mirror prior to use. The residual warmth of the mirror avoids it steaming up from the patient's breath during use. An alternative approach is to ask your patient to breathe through their nose while you take the mirror shot and use a gentle airstream from the 3-in-1 onto the surface of the mirror.

GENERAL PHOTOGRAPHIC TECHNIQUE

It is often easier to recline your patient in the dental chair to take intra-oral photographs. You should ask your patient to move their head towards you to allow you to take your photographs without having to lean over the dental chair. The dental light can be used to allow you to visualize the teeth for framing and focusing the view.

The camera should be held with the body of the camera in your right hand and the lens supported by your left hand. Your arms should be held against your chest to give a stable support (Fig. 4.17).

Angulation is crucially important, as we are evaluating smile elements such as canting and parallelism in relation to the true horizon. Thus, most views should be obtained with the camera held at 90° to the subject (or in the case of occlusal

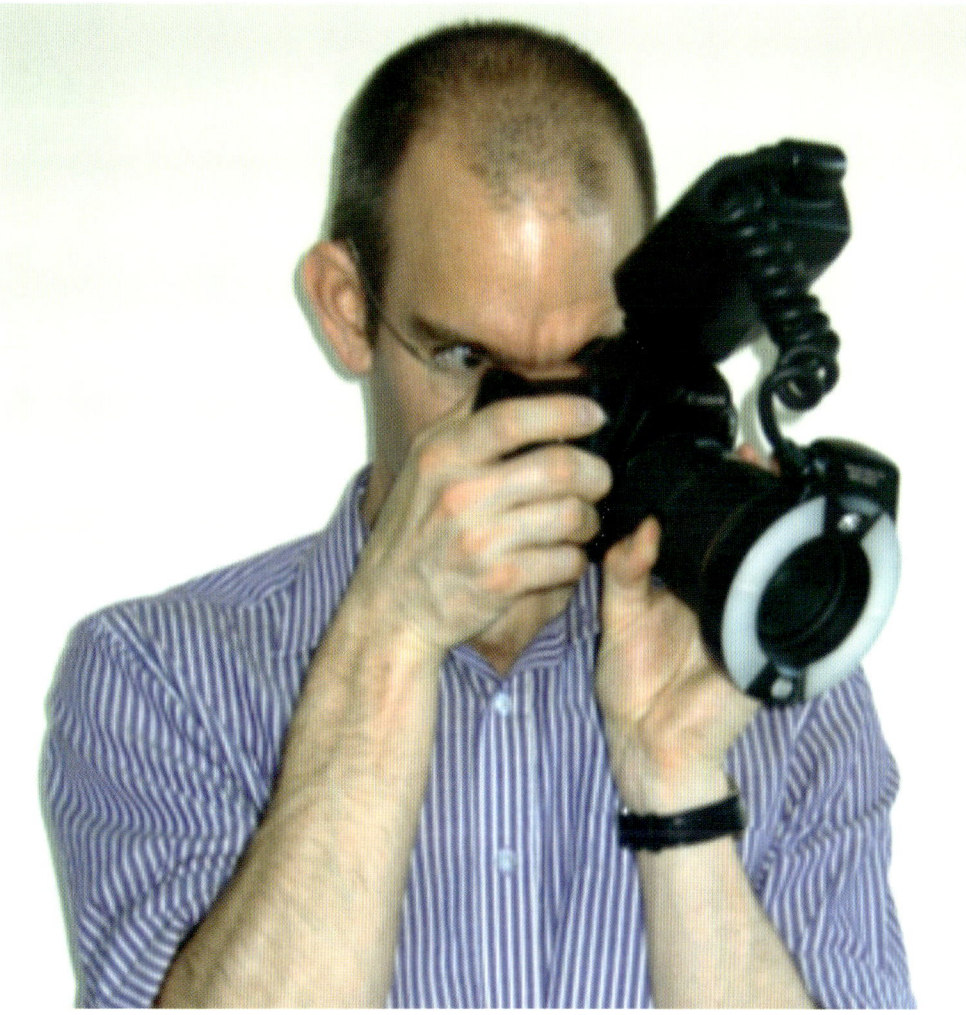

Fig. 4.17 Stable arm and hand position for taking dental photographs.

views, the camera held at 90° to a mirror held at 45° to the occlusal plane). As Figures 4.18 and 4.19 demonstrate, a photograph taken from a low angle will give the false appearance of a reverse smile, where the maxillary canines seem longer than the centrals. It follows that angling the camera from above the subject will exaggerate the curve of the smile. Note that a photograph angled from below can be useful for shade assessment, as the angulation will prevent the flash from drowning out the shade tabs (Fig. 4.19).

The reproduction ratio should be set on the lens according to the standard view you are taking. Focusing is best carried out by setting the camera to manual focusing rather than automatic focusing and then moving the camera backwards and forwards to bring the object into focus. The reason for this approach is to ensure reproducibility of images taken on different occasions. You may need to make minor changes to the focusing to give an ideal coverage for the standard view.

STANDARD PHOTOGRAPHIC VIEWS

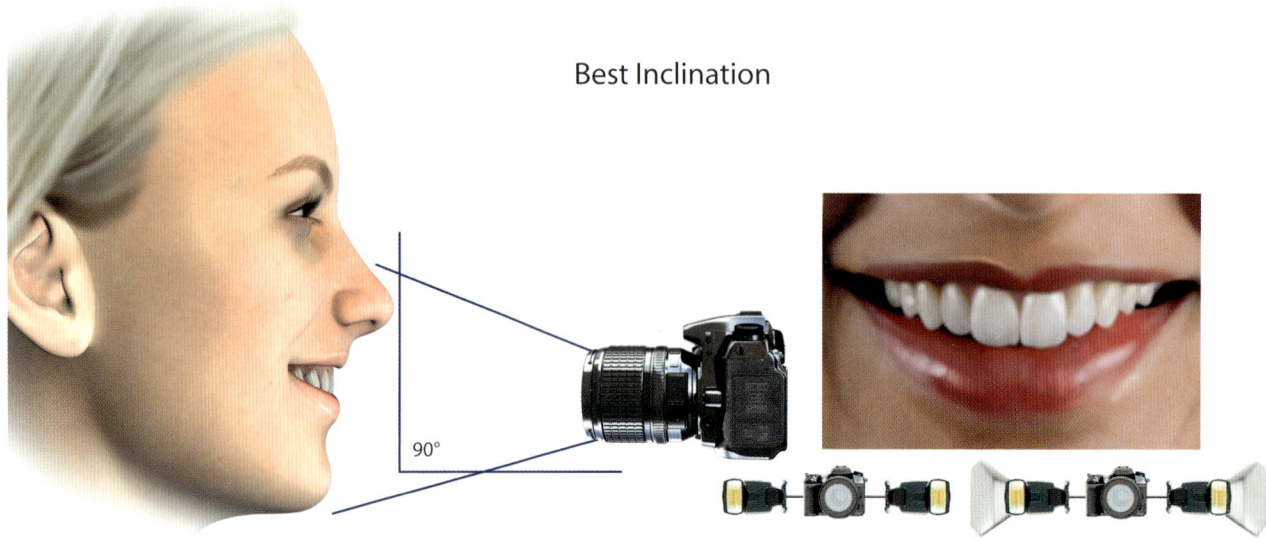

Fig. 4.18 The proper angulation for obtaining a frontal view of the smile.

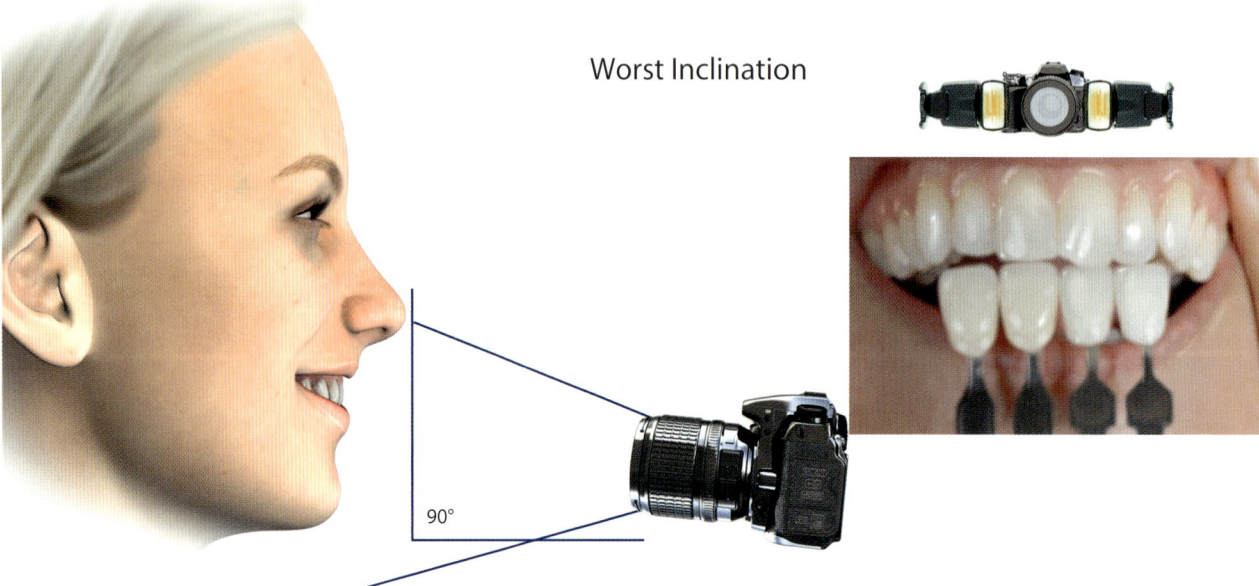

Fig. 4.19 This photograph, taken from a lower angle, falsely gives the appearance of a reverse smile. A photograph taken at this angle can only be used for shade assessment and never for facial analysis.

STANDARD PHOTOGRAPHIC VIEWS

When photographing teeth for esthetic smile design, the American Academy of Cosmetic Dentistry (AACD) recommend obtaining 12 standard views.[16,20] These standard views show a full face view and allow a record of the relationship between the lips and the teeth during smiling, the relationship of the upper anterior teeth to the lower anterior teeth and the posterior teeth and their angulation, and more detailed views of the anterior teeth. The sequence is shown in the clinical cases. Note that the system presented in this book (the 3-step analysis and Aesthetic Evaluation Form) relies heavily on two more views not required by the AACD: full-face profile view at rest (to evaluate nasolabial angle and lip protrusion) and dentofacial view of lips at rest ('emma' position used to assess incisal display with the lips at rest).

FILE TYPES AND DIGITAL WORKFLOW

Digital SLRs will typically save photographs as either a JPEG or alternatively as a RAW image format. JPEGs are a very standard image format; however, as they are a 'lossy' compression file type, they lose detail every time they are opened and saved. For this reason, any manipulation of the image should be done on a copy not the original image. The RAW format has to be converted to a JPEG by software that comes with the camera, but this records all of the information from the camera's sensor and is therefore like a digital negative.[18] RAW file sizes are generally very large, but as they are not directly editable they allow you to keep an unprocessed image.

Once you have taken your photographs you need to think about how you are going to process the images. This is covered by the digital workflow and includes the method of storage, any image manipulation and back-up.[17] The best means of storage or cataloguing photographs is by integration into the practice management software, if possible. Alternatively, commercial products exist to catalogue photographs and categorize photographs.[18] Care is needed with regard to the confidentiality of images when labelling them and must not use patients' names or details.

Simple modifications of images such as removal of red-eye and minor errors in vertical or horizontal axis can be carried out easily with free image editing programs such as Picasa (http://picasa.google.com/). Other modifications or digital simulations can be carried out in a photo-editing program or in commercially available dental imaging software, e.g. SNAP Dental Cosmetic Imaging Software and Cosmetic Imaging Module (Carestream Dental).

Overall, digital dental photography is the most appropriate way to record esthetic dental treatment, giving you both before and after photographs and allowing you to assess the outcomes of treatment. This analysis allows us to evolve as esthetic dentists and to predictably achieve beautiful results for our patients.

CLINICAL CASES

ESSENTIALS

- A digital SLR with a 100 mm macro lens and ring flash is needed for good quality, consistent dental photographs.

- Photographs can be used for treatment planning, patient education and communication, monitoring treatment, and communicating with technicians.

- Three levels of consent can be obtained for dental photographs: dental records, teaching and publication.

- A standard set of photographic views allows a systematic and efficient way of recording your patient's teeth and smile.

CLINICAL CASES

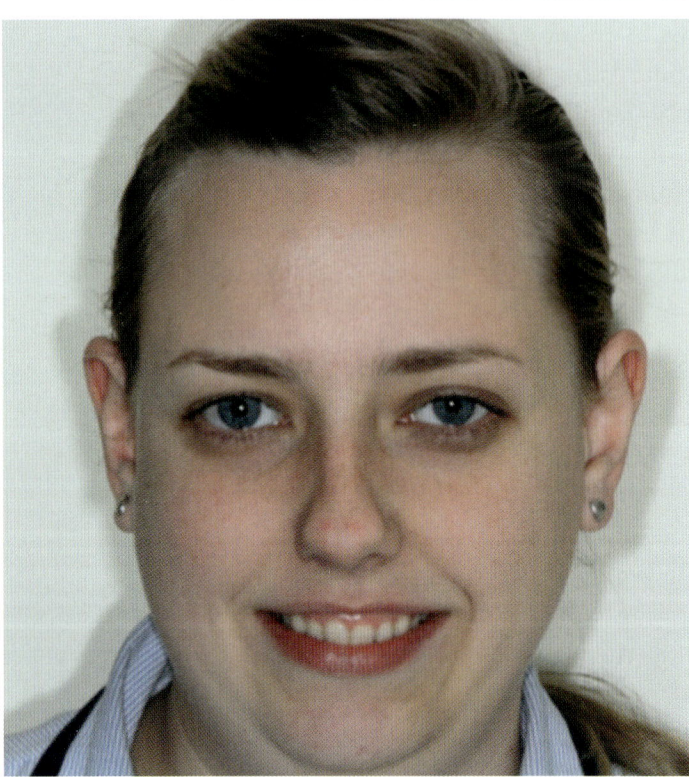

Fig. C4.1 Full face view. This photograph allows the inclination of the incisal plane to be assessed in relationship to the interpupillary line. The macro lens should be set with a reproduction ratio of 1:10 multiplied by the correction for the digital sensor, e.g. 1:15 for a Nikon D7000. Select a shutter speed of 1/200 seconds and an aperture of f11.

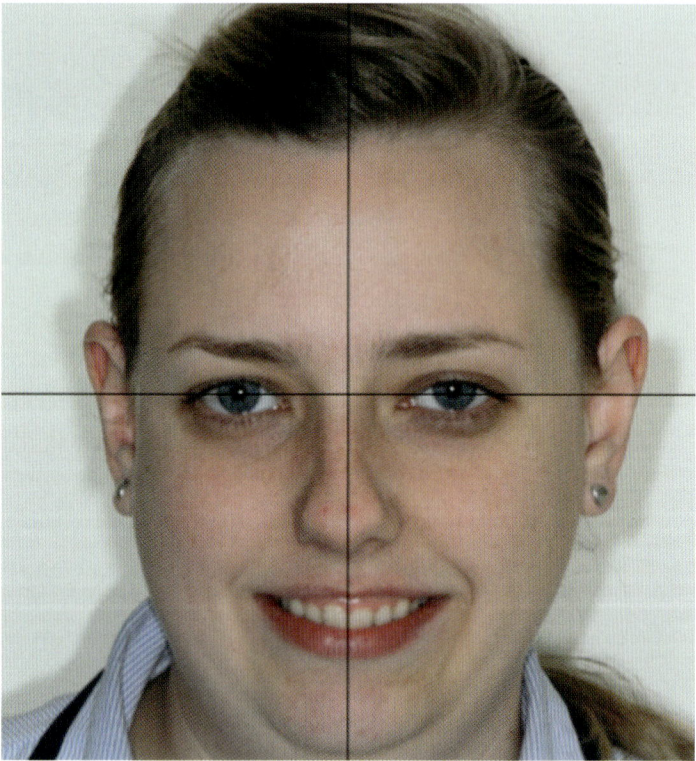

Fig. C4.2 Full face view technique. The patient should be positioned in front of a neutral background with you standing straight in front of them. Hold the camera so that it is at right angles to the face to avoid distortion of the facial proportions. You are aiming to take a photograph that should frame the face from the chin, just above the lower border, to the top of the head, just below the upper border. The patient is then asked to give a relaxed smile. The horizontal plane should run parallel to the interpupillary line and the vertical midline should bisect this line.

Lighting of full face photographs needs care to avoid a shadow behind the patient. This is a potential problem when using the ring flash. It is often convenient to use this flash; however, if you remove it from the end of the camera and hold it to bounce the light off the ceiling, then this can minimize the shadow effect. Another option is to use a standard flash with a diffuser. Alternatively, if you use this view on a frequent basis, a studio set-up can give a more professional look with the use of flashes and flash softboxes.[21]

CLINICAL PHOTOGRAPHY IN ESTHETIC DENTISTRY

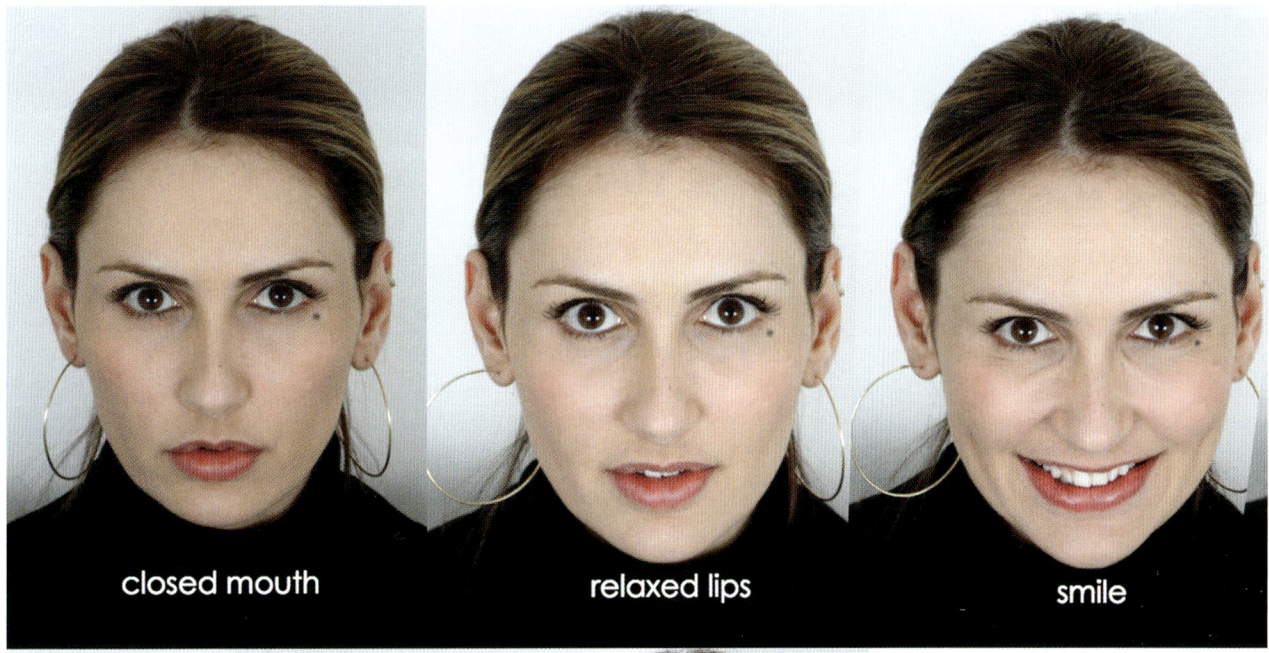

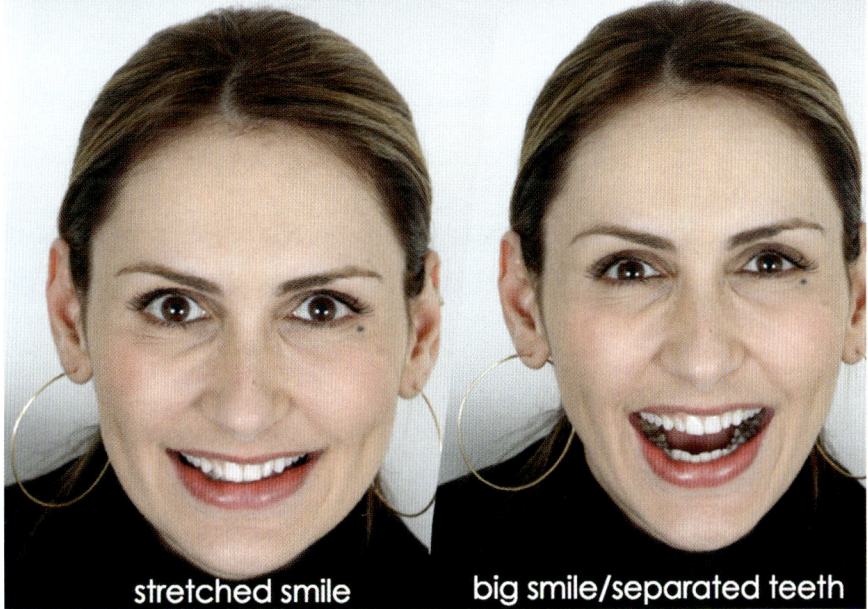

Fig. C4.3 The variety of smiles a patient can be asked to display. These photographs are helpful for diagnosis, as they allow for a detailed analysis of facial symmetry, smile, face shape, muscle tone, lip support, feelings and expressions. Note that the photographs in this figure are taken with the camera held vertically, which is not in line with AACD protocol, but gives a more 'portrait' style of depiction that can be used for marketing or presentations (namely, there is no empty space on either side of the patient and the top of her head is not cropped in this version of the full facial view).

CLINICAL CASES

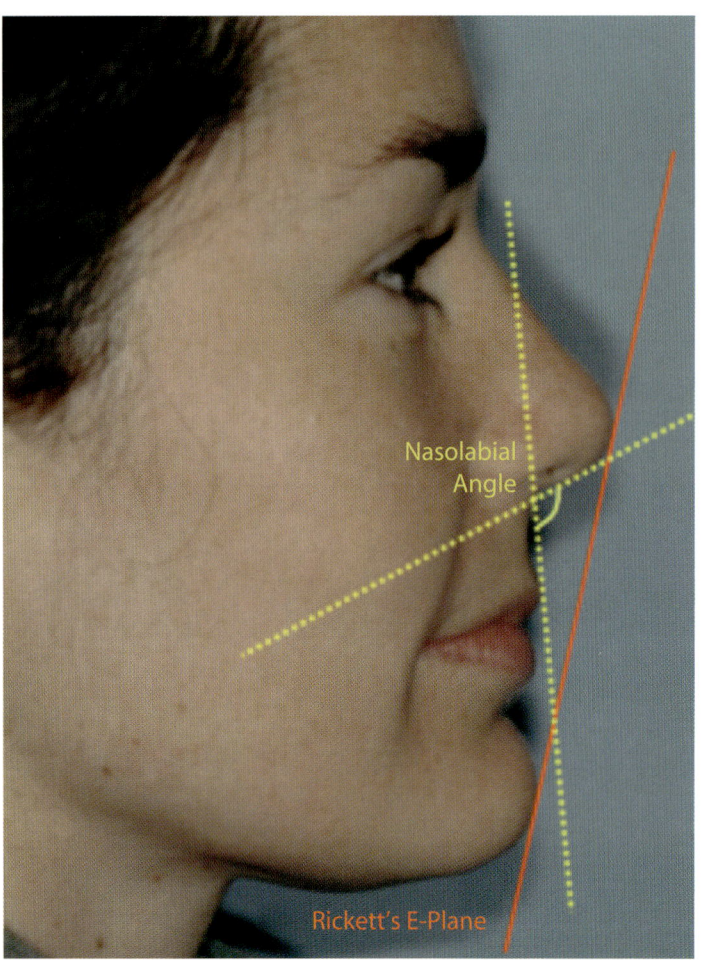

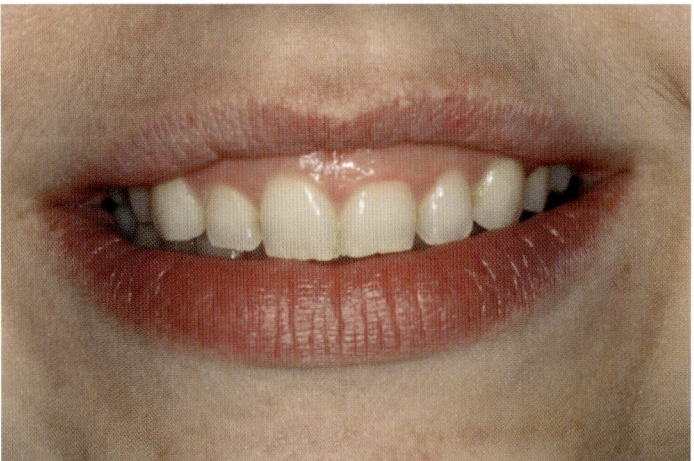

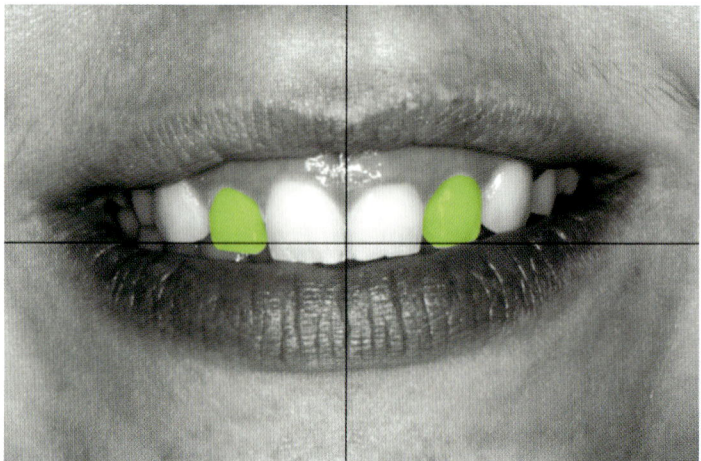

Fig. C4.4 A full-face profile view with lips at rest. While not one of the AACD's standard 12 views, this will allow the clinician to assess Ricketts' E-plane and the nasolabial angle, providing information of where the smile is in relationship to the face. These orthodontic measurements are used in the Aesthetic Evaluation Form, as discussed in Chapter 1, and facially generated treatment planning.

Fig. C4.5 Full natural smile. This photograph allows the amount of teeth and gingiva exposed during a full smile to be viewed. It can be an artificial situation for the patient and so it is important that this is a relaxed full smile.

The macro lens should be set with a reproduction ratio of 1:2 multiplied by the correction for the digital sensor, e.g. 1:3 for the Nikon D7000. Select a shutter speed of 1/200 seconds and an aperture of f29–f32.

Fig. C4.6 Full natural smile technique. Hold the camera so that it is at right angles to the face to avoid distorting the incisal plane. The horizontal plane should run parallel to the interpupillary line so that any incisal cant is accurately recorded and you do not try to inadvertently straighten this by tilting the camera. The horizontal midline should coincide with the incisal edge of the upper incisors. The vertical midline should coincide with the midline of the face in order to correctly record any asymmetries associated with the incisal teeth. You should focus on the lateral incisors; the depth of field should keep everything else in focus.

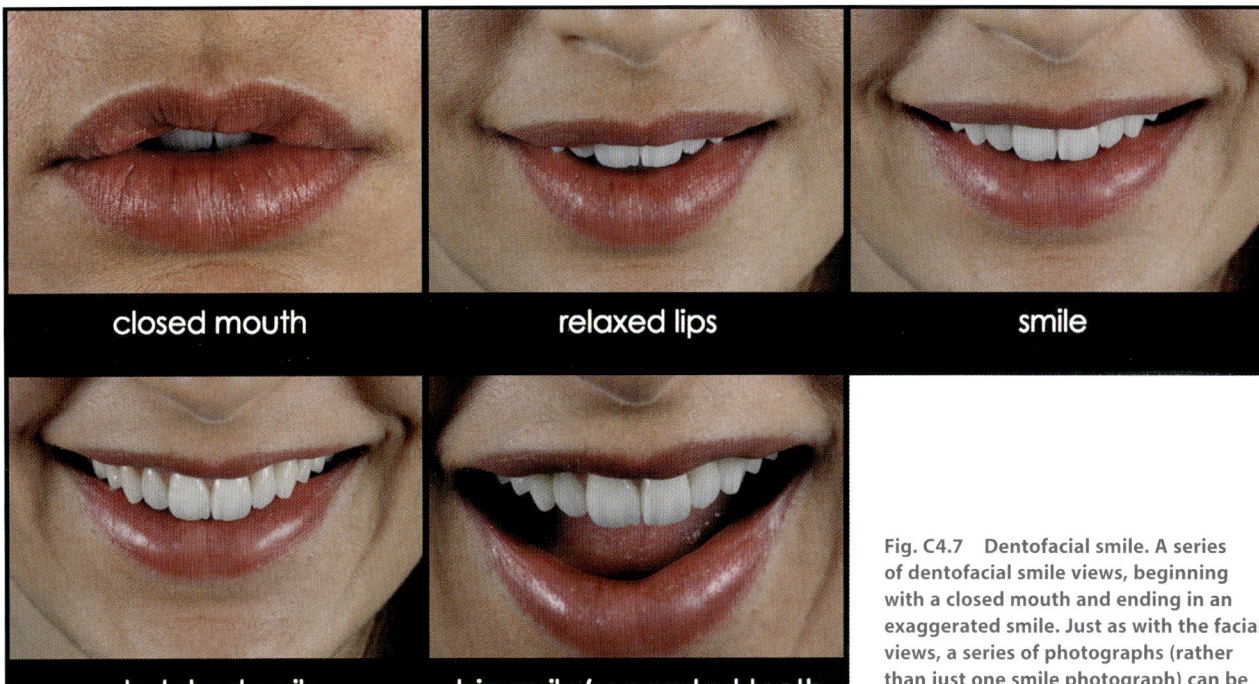

Fig. C4.7 Dentofacial smile. A series of dentofacial smile views, beginning with a closed mouth and ending in an exaggerated smile. Just as with the facial views, a series of photographs (rather than just one smile photograph) can be tremendously helpful with diagnosis.

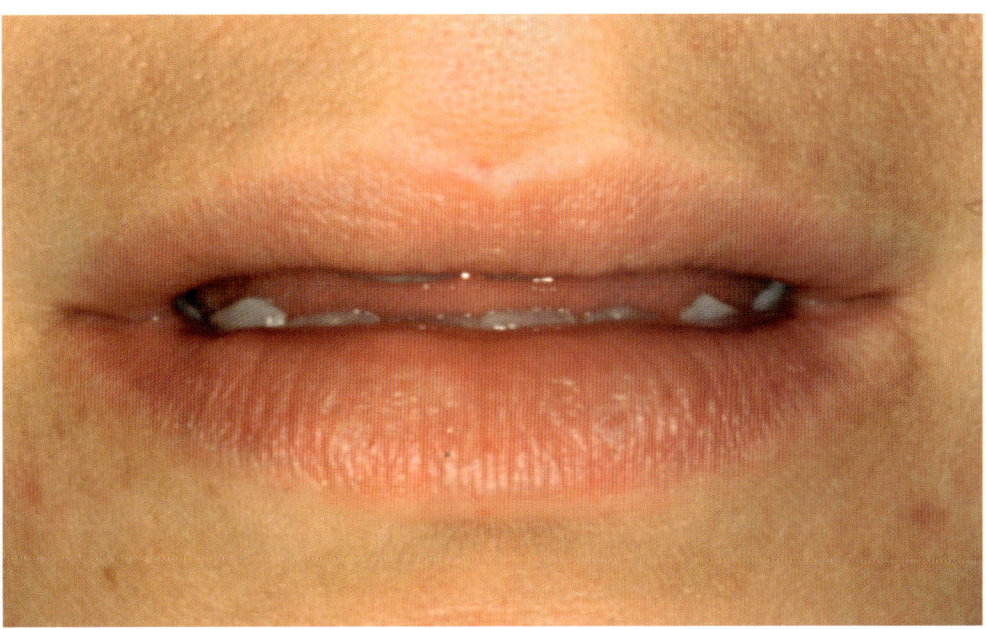

Fig. C4.8 Dentofacial view: lips at rest. A dentofacial view of the lips at rest is critically important, as we must determine whether the degree of incisor display at rest is adequate. A smile displaying unworn, symmetrical incisal edges at rest appears youthful, and thus we will often lengthen the maxillary anterior teeth to achieve this end. Remember that, with our esthetics first and end-in-mind approach, the entire case is planned around the proper placement of the maxillary centrals' incisal edges. To obtain this view the patient is instructed to relax their lips and pronounce the word 'emma' and then freeze.

CLINICAL CASES

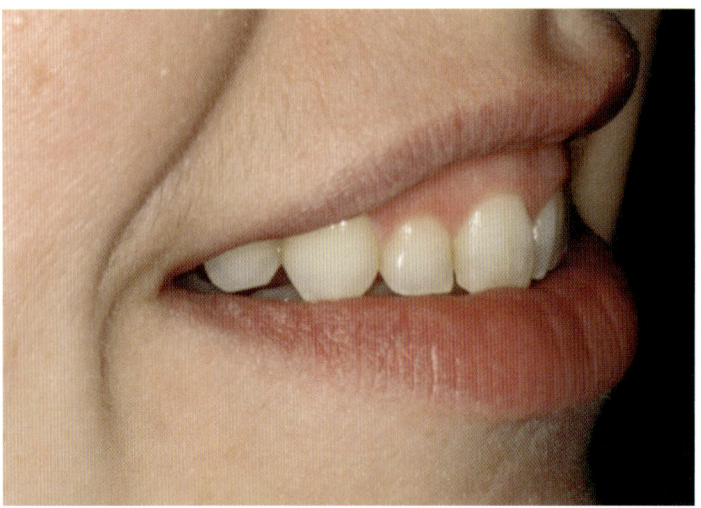

Fig. C4.9 Full natural smile: right lateral view. The lateral views not only allow the amount of teeth and gingiva during a full smile to be viewed, but also gives some indication of the profile of the teeth. It is important that it is a full relaxed smile.

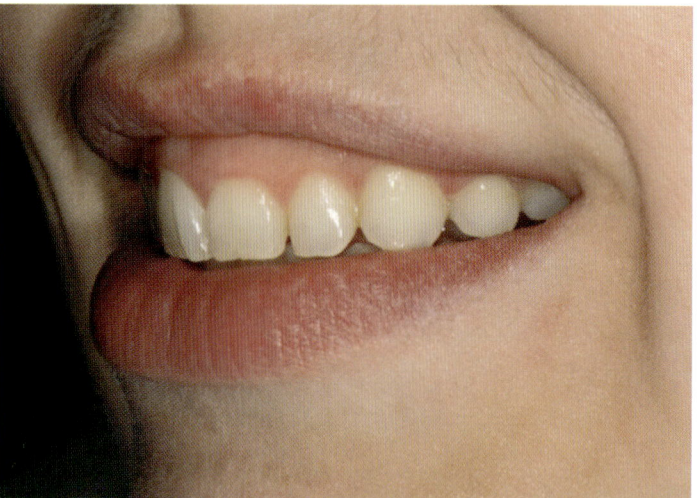

Fig. C4.10 Full natural smile: left lateral view. The macro lens should be set with a reproduction ratio of 1:2 multiplied by the correction for the digital sensor, e.g. 1:3 for the Nikon D7000. Select a shutter speed of 1/200 seconds and an aperture of f29–f32. Note that the easiest method is f-stop 'bracketing', where we take the same photograph with three different f-stop settings (one above and one below the usual number) and assess the depth and exposure.

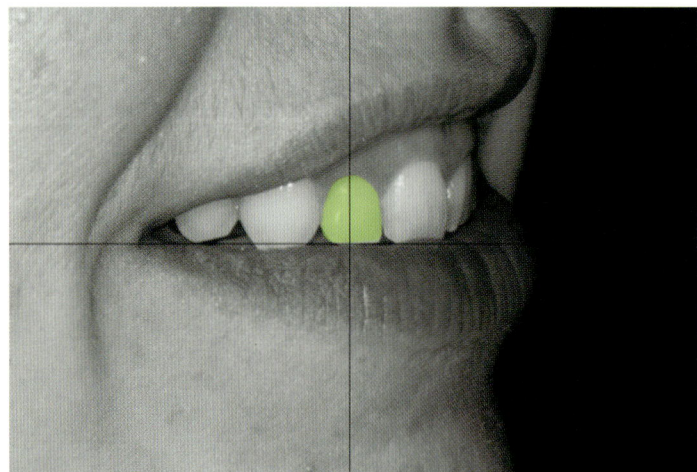

Fig. C4.11 Full natural smile: lateral view technique. Hold the camera so that it is at right angles to the face to avoid distorting the incisal plane. For the AACD view, the lateral incisor should be the centre of the vertical midline with the horizontal midline coinciding with the incisal edge of the upper incisors.[20] You should focus on the lateral incisors; the depth of field should keep everything else in focus. The dark background beyond the cheek is common as a result of the depth of field and the illumination provided by the ring flash.

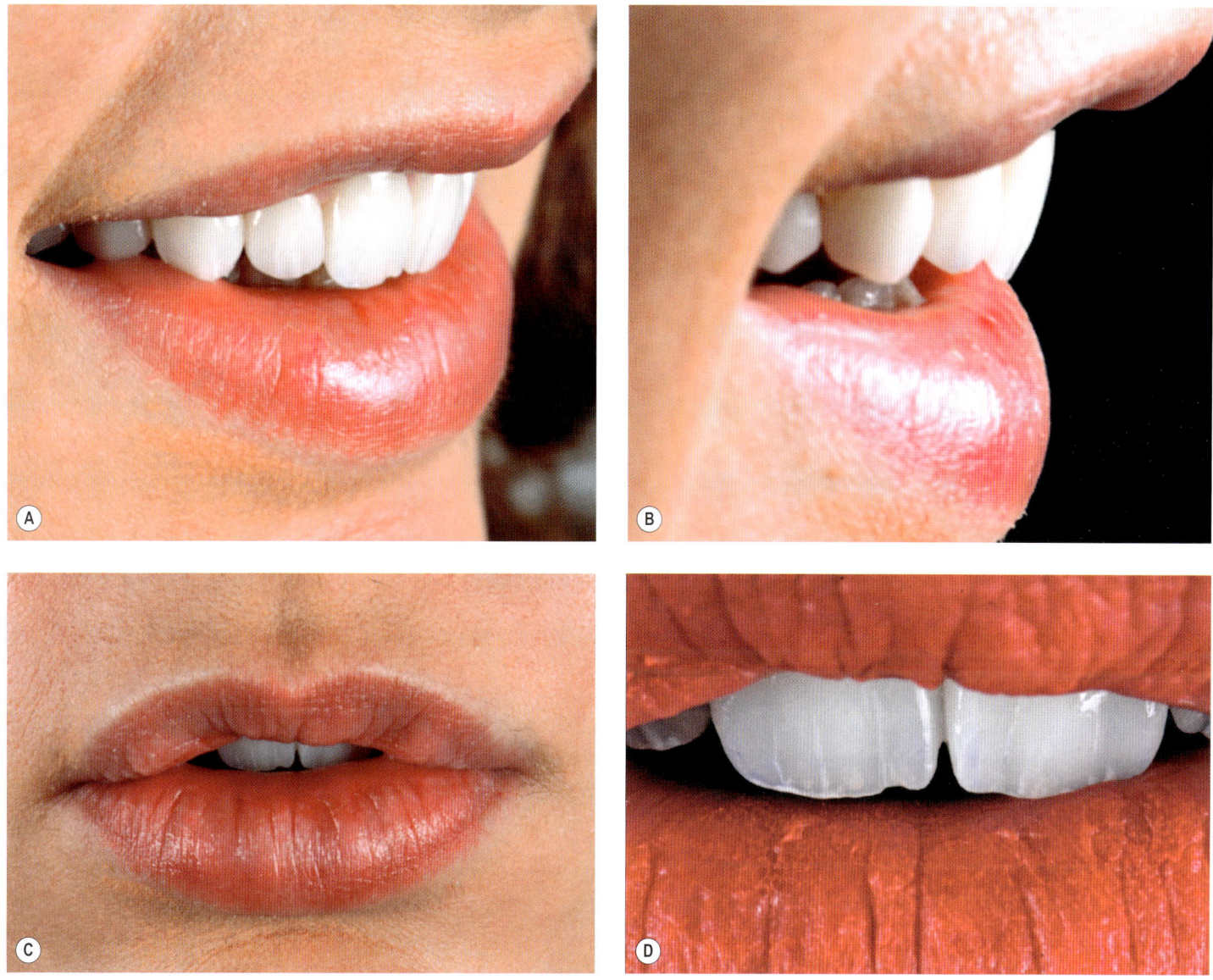

Fig. C4.12A–D Close-up photographs of the lips. These close-up photographs of the lips show the positioning of the incisal edges of the upper teeth in relation to the lower lip.

CLINICAL CASES

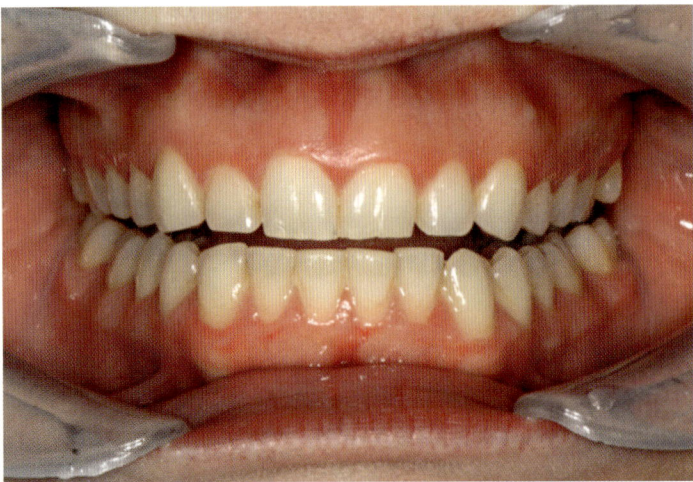

Fig. C4.13 Full dentition (retracted) view. This photograph should show all the dentition and relies on a good depth of field to ensure that all the teeth look in focus. There are two versions of this view. The AACD[20] advocate a teeth-apart view in order to allow both upper and lower incisal edge shape and embrasures to be properly viewed.

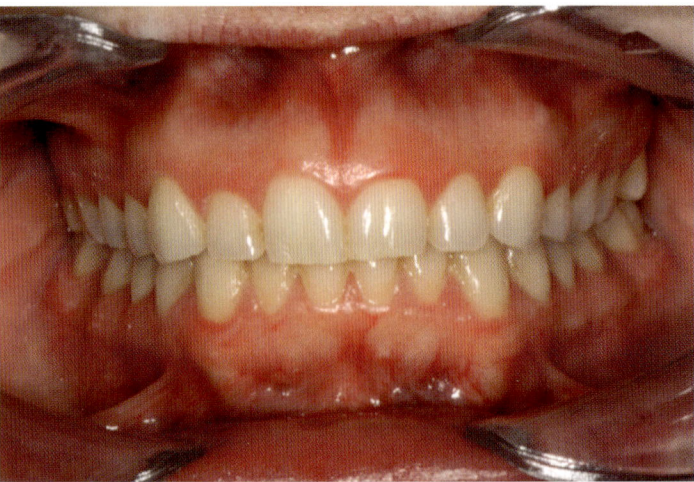

Fig. C4.14 Alternative full dentition (retracted) view. This photograph, which has the teeth together, gives a general view of the interdigitation of the teeth and the gingival shape and contour. The photographic view should not show any of the lips or retractors.

The macro lens should be set with a reproduction ratio of 1:2 multiplied by the correction for the digital sensor, e.g. 1:3 for the Nikon D7000. Select a shutter speed of 1/200 seconds and an aperture of f29–f32.

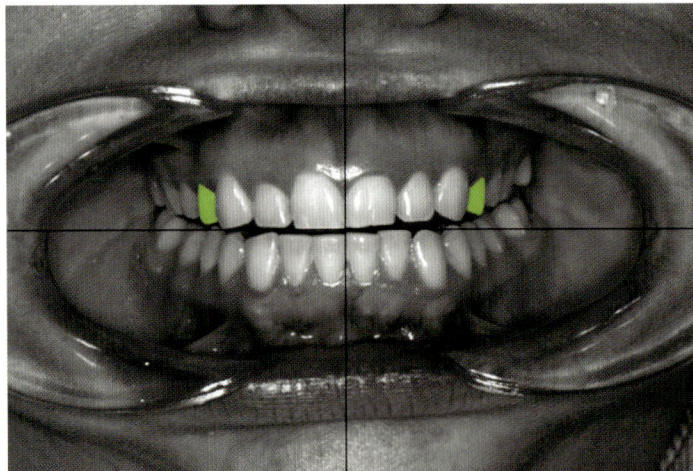

Fig. C4.15 Full dentition (retracted) view technique. Cheek retractors should be moistened and can be held by the patient. The retractors should be pulled laterally and forward away from the teeth. The vertical midline should coincide with the midline of the face in order to correctly record any asymmetries associated with the incisal teeth. The horizontal midline should coincide with the incisal edge of the upper incisors and be perpendicular to the vertical midline. You should focus on the upper 1st premolars; the depth of field should keep everything else in focus.

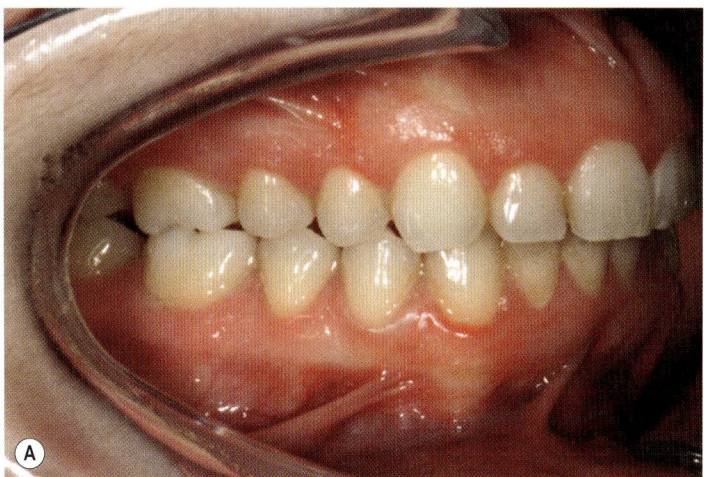 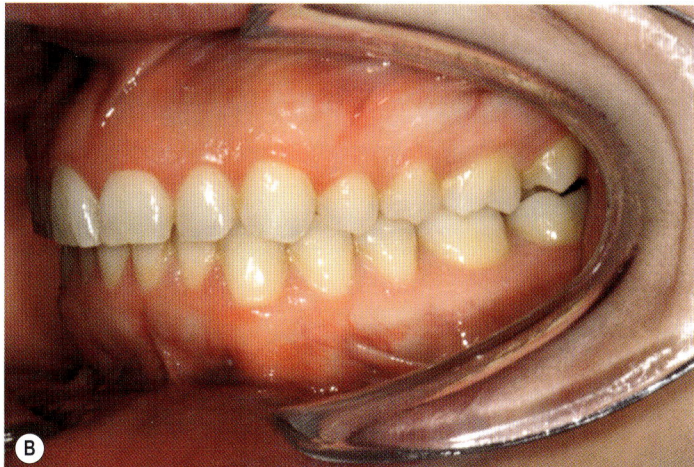

Fig. C4.16A,B General right and left lateral dentition (retracted) view.

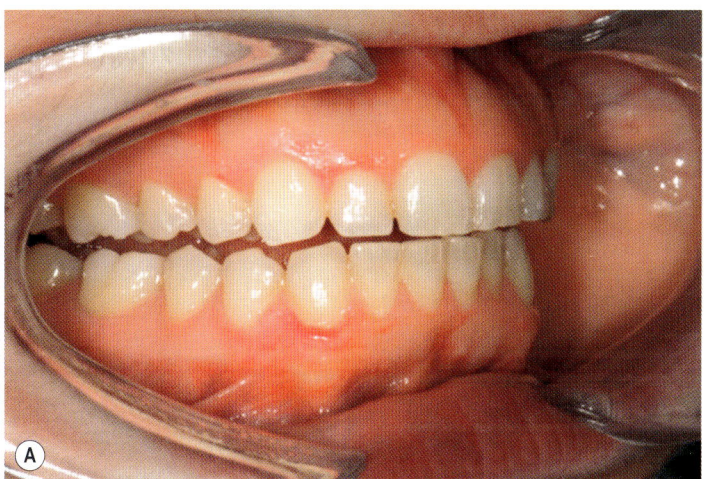 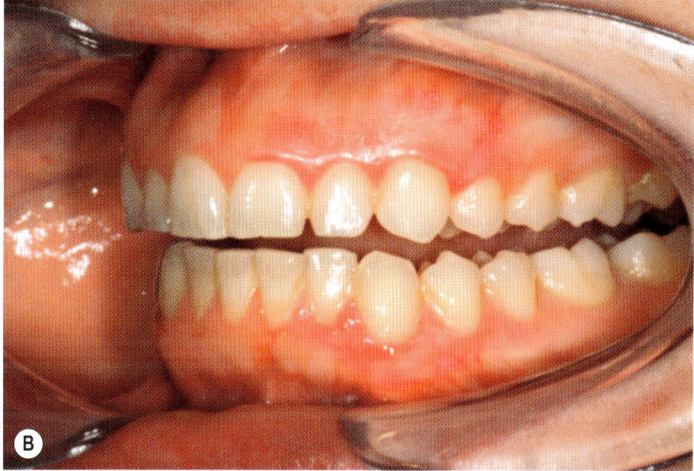

Fig. C4.17A,B Right and left lateral dentition (retracted) views. There are several versions of these views. The photograph has an oblique lateral view but is used as it is easier to take than using a mirror in the buccal vestibule. The AACD[20] advocate a view focused around the anterior teeth with the teeth apart, whereas a more general view focuses on the buccal teeth. These views give further information about the incisal and occlusal plane, the interdigitation of the teeth and the profile of the central incisors.

The macro lens should be set with a reproduction ratio of 1:2 multiplied by the correction for the digital sensor, e.g. 1:3 for the Nikon D7000. Select a shutter speed of 1/200 seconds and an aperture of f29–f32.

Fig. C4.18 Right lateral dentition (retracted) view technique. Cheek retractors can be left in from the full dentition view but pulled laterally on the side you are photographing and relaxed on the opposing side. For the AACD view, the vertical midline passes through the lateral incisors, with the horizontal plane perpendicular at the incisal edge.[20] The more buccal view is centred on the first premolars. The camera is focused on the lateral and first premolars, respectively, and the depth of field should keep everything else in focus.

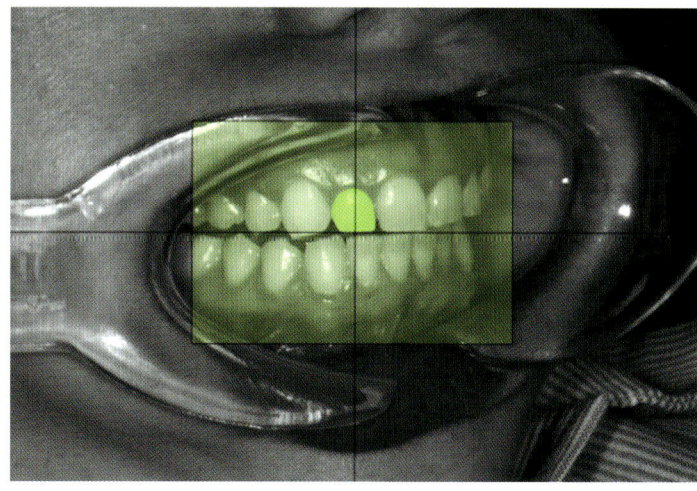

CLINICAL CASES

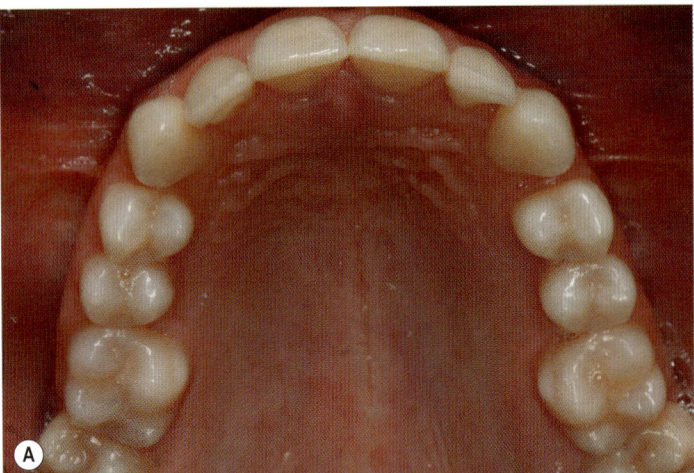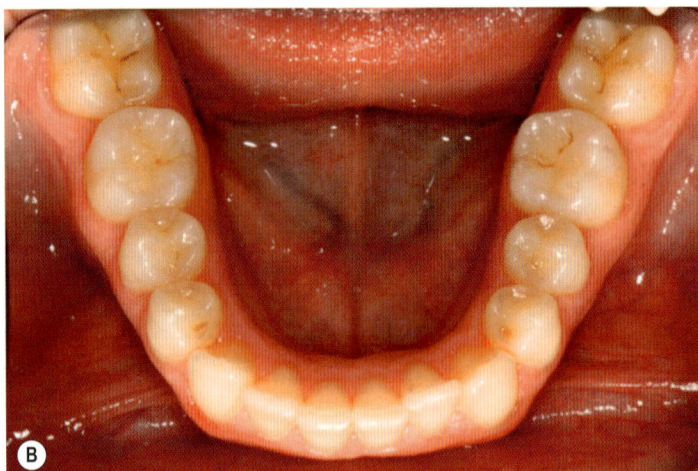

Fig. C4.19A,B Upper and lower occlusal views. These photographs show the whole of the dentition from the central incisors to the second molars and allow the contour of the buccal face of the incisors and general arch form to be viewed. Lips and retractors should be kept out of the photograph as much as possible. These photographs can be flipped digitally about the horizontal plane to show them as viewed in the mouth and not in the mirror.

The macro lens should be set with a reproduction ratio of 1:2 multiplied by the correction for the digital sensor, e.g. 1:3 for the Nikon D7000. Select a shutter speed of 1/200 seconds and an aperture of f22–f29. Exposure compensation should be increased to +2 EV dependent upon the brightness of the image obtained.

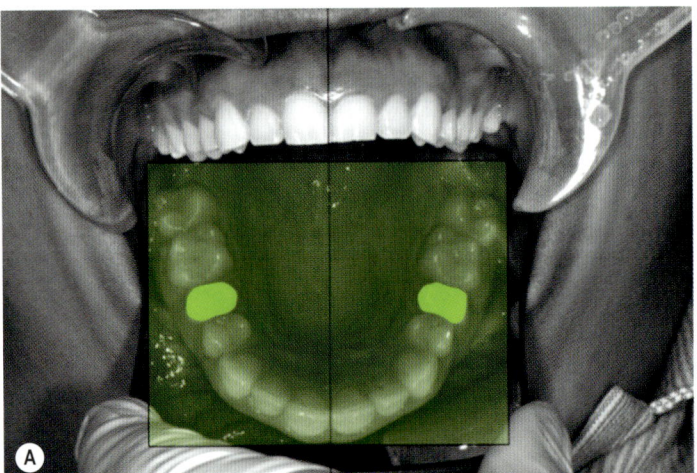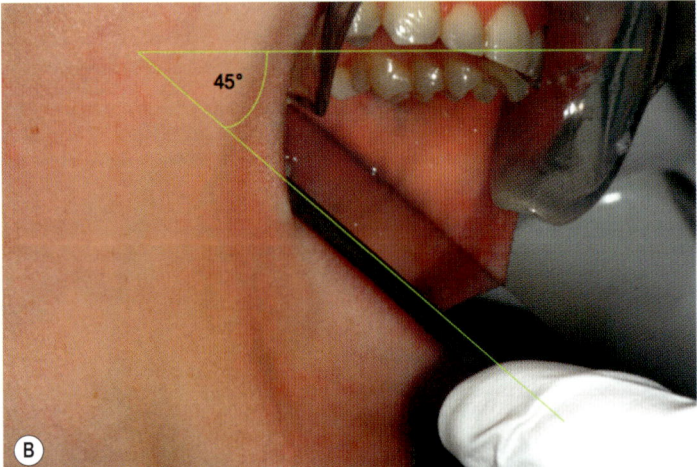

Fig. C4.20A,B (A) Upper occlusal view technique and (B) mirror position for the upper occlusal view. Smaller cheek retractors should be positioned more superiorly and laterally to pull the upper lip upwards and outwards away from the alveolar ridge. The mirror is positioned at 45° to the occlusal plane (B). The camera should be held parallel to the occlusal plane with the vertical midline bisecting the arch, and the patient is asked to rotate their head towards you to prevent angling the camera from either the left or right side. The buccal face of the incisors should be visible and just into the buccal sulcus and you should focus in the premolar region. Try to avoid including the tips of the teeth on the edge of the view. The appropriate angulation of the mirror and depth of field will keep all the teeth in focus.

CHAPTER 4
CLINICAL PHOTOGRAPHY IN ESTHETIC DENTISTRY

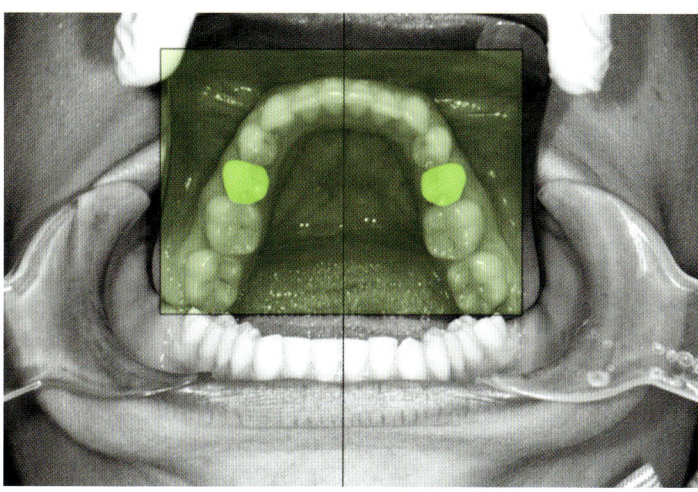

Fig. C4.21 Lower occlusal view technique. Small cheek retractors should be positioned inferiorly and laterally to pull the lower lip downwards and outwards away from the alveolar ridge. The mirror is positioned at 45° to the occlusal plane and the tongue is relaxed in the floor of the mouth. Otherwise, the positioning and framing should be the same as for the upper occlusal view.

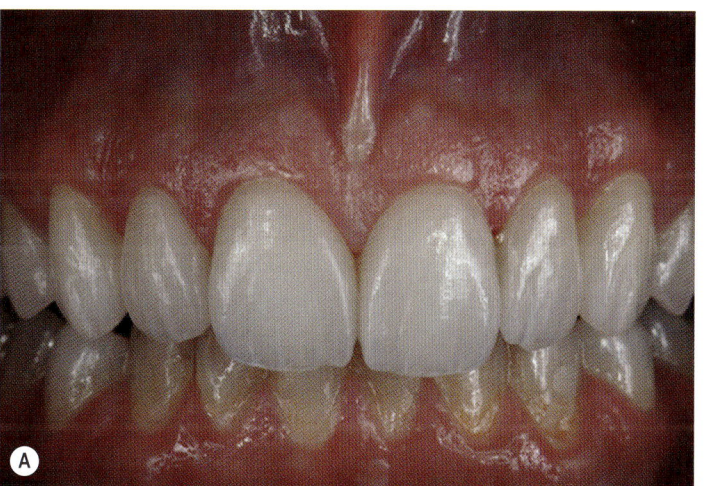
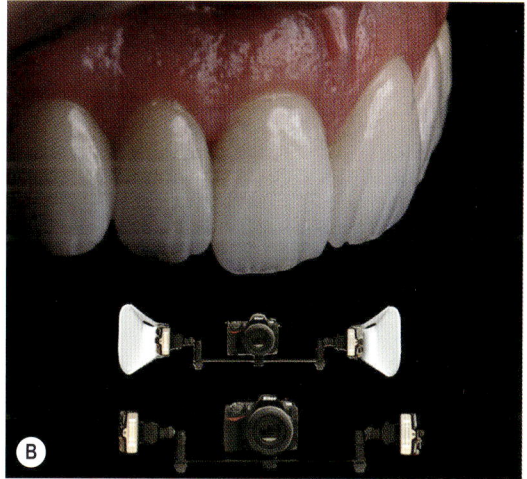
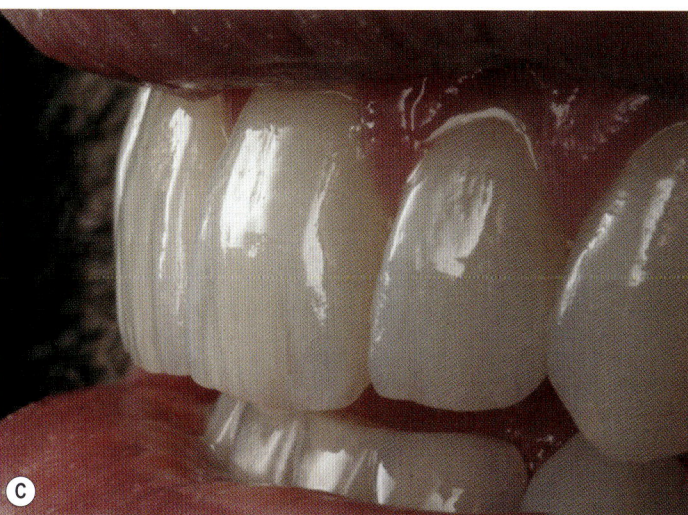

Fig. C4.22A–C Close-up dental photographs. These are used to see all the characteristics of translucency, brightness, value, colour, texture, surface, proportion and harmony of the tooth and the gingiva. We can use side flashes with either direct or indirect light.

CLINICAL CASES

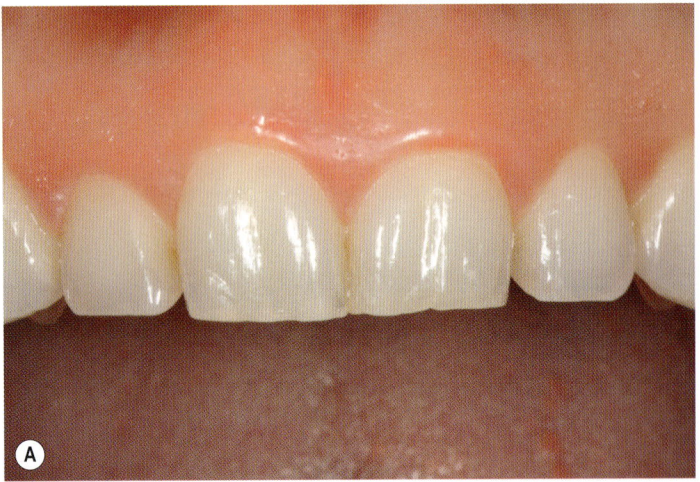

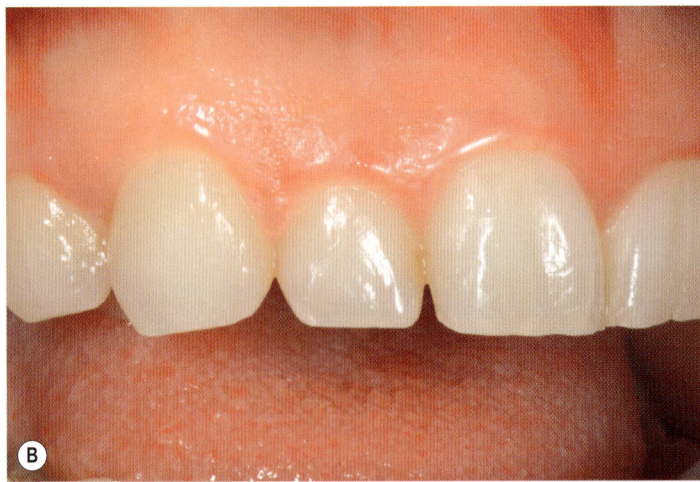

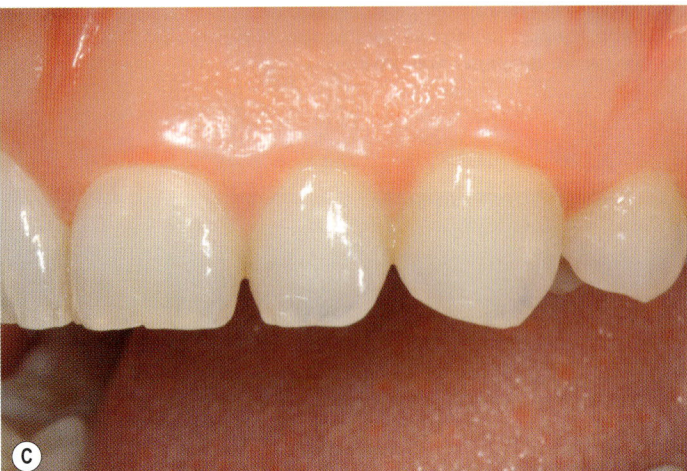

Fig. C4.23A–C Upper anterior teeth: frontal and right and left lateral views. In the AACD views[20], these photographs show a close-up view of central and lateral incisors and some of the canines, and central and lateral incisors and the canine on one side for the lateral view; they generally cover 4–6 teeth. The views should not show the opposing teeth. It often looks cleaner using a contrastor to highlight translucencies in the teeth, which also isolates the teeth making for a dramatic picture. Surface characteristics and texture can also be seen.

The macro lens is set with a reproduction ratio of 1 : 1 multiplied by the correction for the digital sensor, e.g. 1 : 1.5 for the Nikon D7000. Select a shutter speed of 1/200 seconds and an aperture of f29–f32.

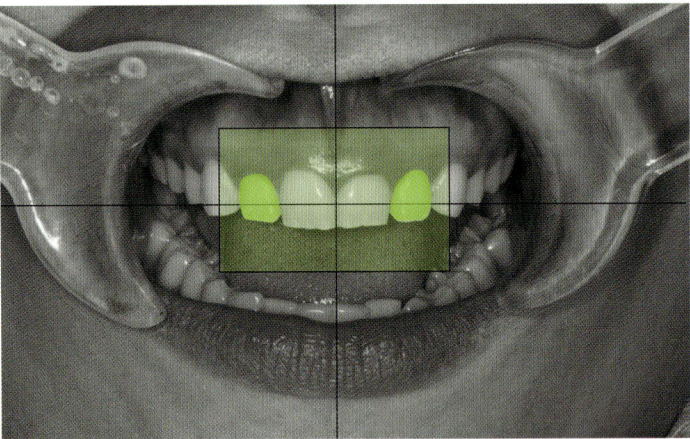

Fig. C4.24 Technique for upper anterior frontal view. Small cheek retractors should be positioned superiorly and laterally to pull the upper lip upwards and away from the alveolar ridge. For the AACD view, the vertical midline should coincide with the contact point of the central incisors.[20] The horizontal midline is perpendicular to this and runs through the midpoint of the contact point of the lateral incisor with the central incisor and canine. It often helps to consider composing the picture with the teeth in the middle third of the photograph. The camera should be focused on the lateral incisors and held so that it is at right angles to the labial face of the teeth.

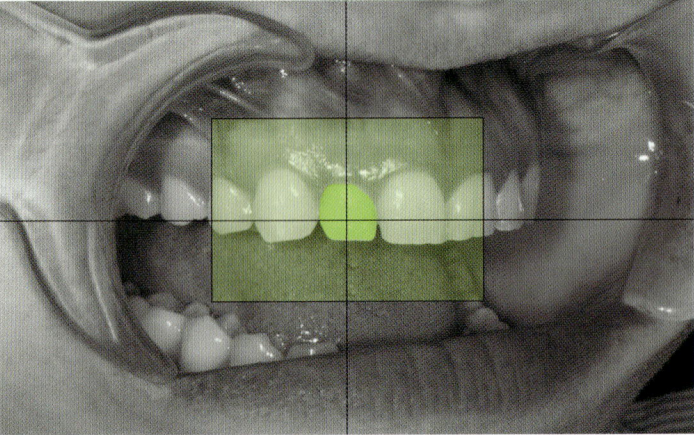

Fig. C4.25 Technique for upper anterior lateral view. Small cheek retractors are positioned in the same way as for the upper anterior frontal view. For the AACD view, the vertical midline should bisect the lateral incisor.[20] The horizontal midline is perpendicular to this and runs through the midpoint of the contact point of the lateral incisor with the central incisor and canine. The camera should be focused on the lateral incisors.

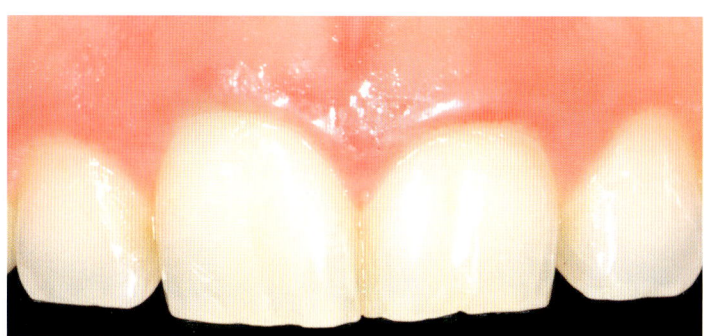

Fig. C4.26 Upper anterior teeth: frontal view with contrastor. This is a 1:1 photograph with a contrastor placed behind the upper anterior teeth. This shows how the contrastor acts to isolate the incisors and concentrate the nuances of these teeth.

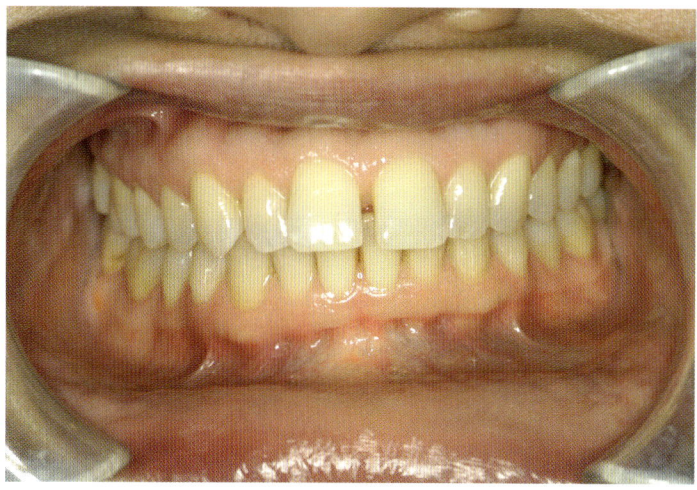

Fig. C4.27 Common faults in retracted full dentition view. This view shows that the horizontal plane of the camera has been tilted down to the patient's left with the left retractor position failing to fully retract the cheek. The centre of the photograph is more or less correct with this patient, as the contact point of the lower central incisors is on the midline of the face. This shows the importance of not inadvertently correcting centre lines of the upper incisor teeth when assessing esthetics. In general, there is too much view of the lower alveolar mucosa compared to the upper alveolar mucosa.

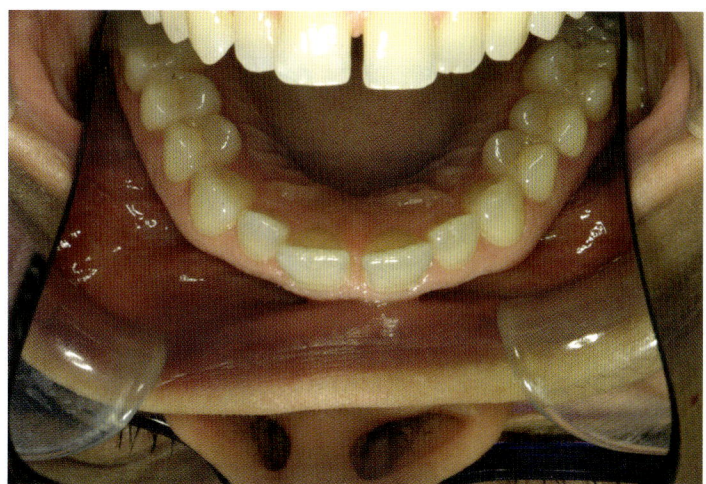

Fig. C4.28 Common faults in a mirror view. This view has occurred because the mirror was not placed far enough back in the mouth and the patient has not opened sufficiently wide to allow it to be positioned at 45° to the occlusal plane. The camera has been positioned at an angle to the occlusal plane in order to try and record some of the occlusal surfaces of the teeth. This has resulted in the upper anterior teeth being visible both directly and in the mirror. The view should also not include any aspect of the nose in the photograph. Finally, the mirror has not been warmed sufficiently as it is starting to fog on the right-hand side of the patient's mouth.

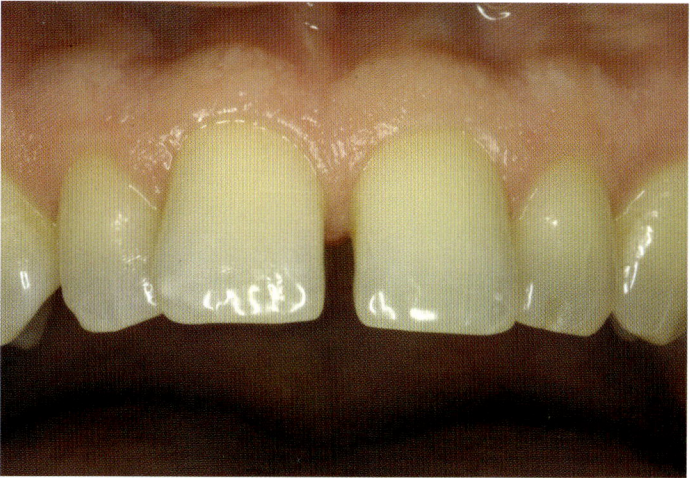

Fig. C4.29 Common faults in the upper anterior teeth view. In the upper anterior view, the camera needs to be at right angles to the facial surface of the teeth. The most common problem with this view is either having the camera angled from above or below the incisors. For example, the photograph has been taken from below leading to a shortened perspective of the incisors. This angle of view also shows the palatal cusps of the first premolars becoming visible. Neither of these elements lead to a natural looking, or diagnostically valuable, photograph. These problems can be avoided by positioning the patient's head correctly and holding the camera at right angles to the surface of the incisors.

Seminal literature

Ahmad I. Digital dental photography, part 7: extra-oral set-ups. Br Dent J 2009;207(3): 103–10.

This article provides useful information on different lighting conditions and studio set-ups for taking high quality full-face views of patients.

Moore S, Young S, Jones B, et al. IMI National Guidelines – Consent to Clinical Photography. London: Institute of Medical Illustrators, 2006. Available at: http://www.imi.org.uk/file/download/2143/IMINatGuidelinesConsentMarch_2007.pdf [accessed 12 December 2014].

This guideline, which can be downloaded from the Institute of Medical Illustrators, gives a very clear summary of the issues of consent and will help any practitioner develop their own consent policy.

Terry DA, Snow SR, McLaren EA. Contemporary dental photography: selection and application. Compend Contin Educ Dent 2008;29(8):432–6, 438, 440–2; quiz 450, 462.

A more in-depth discussion is provided on the selection of a digital SLR and flash system together with some coverage of digital imaging.

REFERENCES

1. Mack MR. Perspective of facial esthetics in dental treatment planning. J Prosthet Dent 1996;75(2):169–76.

2. Griffin JD. Using digital photography to visualize, plan, and prepare a complex porcelain veneer case. Pract Proced Aesthet Dent 2008;20(1):39–45, quiz 47.

3. Richelme J, Casu JP. Apport de la nouvelle céramique IPS e.max dans les plans de traitement esthétiques. Stratégie Prothétique 2006;6(5):325–37.

4. Almog DM, Meitner SW, Even-Hen N, et al. Use of interdisciplinary team approach in establishing esthetic restorative dentistry. N Y State Dent J 2005;71(5):44–7.

5. Almog D, Sanchez Marin C, Proskin HM, et al. The effect of esthetic consultation methods on acceptance of diastema-closure treatment plan: a pilot study. J Am Dent Assoc 2004;135(7): 875–81, quiz 1035–6, 1038.

6. Morse GA, Haque MS, Sharland MR, Burke FJ. The use of clinical photography by UK general dental practitioners. Br J Dent 2010;208(1):E1, discussion 14–15.

7. Derbabian K, Marzola R, Arcidiacono A. The science of communicating the art of dentistry. J Calif Dent Assoc 1998;26(2):101–6.

8. Derbabian K, Chee WW. Simple tools to facilitate communication in esthetic dentistry. J Calif Dent Assoc 2003;31(7):537–42.

9. Terry DA, Snow SR, McLaren EA. Contemporary dental photography: Selection and application. Compend Contin Educ Dent 2008;29(8):432–6, 438, 440–2; quiz 450, 462.

10. Chu SJ, Trushkowsky RD, Paravina RD. Dental color matching instruments and systems. Review of clinical and research aspects. J Dent 2010;38(Suppl. 2):e2–16.

11. Bengel WM. Digital photography and the assessment of therapeutic results after bleaching procedures. J Esthet Restor Dent 2003;15(Suppl. 1):S21–32, discussion S32.

12. Wander P. Zoom in on dental photography. Vital 2011;8:32–3.

13. Hood CA, Hope T, Dove P. Videos, photographs, and patient consent. BMJ 1998;316(7136): 1009–11.

14. Moore S, Young S, Jones B, et al. IMI national guidelines – consent to clinical photography. London: Institute of Medical Illustrators; 2006. Available at: <http://www.imi.org.uk/file/download/2143/IMINatGuidelinesConsentMarch_2007.pdf>; [accessed 12 December 2014].

15. Christensen GJ. Important clinical uses for digital photography. J Am Dent Assoc 2005;136(1):77–9.

16. Lowe E. Digital Photography: The AACD Series – Part One. J Cosm Den 2010;26(1):25–30.

17. Sharland MR. An update on digital photography for the general dental practitioner. Dent Update 2008;35(6):398–400, 402–4.

18. Farrell I. Complete guide to digital photography. London: Quercus Publishing Plc; 2011.

19. McLaren EA, Terry DA. Photography in dentistry. J Calif Dent Assoc 2001;29(10):735–42.

20. American Academy of Cosmetic Dentistry. Photographic documentation and evaluation in cosmetic dentistry: a guide to accreditation photography. Madison, WI: AACD; 2009.

21. Ahmad I. Digital dental photography, part 7: extra-oral set-ups. Br Dent J 2009;207(3): 103–10.

CHAPTER 5

Periodontal Factors

KIA REZAVANDI

Gingival recession 124
Implant esthetics 129
The interdental papilla 133
Long-term maintenance of soft tissue esthetics . . . 135
Clinical case 5.1 136
Clinical case 5.2 141
Clinical case 5.3 143

Achieving an esthetically pleasing gingival architecture is an integral part of esthetic treatment planning. Over the years a number of techniques have been proposed to deal with poor soft tissue esthetics and gingival recession. In addition, an ever increasing number of patients are now receiving dental implants in the esthetic zone, where a discrepancy of 1–2 mm in the gingival outline between the implant crown and the adjacent teeth can have a dramatic effect on the success of treatment. Hence, gingival augmentation procedures form an important part of the armamentarium used by clinicians to correct recession defects, to alter the gingival biotype and to improve the emergence profile of implant-supported restorations.

GINGIVAL RECESSION

Gingival recession can be defined as the displacement of the marginal tissue apical to the cemento-enamel junction (CEJ) (see *AAP Glossary of Terms*).[1] It can be generalized or localized and a number of causative factors have been suggested that include:

- Tissue trauma caused by vigorous tooth brushing and tangential forces due to parafunctional habits.
- Tooth position.
- Plaque induced inflammatory lesions.
- Iatrogenic factors related to restorative and periodontal treatment procedures.
- Recession associated with generalized forms of destructive periodontal disease.
- Previous surgical procedures.

The gingival morphology and tissue biotype have an influence on the likelihood of recession occurring. In general, flat gingiva are related to square teeth and a scalloped gingival morphology is associated with tapering teeth. The highly scalloped gingiva appears to be thinner with the gingival margin at or apical to the CEJ. Furthermore, the anatomy of the underlying bone dictates the gingival contour with the presence of bone dehiscence and fenestration more likely in individuals with a highly scalloped gingival outline.[2] Buccal recession is commonly found for teeth with thin or absent alveolar bone and where the gingival tissue is thin.

Histological studies using animal models have suggested that the inflammatory lesion formed as a result of trauma or plaque seldom extends more than 1–2 mm laterally or apically. However, in thin gingiva this may be sufficient to include the entire connective tissue (CT). Epithelial proliferation into the degraded CT may therefore bring about a subsidence of the epithelial surface that is seen clinically as recession of the marginal tissues.[3]

It is also important to distinguish between buccal recession caused by trauma or inflammation affecting the marginal gingiva and recession observed as the result of destructive periodontal disease. The latter generally includes the interdental regions and the techniques described to date are not aimed at correcting such defects.

TREATMENT OF RECESSION

The use of periodontal plastic surgery techniques in the treatment of recession is widely accepted. These techniques can be broadly divided into two categories:

- Free gingival grafts.
- Pedicle soft tissue grafts. This includes rotational and coronally advanced flap procedures that can be combined with a subepithelial CT graft or used in combination with regenerative techniques.

Miller[4] proposed a classification system for recession that has an influence on the success of surgical procedures:

- Class I: recession not extending to the MGJ. No loss of interdental bone or soft tissue.
- Class II: recession extends to or beyond the MGJ. No loss of interdental bone or soft tissue.
- Class III: recession extends to or beyond the MGJ. Loss of interdental bone or soft tissue that is coronal to the apical extent of the marginal tissue recession.
- Class IV: recession to or beyond the MGJ. Loss of interdental tissue to a level apical to the recession.

Complete root coverage can be achieved in Class I and II defects with only partial coverage possible in Class III. However, Class IV defects cannot be successfully treated. It therefore appears that the level of interproximal periodontal tissue is the critical clinical variable in determining the outcome of a root coverage procedure.

CLINICAL TIPS

Factors affecting predictability of surgery in treating recession defects:

- Technique sensitivity.
- Characteristics of the defect.
- Thickness, quality and maturation of the tissues at the recipient site.
- Ability to achieve blood supply.
- Systemic conditions affecting healing.
- Smoking has an adverse effect on healing.

FREE GINGIVAL GRAFT

The earliest technique devised for root coverage was the free gingival graft. This involved preparation of a 3–4 mm wide recipient bed, apical as well as lateral to the defect, by removal of the surface epithelium. A 2–3 mm thick epithelialized palatal graft is then placed over the recipient bed and immobilized with interrupted and sling sutures.[5] Although successful, especially on deep and narrow defects, the esthetics is not ideal and the grafted tissue is not always a good match in colour and consistency when compared to the adjacent gingiva. In addition, protecting the blood supply can be difficult until vascularization has occurred approximately a week later (Figs 5.1–5.5).

CONNECTIVE TISSUE GRAFT

The problem of poor appearance and blood supply is not generally encountered with the pedicle flaps that appear esthetically superior. Hence, when a change in thickness of the gingiva is required, the subepithelial grafts combined with a rotational or advanced flap have become the most commonly used technique. This involves harvesting a free CT graft of 1.5–2 mm in thickness from the mucosa of the hard palate. The graft may be harvested using several different methods. Langer and Langer[6] described the use of a trapdoor approach and Harris[7] introduced the parallel double-blade scalpel. However, the overall principal is based on securing the free graft to the recipient CT bed that is then covered by the pedicle flap. A meticulous surgical protocol should be followed with adaptation of the flaps and careful suturing.[8] Since the characteristics of the overlying epithelium are dependent on the underlying CT, this will lead to an increase in the width of attached keratinized gingiva and a thicker biotype.[9]

CHAPTER 5
PERIODONTAL FACTORS

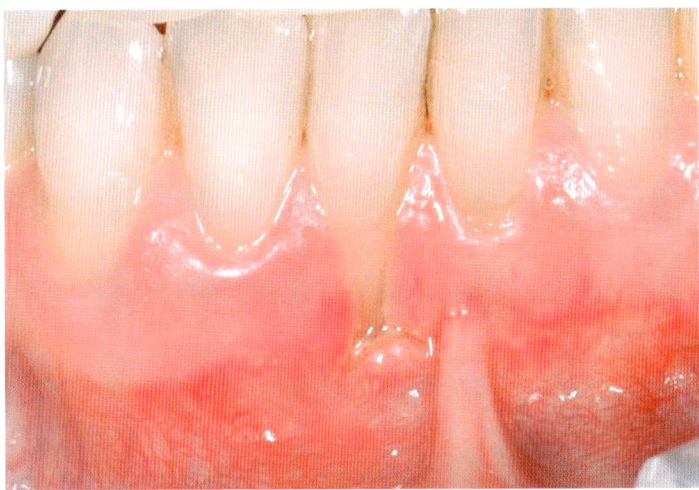

Fig. 5.1 A deep narrow Miller Class II recession defect affecting the lower right central incisor tooth with an associated high fraenal attachment.

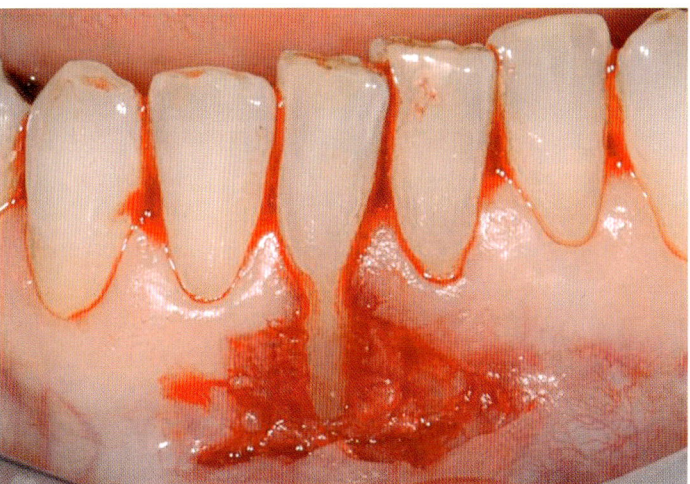

Fig. 5.2 The root surface is debrided and a recipient bed is prepared by removing epithelium laterally as well as apically. The movable tissue is separated from the periosteum, so that the graft is more likely to be stable during healing.

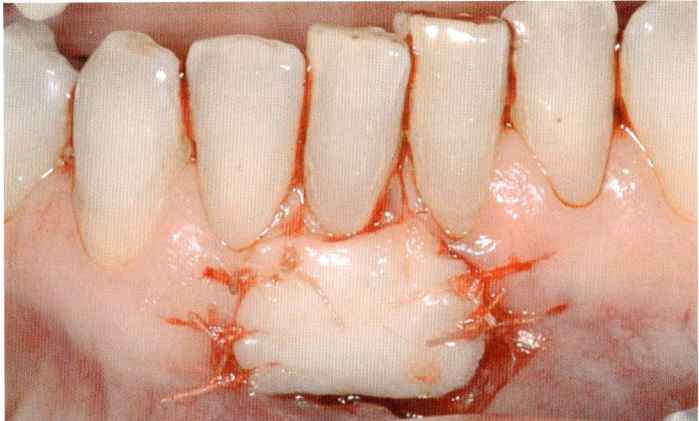

Fig. 5.3 The free gingival graft is sutured into position over the denuded root surface and the connective tissue bed.

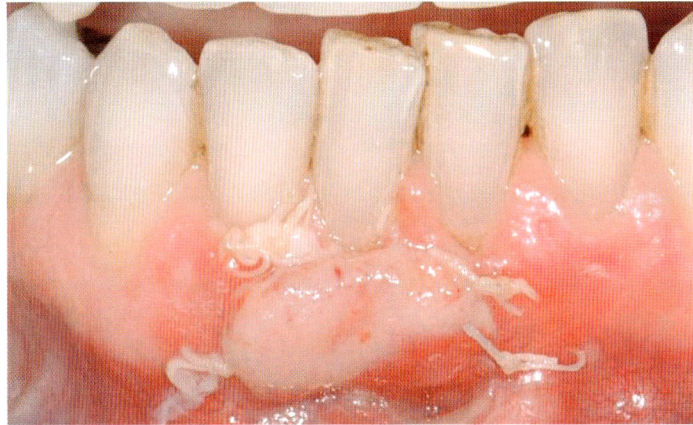

Fig. 5.4 A 1-week postoperative picture indicating successful integration of the graft and the underlying recipient connective tissue.

CLINICAL TIPS[10]

- A coronally advanced flap can result in a reduction in recession generally and in many instances complete root coverage is observed.
- The addition of enamel matrix derivative or CT graft can improve clinical outcome.

GINGIVAL RECESSION

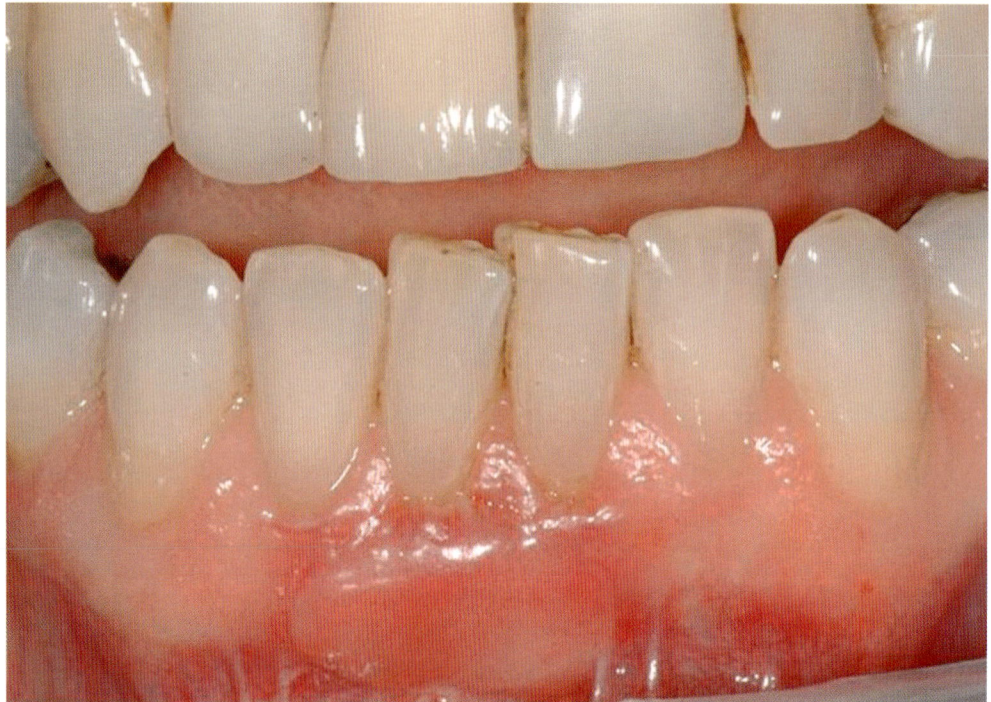

Fig. 5.5 At 3 months postoperatively, the outline of the graft is still clearly visible and it fails to match the surrounding tissue. However, this is of minor significance in this region and if necessary it is possible to re-contour the tissues by gingivoplasty at a later date.

PATIENTS' FAQS[11,12]

Q. What are the most commonly occurring postoperative complications associated with periodontal plastic surgery procedures?

A. Postoperative pain is unlikely to be any different from any other oral surgical procedure. However, there is an increased likelihood of swelling with the coronally advanced flap.

Q. What is the chance of complete root coverage?

A. Data in the literature is rather variable. However, in Miller Class I and II defects the use of a coronally advanced flap together with a CT graft or enamel matrix derivative appears to show the best results. A mean percentage root coverage of over 80% has been reported.

Q. How predictable are the results in the long term?

A. Zucchelli and De Sanctis[11] reported on 5-year follow-up of 73 defects treated in 22 patients. Maintenance of soft tissue was observed in 94% of defects and 85% of sites showed complete coverage at 5 years. The average increase in keratinized tissue from baseline amounted to 1.38±0.90 mm after 5 years.

IMPLANT ESTHETICS

Esthetically pleasing implant-supported restorations imitate the appearance of the natural teeth. The level, colour and texture of the peri-implant soft tissue should be in harmony with the soft tissue profile of the adjacent teeth. Although a variety of techniques have been suggested to increase the width of keratinized tissue and improve soft tissue esthetics around dental implants, these are, by and large, in the form of case reports or expert opinions. However, augmentation of peri-implant soft tissue can be considered an important addition to our armamentarium, as clinicians, in dealing with esthetic complications in implant dentistry.

IMPLANT POSITION (Figs 5.6–5.8)

The most important factors in achieving excellent soft tissue esthetics are the position of the implant and the gingival biotype. Hence, 3-dimensional planning of implant position is a prerequisite to provision of implant-supported restorations in the esthetic zone. A thorough assessment is required prior to implant surgery since correction of esthetic complications due to poor positioning is extremely difficult to manage. The most commonly found errors in implant positioning in the anterior region are poor axial inclination and buccolingual position. These can be the consequence of a lack of bone volume for ideal implant positioning (i.e. ridge defects) leading to a long looking crown, which in a patient with a high lip line can be esthetically disastrous. Unfortunately there is little that can be done, as far as manipulation of the soft tissue is

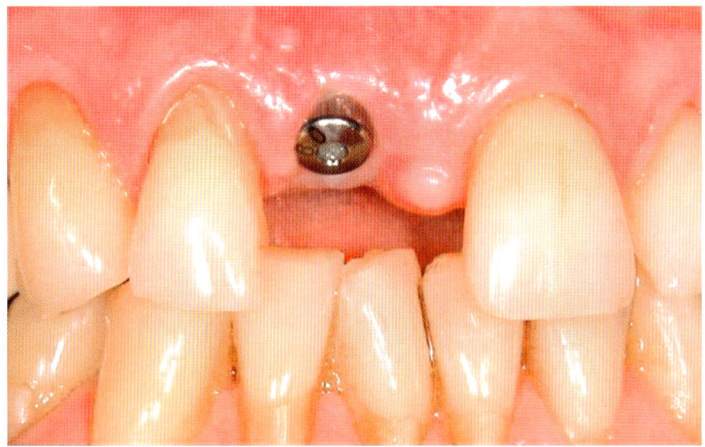

Fig. 5.6 Careful planning of implant position is a key factor in success. In this case the contour of the adjacent natural central incisor tooth dictates an implant position that is slightly distal to the midline as opposed to being in the middle of the edentulous space.

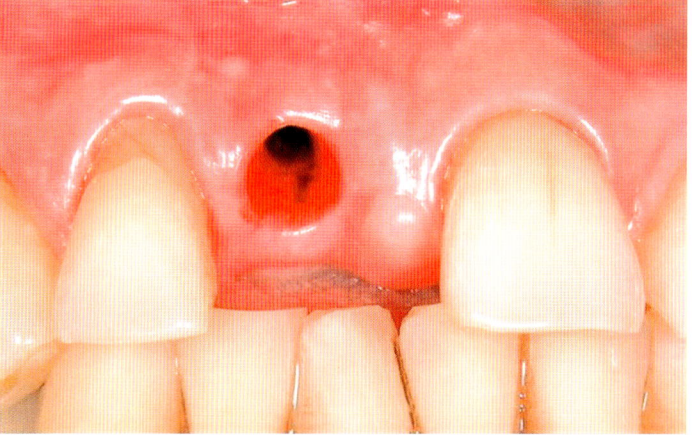

Fig. 5.7 The thick gingival biotype seen in this case provides a better opportunity for recreating good soft tissue esthetics. Implant position becomes critical in the individual with a thin scalloped gingival biotype.

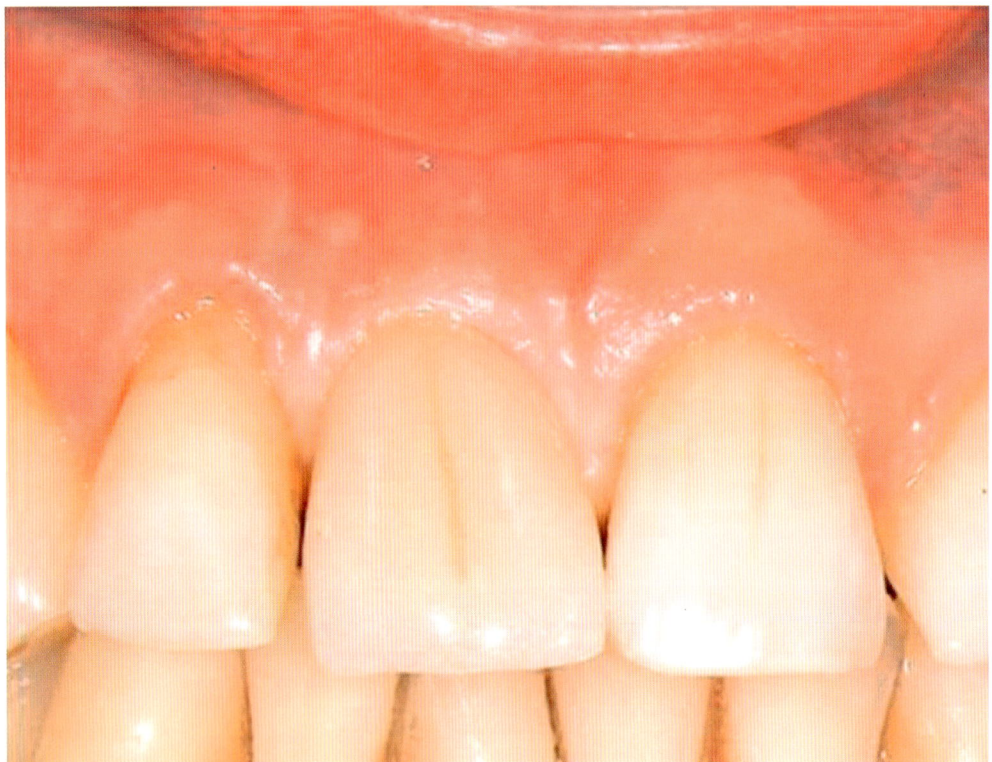

Fig. 5.8 The final implant supported crown shows that individual tooth characteristics, including morphology, shape, colour and surface characteristics of the natural dentition, have been well reproduced.

concerned, to create an even gingival contour if an implant is too buccally placed.

Implants should be placed in the same long axis as the crown. However, angles of between 20° proclined and 10° retroclined are acceptable. Buccal orientation would cause pressure from the abutment on the buccal soft tissues, which results in apical migration of the peri-implant mucosa. It may be possible to correct minor errors in axial inclination by the use of angled abutments and modification of healing abutments to reduce pressure on the buccal soft tissue.

The vertical position of the implant head is important in allowing a smooth transition profile. The emergence profile is dependent on the size of the crown, the diameter of the implant, and the distance between the implant head and the crown cervical margin. For example, in the case of a central incisor (7–8 mm mesiodistal width and a 6 mm buccopalatal measurement) being replaced by a 4 mm diameter implant, the implant margin should be placed 3–4 mm apical to the soft tissue level of the adjacent teeth. As a general guide, a minimum of

3 mm should be allowed between the implant head and the CEJ of the adjacent teeth. However, where the gingival biotype is thin it may be appropriate to place the implant in a more apical position.

Lack of bone in the vertical or horizontal directions that interferes with proper implant positioning should indicate the use of hard tissue augmentation techniques. These would either involve provision of block grafts for the more severe cases or guided bone regeneration where defects are considered to be mild to moderate.

Soft tissue grafts have in the past been widely used in correction of ridge defects in pontic areas. These have included free gingival onlay grafts to increase height, and subepithelial CT grafts to increase ridge width. However, the use of these techniques is limited in implant dentistry to mild horizontal defects. The pattern of bone remodelling that occurs following tooth loss usually results in the loss of the coronal aspect of the buccal bone. This can then lead to a mild horizontal defect that, although it has no effect on proper positioning of the implant, will influence the emergence profile of the restoration by the presence of an indentation at the cervical margin. Such defects can be addressed using subepithelial CT grafts in implant dentistry. Consequently the defect is corrected and the thickness of the soft tissue increased. It has been suggested that this would make the site more resilient to future recession by altering the gingival biotype.

THE PERI-IMPLANT MUCOSA

The peri-implant mucosa, like its natural teeth counterpart, comprises similar histological components and dimensions. There is a well keratinized oral epithelium and a junctional epithelial attachment of 2 mm. This is separated from the bone by CT that is approximately 1 mm in height. There is therefore an interaction between the implant surface and the supra-alveolar CT that is maintained following abutment connection. In addition, the peri-implant mucosa comprises epithelium and CT that form a barrier between the oral environment and the bone.[13,14]

There are, however, distinct differences in the histological appearance of periodontal and peri-implant tissues. In the natural dentition, the supra-alveolar collagen fibres project from the cementum on the tooth surface in lateral, coronal and apical directions. However, these fibres appear to be parallel to the implant surface projecting from the periosteum or present as coarse bundles that are parallel to the surface of the underlying bone. Observation of the composition of the supra-alveolar CT around implants also reveals tissue that is rich in collagen with few fibroblasts; hence, resembling scar tissue rather than gingival CT. In addition, gingival blood supply is from the supraperiosteal blood vessels and from the vascular plexus of the periodontal ligament. The blood supply for the peri-implant mucosa is solely from supraperiosteal vessels. Therefore, the CT apical to junctional epithelium (JE) is almost devoid of vessels.[15]

It is due to differences in the orientation of supracrestal fibres, vascular distribution and composition of peri-implant mucosa that coronal advancement of the buccal flap (with or without a CT graft carried out after abutment connection and placement of the restoration) is rather unpredictable. Although the clinical appearance of the soft tissue around natural teeth and dental implants is similar, a different approach is necessary when tissue is found to be lacking or of too thin a biotype to achieve optimal implant soft tissue esthetics. The timing of the procedure is therefore critical for its success. It can be considered at the time of implant placement or at the time of implant exposure, as in these situations the graft is completely submerged below the buccal flap and more likely to receive an adequate blood supply.

PERIODONTAL PLASTIC SURGERY PROCEDURES IN THE TREATMENT OF RIDGE DEFECTS

A frequently encountered problem in the esthetic zone is the presence of ridge defects that occur following tooth loss and result in gingival disharmony and poor soft tissue esthetics of the implant-supported crown if left uncorrected. These defects appear to stem from the loss of the coronal portion of the buccal alveolar bone crest that results in a buccopalatal reduction in ridge width. Araújo and Lindhe[16] reported that the coronal part of the buccal plate comprises bundle bone that loses its function following tooth extraction and is therefore resorbed. As the contour of the soft tissue is determined by the form of the underlying bone, a ridge defect is observed buccopalatally that would have an adverse effect on the emergence profile and soft tissue esthetics around the implant crown. The careful extraction of teeth, performed with minimal trauma to the bone or the surrounding soft tissue, and the recent use of various socket preservation techniques can reduce volumetric alterations of the extraction socket. Nevertheless, some ridge alteration is likely, which in the esthetic zone may necessitate the use of hard or soft tissue augmentation techniques.

It is obvious that the problem of the edentulous ridge defect is not exclusive to implant dentistry. Various esthetic surgical procedures have been described in the literature, since the late 1970s, as being used in situations where patients have lost teeth due to periodontal disease, failed endodontic treatment or traumatic injuries to the alveolar structures. Soft tissue surgical techniques can be used to correct mild defects of 3 mm or less in the buccopalatal direction. The most widely used and predictable soft tissue esthetic surgical technique to correct such defects in implant dentistry is the subepithelial CT graft. This graft is secured to the buccal flap leading to a thicker gingival biotype, which in effect fills the buccal defect. In addition the alteration of gingival biotype makes the site more resilient to future recession.

THE INTERDENTAL PAPILLA

In the esthetic zone, the loss of interdental papilla height can be unsightly. Although labial gingival contour and biotype can be successfully altered surgically, a surgical technique that can deal predictably with the presence of black triangles has been elusive. This is due to the fact that it is extremely difficult to protect the blood supply of the interdental tissues during surgery.

A number of techniques have been proposed which generally involve soft tissue augmentation through a partial thickness semilunar incision at the base of the papilla, thus building the papilla with a graft that may be nourished from the underlying periosteum as well as the overlying mucosa. These procedures have been limited to areas where a wide embrasure space is present, hence allowing coronal mobilization of the interdental papilla without damaging it. However, more recently dermal fillers have been used, which is a promising concept that at present is largely experimental.

The two most frequently quoted factors influencing the papilla height are the gingival biotype and the position of the contact point. Not surprisingly, when a number of teeth are being replaced by either implant or tooth supported bridgework, it is easier to create the illusion of an interdental papilla in patients where the mucosa is thick and there is minimal gingival scallop. When these conditions are met it may also be possible to use temporary restorations and pontics that apply pressure to the underlying mucosa, shaping the soft tissue accordingly.

The formation of an interimplant papilla is also extremely difficult. Nevertheless, a number of surgical procedures have been proposed to reconstruct the interimplant papilla at the time of implant exposure. Palacci[17] (Fig. 5.9A–C) suggested a method of rotating a pedicle flap to the mesial side of the healing abutment using a semilunar bevelled incision. More recently, Shahidi et al[18] described a technique without the need for suturing. This involved a U-shaped incision in the soft tissue over the implant; following its elevation and the connection of a healing abutment, this tissue is moved to the interimplant region.

It has been shown in a number of studies that the position of the contact point in relation to the alveolar bone crest determines the interdental papilla height.

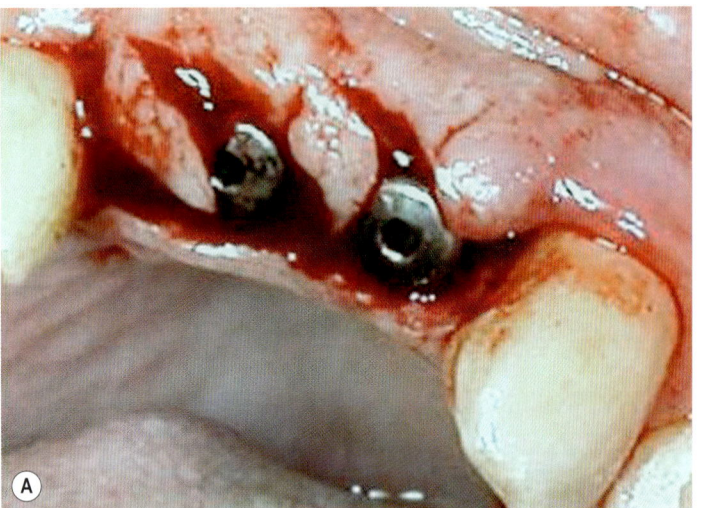
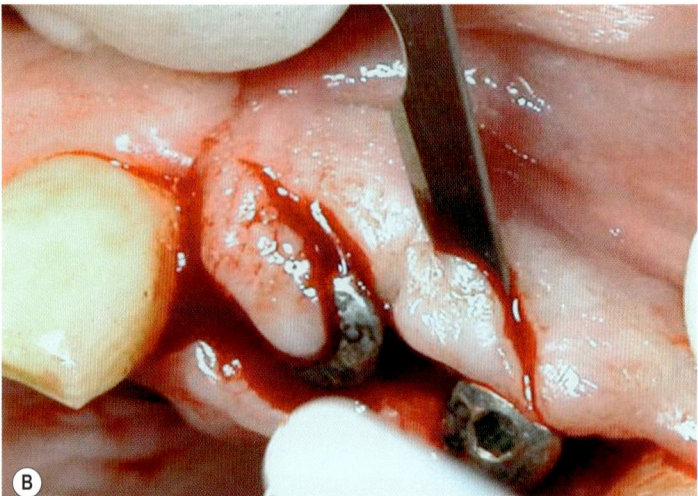
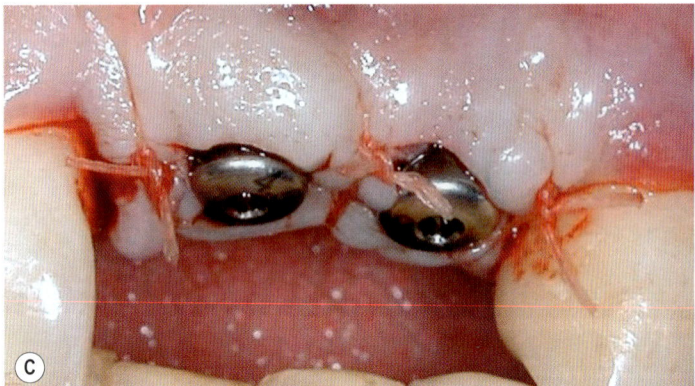

Fig. 5.9A–C The semilunar incision proposed by Palacci to increase the thickness of the mucosa in the interimplant region.

Restorative techniques can therefore be utilized in altering the contact points and hence eliminating the black triangles. A distance of up to 5 mm between the contact point and the interdental bone crest is often reported as the requirement for achieving a full interdental papilla height. When the distance is greater, the chance of soft tissue fill is reduced, according to a study by Tarnow et al.[19] Choquet also reported similar distances in relation to papilla height adjacent to single tooth implant restorations.[20]

In a more recent study Palmer et al[21] reported that the critical measurement for a complete papilla is 6 mm from the tooth bone crest and 8.5 mm from the implant bone crest to the contact point. Interestingly a number of subjects presented with no contact points; however, in the majority of cases a normal papilla height was observed. Palmer et al explained that the differences in their study compared to previous reports could be due to more accurate measurements and

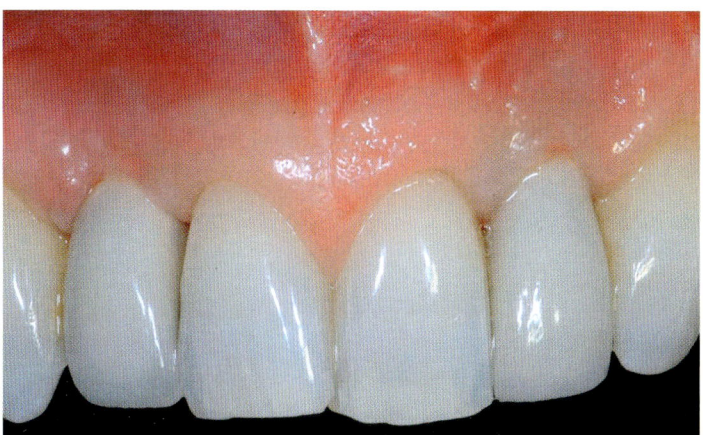

Fig. 5.10 Implant supported crowns replacing the lateral incisor teeth immediately after provision of the definitive restorations. Although the emergence profile and labial gingival contour are satisfactory, the papilla height does not match that observed adjacent to the natural teeth.

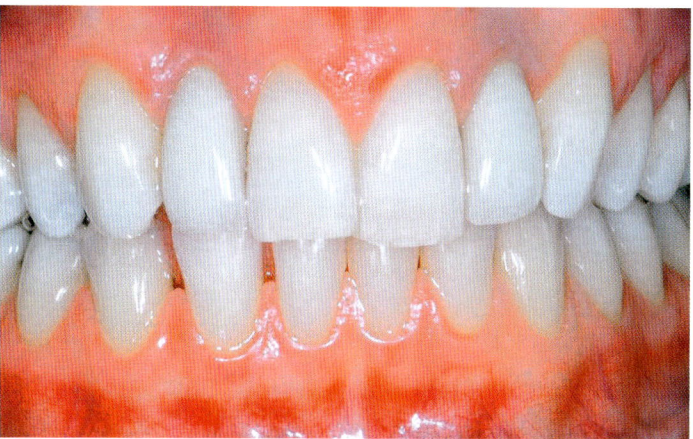

Fig. 5.11 One year following the provision of crowns, there has been an obvious improvement in papilla height resulting in a harmonious soft tissue appearance. This is expected since the adjacent teeth presented with good attachment levels and care was taken during the fabrication of the crowns to ensure correct positioning of contacts.

greater numbers of subjects with good periodontal support on the adjacent teeth. The latter is a key factor in determining papilla height in relation to single tooth implant restorations (Figs 5.10 and 5.11).

LONG-TERM MAINTENANCE OF SOFT TISSUE ESTHETICS

As the two most common causes of gingival recession are plaque induced inflammation and trauma to the marginal tissues from tooth brushing, it is important for patients to follow an effective and atraumatic plaque control regime.

Plaque induced inflammation can lead to bone loss and, as the maintenance of the soft tissue architecture is dependent on the stability of the underlying bone levels, this will result in recession and the loss of the interdental papilla height around both natural teeth and implants. In addition, the negative impact of smoking on periodontal health is well documented.[22–24] Smoking has been associated with significantly higher levels of marginal bone loss[25] and impaired healing following soft tissue surgical procedures, which can lead to a compromised esthetic result.[26] Therefore, the control of these factors is important in preventing the development of recession defects and in achieving predictable long-term results.

Good gingival esthetics is largely dependent on implant positioning and the patient's gingival biotype. It is generally easier to achieve a harmonious gingival contour and emergence profile in patients with thick gingiva and, conversely, those with a thin gingival biotype are more likely to suffer from recession. However, there is evidence that the esthetic outcome for single tooth implants can improve significantly during the first year of function.[21] This of course is dependent on the final restoration being fabricated in such a way as to be conducive to the patient's plaque control regime and the crown emerging with proper morphology to support ideal soft tissue esthetics.

CLINICAL TIPS[27]

- There is evidence that the soft tissue esthetic outcome for single tooth implant-supported restorations can improve significantly during the first year of function.
- This also includes the interdental papillae.

ESSENTIALS

- Successful root coverage is possible with periodontal plastic surgery techniques for Miller Class I and II defects.
- Although these procedures can be highly technique sensitive it is possible to achieve significant re-coverage of the denuded root surface using pedicle flaps together with CT grafts.
- Stability of the graft during initial healing, degree of coverage of the graft and the ability to achieve an adequate blood supply all influence the success of re-coverage procedures.
- Implant position is of paramount importance in achieving esthetically pleasing soft tissue architecture.
- A satisfactory result is dependent on the attachment levels of the adjacent teeth and the gingival biotype.
- Subepithelial CT grafts can be used to improve the peri-implant soft tissue profile.
- Improvement in esthetics can be expected following the provision of final restoration and soft tissue maintenance is dependent on underlying bone architecture.

CLINICAL CASE 5.1

The presence of a deep recession defect approaching the mucogingival junction is evident and affecting the UR3. In addition, a large Class V restoration is present. The lack of attached gingiva on the buccal aspect of the tooth makes the advancement of a coronal flap impossible. However, the tissues adjacent to the defect appear thick and mature. In addition, the interdental papillae are intact. Hence, a decision was made to correct the defect using a double papilla flap that utilizes this tissue, and a connective tissue graft was deemed necessary to increase the thickness of the gingiva.[28]

KEY CLINICAL TECHNIQUES

A number of factors should be considered prior to surgery. These include:

- Depth and width of recession defect.
- Availability of donor tissue adjacent to the defect.
- Anatomy and thickness of palatal tissue.
- Presence of muscle attachments.
- Presence of fraenum.
- Root surface, prominence and restorations.

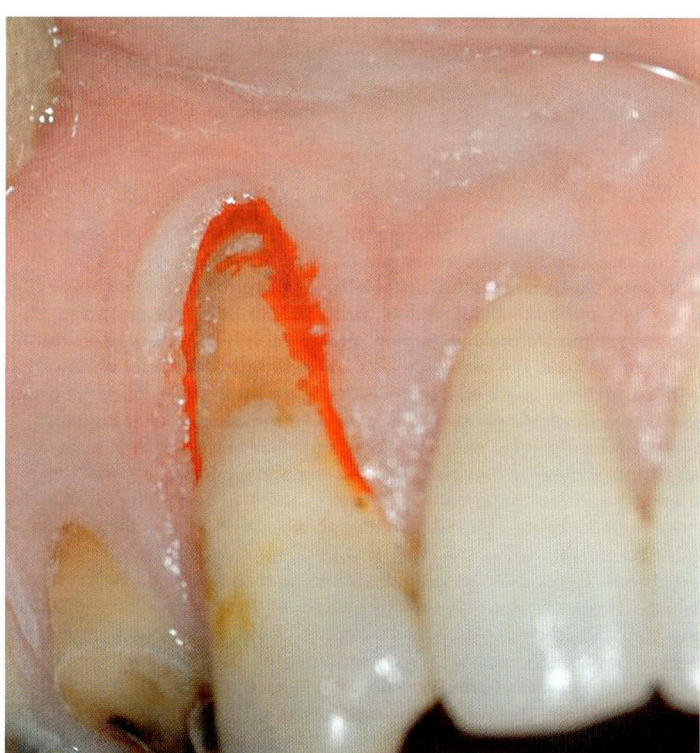

Fig. C5.1.1 The restoration is removed and reshaped coronally at a level that corresponds to the CEJ. The pocket epithelium is also excised and the root surface is debrided prior to flap elevation. Instrumentation of the root surface should be performed prior to any incisions being made so as to avoid inadvertent damage to healthy periodontal tissues, which may occur if the tooth is scaled after flap elevation. It may be necessary in some cases to flatten the convexity of the root surface with burs if the root seems prominent.

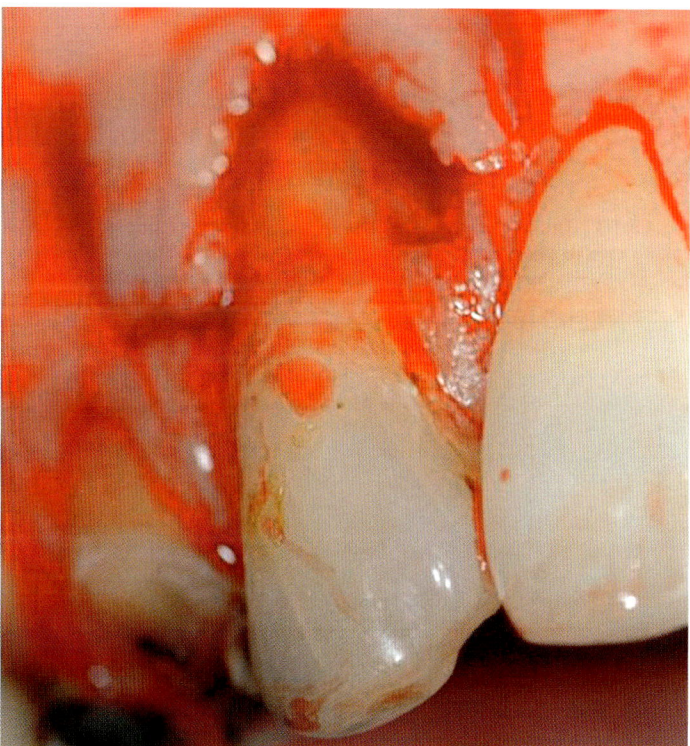

Fig. C5.1.2 Horizontal incisions are made slightly coronal to the level corresponding to the desired future gingival margin on the buccal aspect of the tooth being treated. This is followed by two vertical relieving incisions extending beyond the mucogingival junction that allow for elevation of partial thickness flaps. Hence, the flap elevation can be split thickness adjacent to the vertical incisions but must be kept at full thickness in parts of the flap that will be used to cover the defect.

CLINICAL CASE 5.1

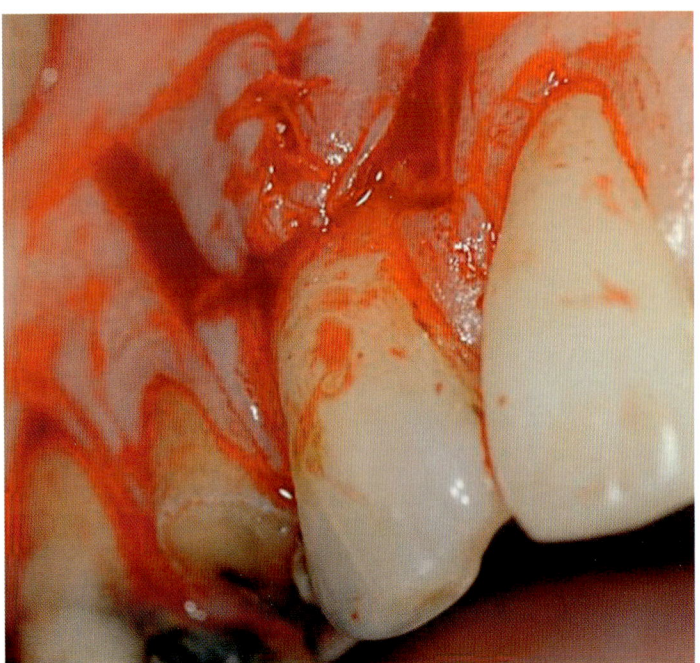

Fig. C5.1.3 The two parts of the flap are sutured using a fine material and taking care to avoid damaging the tissues. The flap must be stable and free of any tension that may cause apical migration during healing.

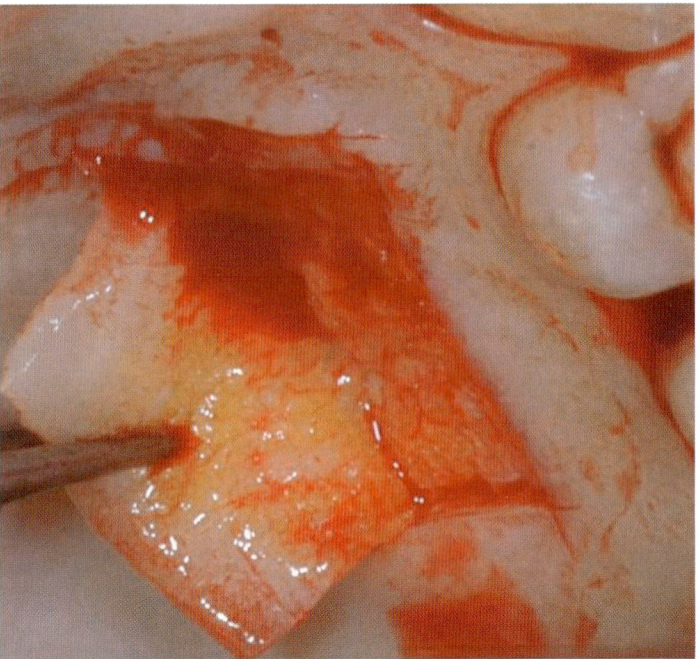

Fig. C5.1.4 The graft may be harvested using several different methods. In this case a trapdoor approach is used to obtain a graft of 1.5–2.0 mm thickness. The donor site usually selected is the palatal vault region of the premolars and first molars, midway between the gingival margin and midline raphae. Before any incisions are made, it is important to establish the dimensions of the required graft, which is done by measuring the width and depth of the recipient bed using a periodontal probe. The graft should be slightly larger than the required dimensions at the recipient site. A horizontal incision is made perpendicular to the underlying bone and approximately 3 mm away from the palatal gingival margin of the premolar and first molar teeth. The length of this incision is determined by the size of the graft required. Vertical relieving incisions can be made to facilitate the removal of the graft. However, care must be taken to ensure that these incisions do not extended down to the bone, especially distally, and inadvertently injure the palatal vessels. In this case, access is difficult, due to the limited opening of the patient's mouth, and relieving incisions are required. An incision is then placed from the line of the first incision and directed apically to perform a split incision of the palatal mucosa, which essentially elevates a split thickness flap.

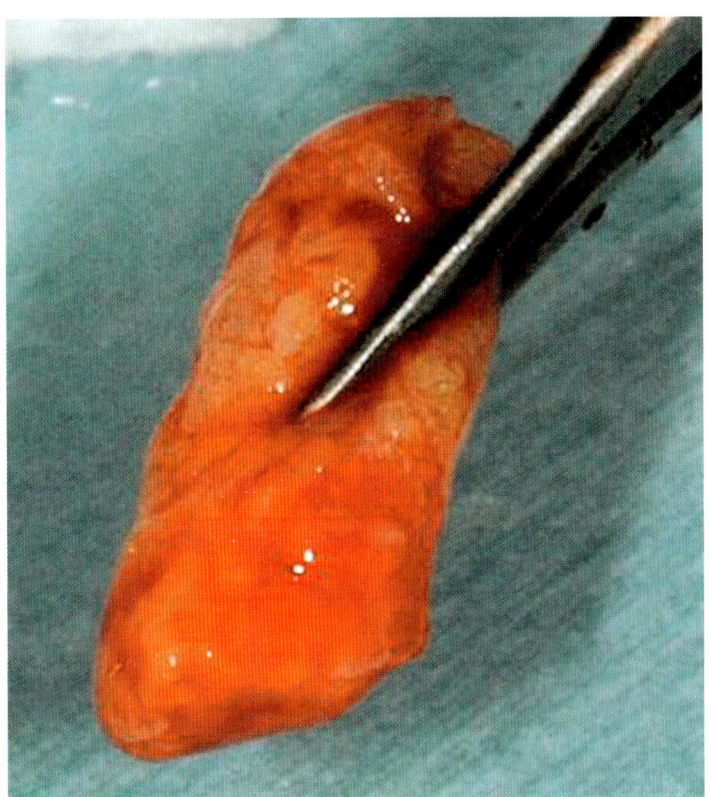

Fig. C5.1.5 The underlying CT is then released from the periosteum using a periosteal elevator followed by careful dissection with a scalpel. To avoid the palatal artery the thicker portion of the graft should be taken from the premolar region.

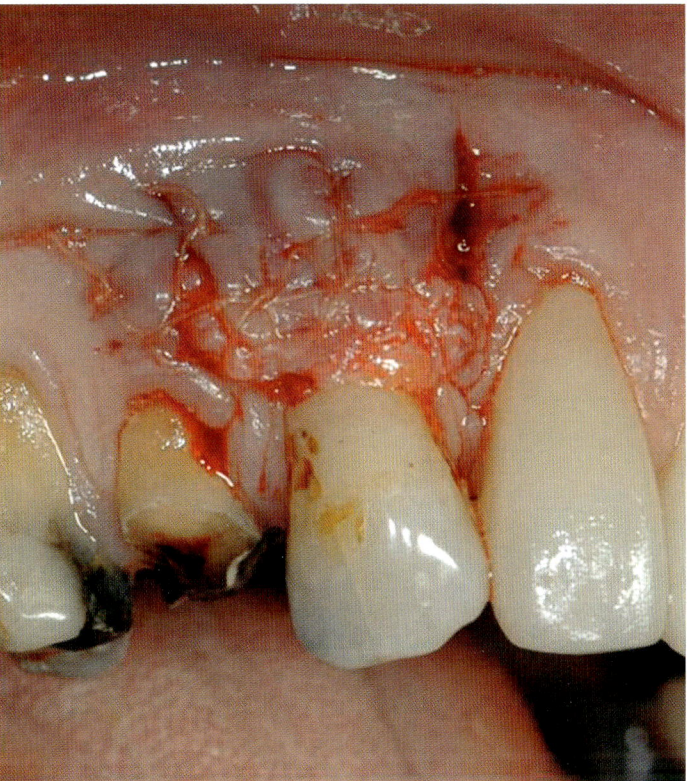

Fig. C5.1.6 The graft is placed immediately on the recipient bed level with the CEJ. It should extend 3–5 mm beyond the area being covered apically, mesially and distally. Over 50% of the graft should be covered by the overlying flap. The survival of the graft is determined by its ability to establish a new blood supply, which is influenced by the thickness of the graft as well as the degree of its coverage by the overlying flap. The graft and the overlying flap are sutured laterally along the wound of the vertical incisions through the periosteum and the attached gingiva, as well as in the interdental papilla region. Suspensory sutures are placed around the tooth to immobilize the flap and pressure is applied for a number of minutes to eliminate blood and exudate. This is important in order to avoid the formation of blood clots that compromise nutrient supply to the graft. The donor site is also sutured using interrupted sutures to achieve haemostasis. In addition to the routine postoperative instructions, the patient is advised to avoid pulling their lip and inspecting the site as this may disturb the stability of the surgical wound.

KEY CLINICAL TECHNIQUES

- The graft should be placed in the recipient bed immediately to avoid loss of vitality.
- Suturing of thin tissues can be difficult without magnification and fine suture materials. However, the use of microsurgical techniques has improved the success rate with such procedures.
- Care should be taken when suturing to avoid tears or damage to the flap as this can have disastrous consequences.
- Application of pressure for 5 minutes using moist gauze is of paramount importance.

CLINICAL CASE 5.1

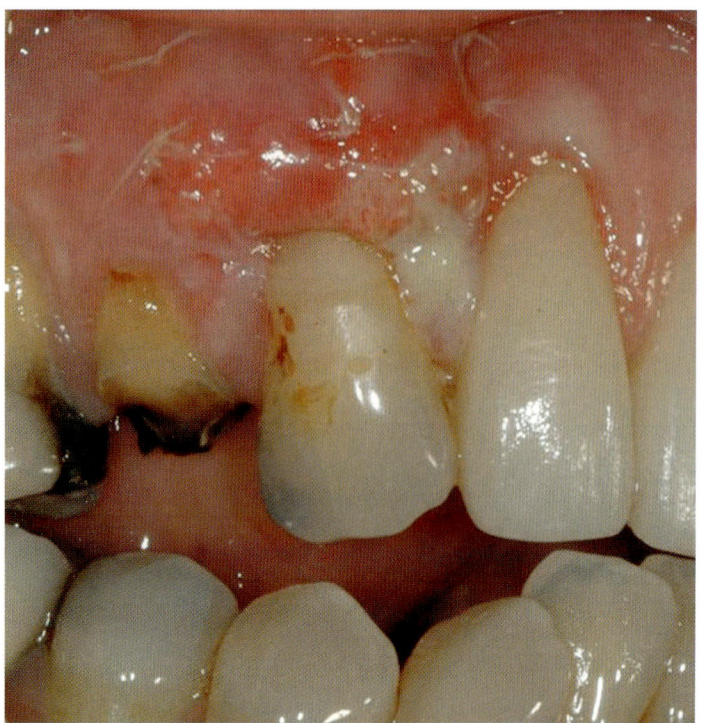

Fig. C5.1.7 The postoperative view at 1 week shows excellent healing with evidence of formation of blood vessels. In the initial phase of healing (0–3 days) the graft survives with an avascular plasmatic circulation. During the following 2–11 days revascularization occurs. Anastomoses are established between vessels in the recipient bed and those in the graft, and a dense network of vessels form within the graft. A fibrous union between the graft and the underlying CT can be seen, as well as re-epithelialization of the graft in parts not covered by the mucosa of the recipient site after surgery.

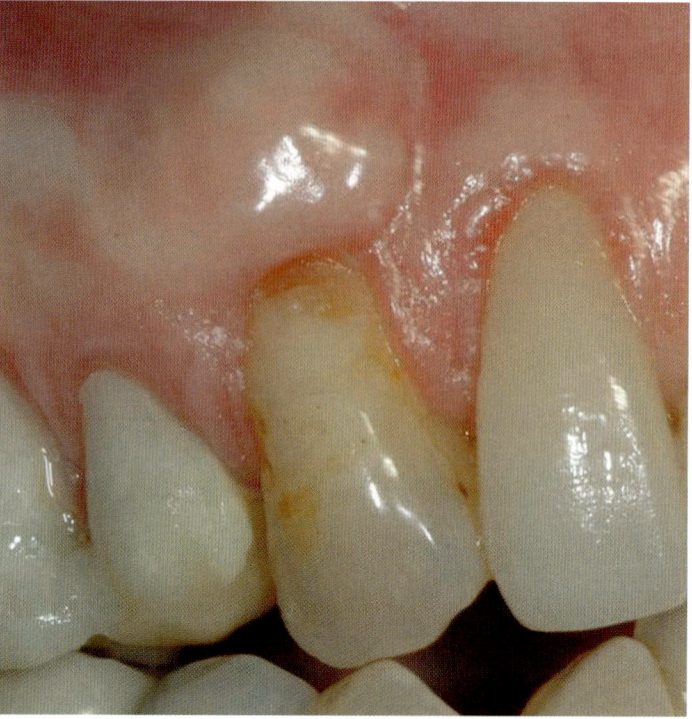

Fig C5.1.8 At 1 month after surgery the treated area shows successful integration of the graft and healthy marginal tissues. During this phase, tissue maturation occurs with a reduction in the number of vessels and epithelial maturation. Although the graft still appears bulky and the contour is not ideal at this stage, the colour of the gingiva at the grafted site closely matches the adjacent tissue.

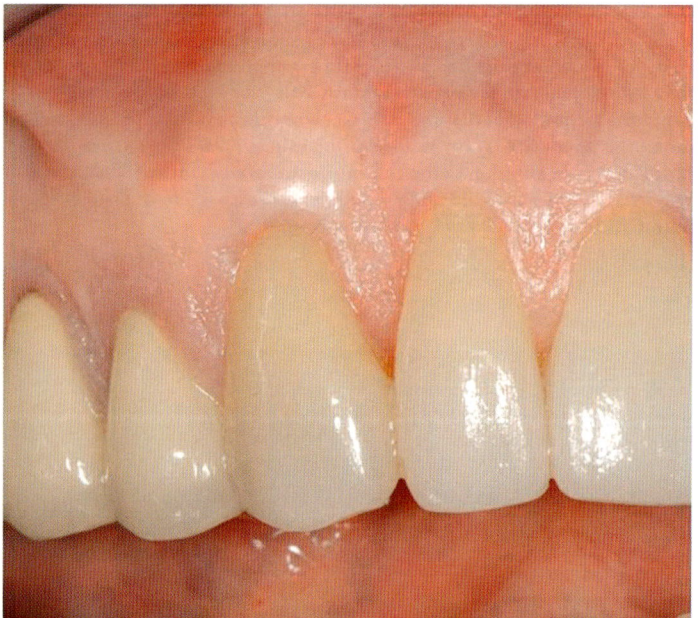

Fig. C5.1.9 Two years after surgery there is no evidence of further recession and the colour and contour of the marginal tissues at the grafted site closely resemble that of the adjacent soft tissue. A gingivoplasty was performed 3 months postoperatively to achieve a satisfactory appearance of the grafted area. The limited histological data suggest that new CT attachments are formed in the apical and lateral parts of the defect and an epithelial attachment is formed coronally and on the mid-buccal aspect.[29]

CLINICAL CASE 5.2

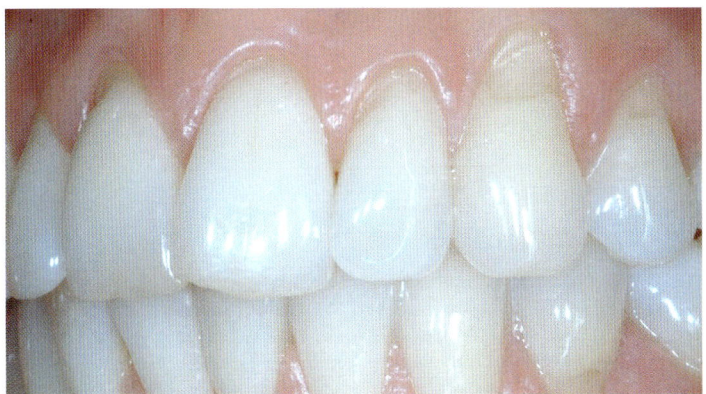 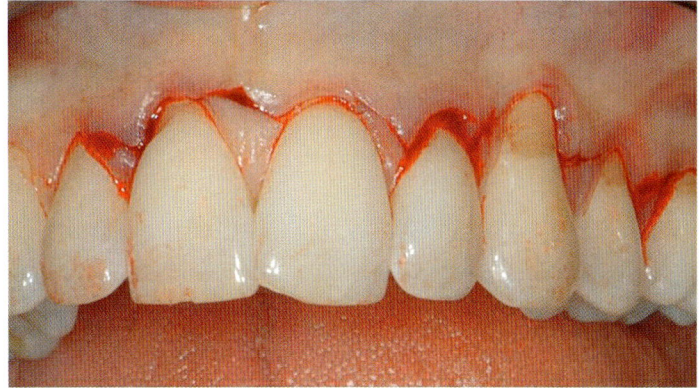

Fig. C5.2.1 Multiple Miller I recession defects are evident and affect the first premolar, canine and incisors. The attached gingiva is of adequate width apical to the defects. The interdental papillae are intact and the gingiva is of reasonable thickness and appears firm and mature. The presence of multiple recession defects dictates the selection of a surgical procedure that allows all gingival defects to be corrected simultaneously. The modified coronally advanced flap has been designed specifically for this purpose. Of particular interest is the absence of any vertical relieving incisions that may result in scarring and a compromised final esthetic result. This technique is simple to perform and leads to excellent esthetic results. It has been shown to be effective in obtaining complete root coverage with results indicating long-term stability.[30]

Fig. C5.2.2 Recession defects are thoroughly scaled prior to flap elevation. In the interdental regions split thickness oblique submarginal incisions are made starting at the CEJ of the affected teeth and extending to the most apical point of the gingival margin of the adjacent teeth. These incisions are converging on the lateral incisor, which is the middle tooth within the surgical field. Papillae incisions are made placing the scalpel parallel to the long axis of the tooth in order to create a connective surface that may support the coronal displacement of the flap and are continuous with intrasulcular incisions that allow for the full thickness elevation of tissues apical to the recession defects. The absence of any vertical relieving incisions dictates the need to extend the intrasulcular incisions to include at least one tooth adjacent to the recession defects in both mesial and distal directions. The tissues apical to the oblique incisions form the future interdental papillae.

CLINICAL CASE 5.2

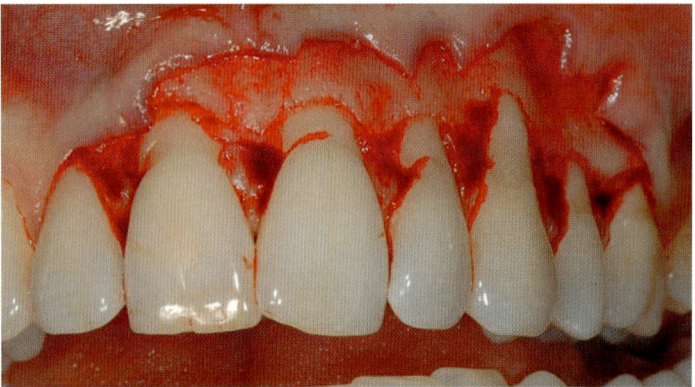

Fig. C5.2.3   Split-full-split flap incisions are performed in a coronal–apical direction. Gingival tissue adjacent to the defect is raised full thickness, whereas the most apical portion of the flap is split thickness to allow coronal repositioning of the flap without tension. The flap is moved coronally by a sharp dissection of the buccal mucosa with the first incision on the periosteum and the elimination of muscular insertions with more superficial incisions. The flap has to be free of tensions that are created by the movement of the lips and peri-oral muscles. Flap mobilization is considered adequate when the marginal portion of the flap is able to passively reach a level coronal to the CEJ of the teeth and when surgical papillae cover anatomical papillae passively. The flap should be stable in its final position without sutures. Anatomical interdental papillae need to be carefully de-epithelialized to improve CT beds and to eliminate epithelia that may interfere with the healing of the two connective surfaces of the new papillae.

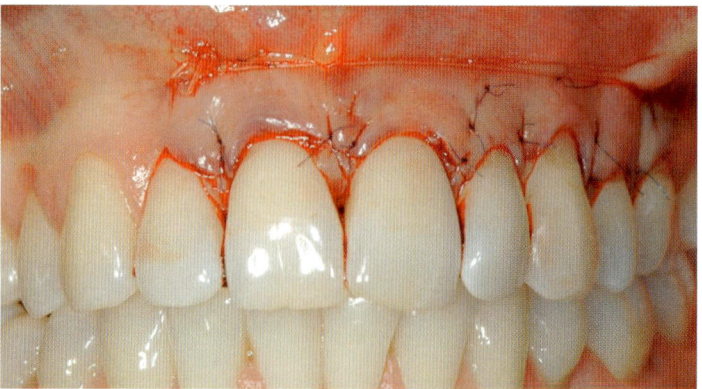

Fig. C5.2.4   When the flap is advanced coronally, surgical papillae are rotated and placed over the prepared CT beds of the anatomical papillae. The surgical papillae located mesial to the lateral incisor tooth are rotated in a mesial and coronal direction while the papillae distal to the tooth are moved in a distal coronal direction. The gingival margin on the apical portion of the defects is therefore moved coronally towards the CEJ. Sling sutures and vertical mattress sutures are placed for the precise adaptation of the flap around the teeth and to stabilize every single surgical papilla over the interdental connective surface. First sutures that have to be placed are the ones that stabilize the peripheral area of the flap; the central area is sutured last. In addition, a further mattress suture is placed at the level of the mucogingival junction. This further ensures that the flap remains stable during healing and is free of tensions produced by movements of the lips and associated muscles. The patient is instructed to avoid mechanical cleaning or inspection of the surgical site. To ensure plaque control is maintained, chlorhexidine mouthwash is prescribed for use three times a day.

KEY CLINICAL TECHNIQUES

- It is possible to combine the modified coronally advanced flap with a subepithelial CT graft if it is deemed necessary to increase the thickness of the gingiva.[31] In fact, this flap design can also be used in combination with regenerative techniques.[32]

- The absence of any tension in the flap in its new coronal position is a key factor in the success of this procedure.

- Sling sutures are placed to engage both the buccal and palatal tissues interdentally to achieve stability.

CHAPTER 5
PERIODONTAL FACTORS

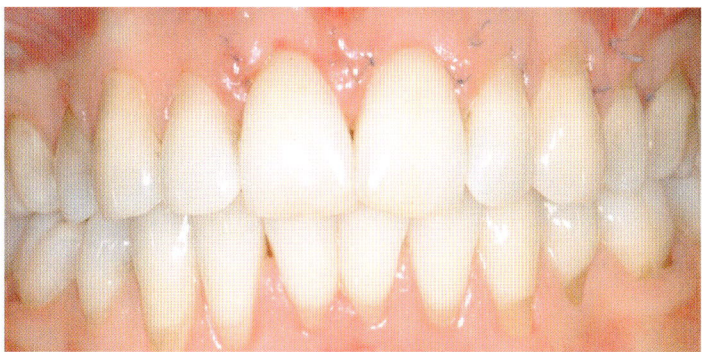

Fig. C5.2.5 Sutures are removed 10 days after surgery. Healing has been uneventful and complete coverage of all defects involved has been achieved. The patient is advised to continue with a chlorhexidine rinse for a further 2 weeks and instructions are given for plaque control using a postsurgical soft toothbrush and a roll technique.

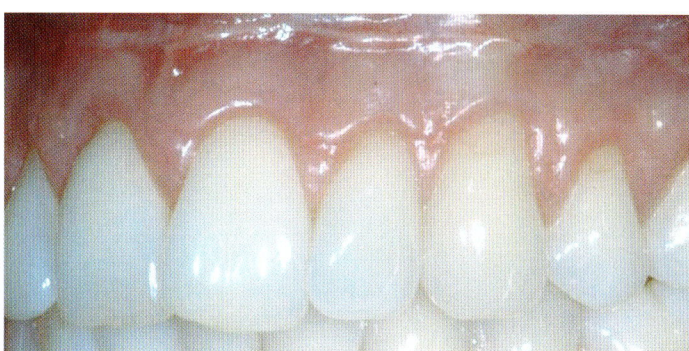

Fig. C5.2.6 One year following surgery, the marginal tissues appear pink and mature. The position of the gingival margins has remained stable with no further recession.

KEY CLINICAL TECHNIQUES

- Patients should be warned of the possibility of swelling that can be quite pronounced. This occurs following fenestration of the periosteum and dissection of muscular insertions.

- The degree of stability in the flap during early wound healing significantly affects the success of this procedure. Patients must therefore avoid inspecting the wound as this may exert indirect tension by movement of the lips.

- It is important to instruct the patient on an atraumatic brushing technique that ensures long-term stability by avoidance of future trauma to the marginal tissues.

CLINICAL CASE 5.3

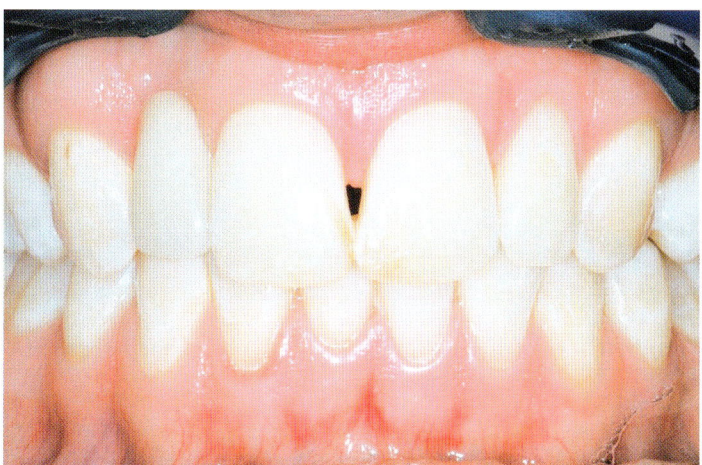

Fig. C5.3.1 The upper right lateral incisor has been lost due to a traumatic injury and the patient has been provided with a removable partial denture.

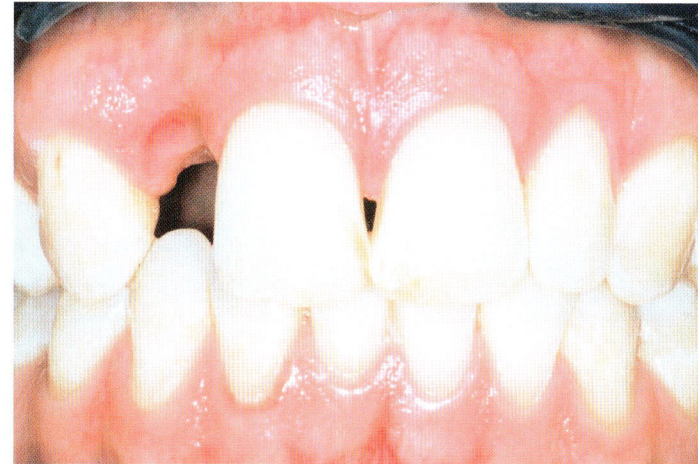

Fig. C5.3.2 The trauma has clearly resulted in loss of alveolar bone crest on the buccal aspect of the tooth creating a mild ridge defect. This could have an impact on the emergence profile of the implant-supported restoration planned for the definitive replacement of the tooth. This type of defect is common in the esthetic zone and can be resolved by the use of a subepithelial CT graft.

CLINICAL CASE 5.3

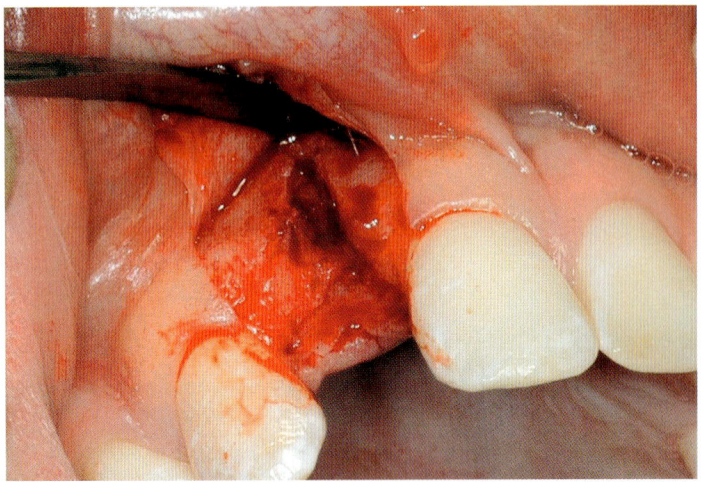

Fig. C5.3.3 A simple flap is elevated with relieving incisions along the distal line angle of the central incisor and the mesial line angle of the canine. At 3 months post-tooth loss, a bone defect is visible with extensive loss of buccal bone.

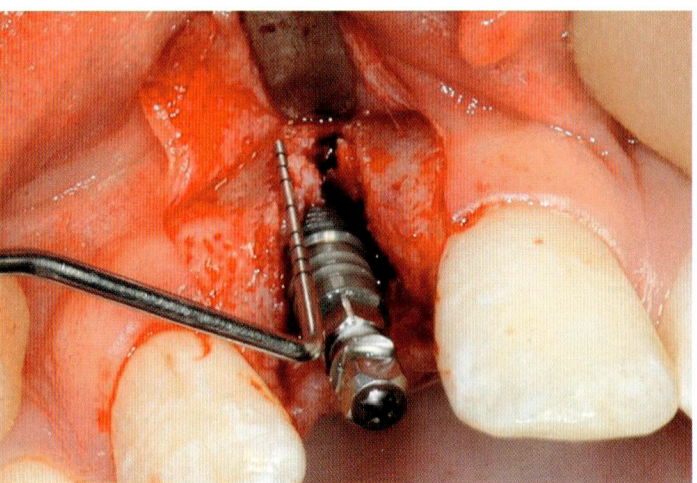

Fig. C5.3.4 Although there has been significant alveolar bone loss, this has little impact on the provision of a stable implant as adequate bone volume was available palatally. The resulting 2- and 3-wall intrabony defects respond well to repair as there is sufficient space available for any graft material, which would remain stable within the defect and be well protected by the overlying tissues.

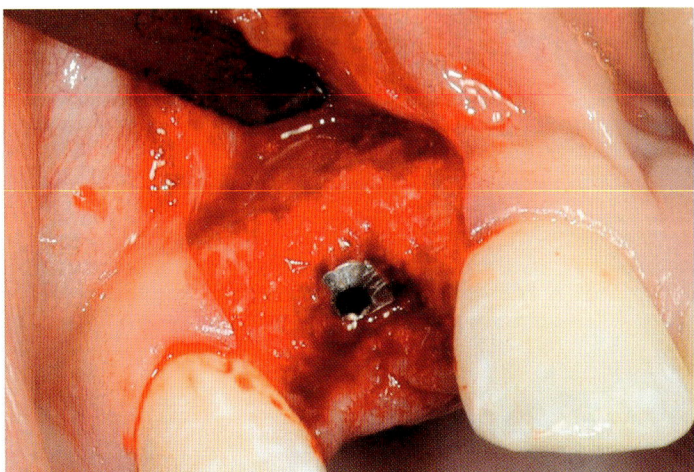

Fig. C5.3.5 The bone defect is repaired using bone chips and osseous coagulum collected during site preparation.

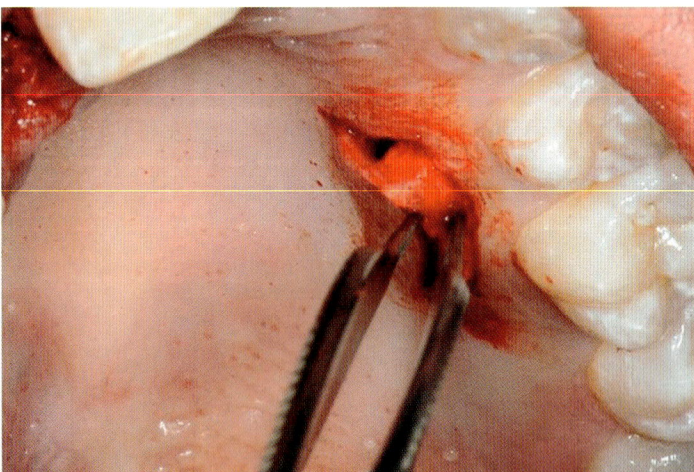

Fig. C5.3.6 To increase thickness of the keratinized tissue, a subepithelial CT graft is harvested from the palate using a technique by Hürzeler et al.[33] This involves a single horizontal incision with the blade at 90° to the bone, 2 mm from the gingival margin, and down to the bone level. The length of this incision is dependent on the size of the graft required. A second incision is made along the line of the initial incision with the scalpel blade angled to 135° and undermined in the forward direction. The CT is now carefully dissected from the bone.

KEY CLINICAL TECHNIQUES

- The harvesting technique described is the preferred method for obtaining the graft, as healing will be much easier and less uncomfortable for the patient with a single incision line.

- Although it is possible to correct such mild defects during exposure of the implant, more healing time is required prior to provision of the implant-supported crown as the tissues need to mature.

- The survival of the graft in these circumstances is more predictable than when used in a root coverage procedure. This is due to the better blood supply with the graft fully submerged as opposed to lying partially on a hard and avascular root surface.

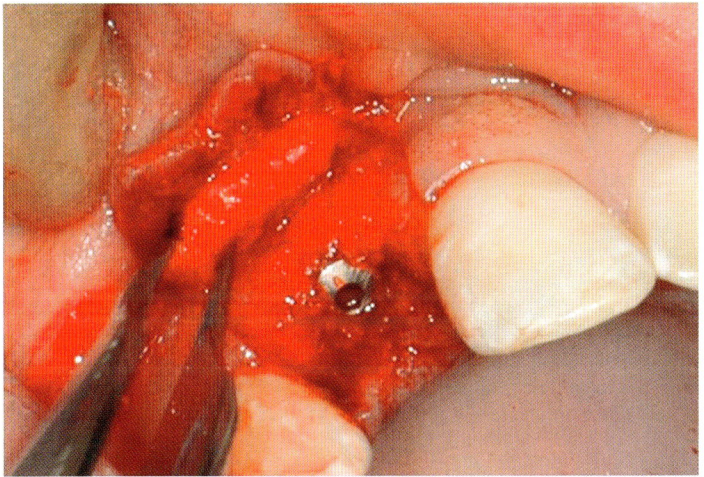

Fig. C5.3.7 The graft is secured to the buccal flap using a single suture.

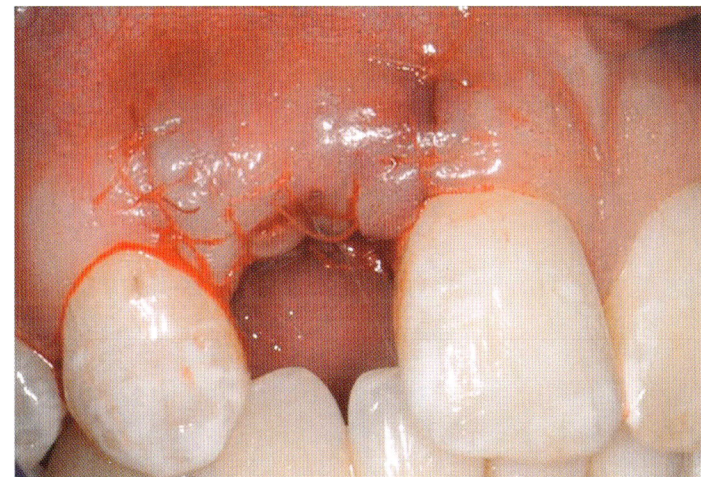

Fig. C5.3.8 The wound is closed using simple interrupted sutures. It is important to achieve primary wound closure to avoid implant exposure.

KEY CLINICAL TECHNIQUES

- If the patient has a partial denture as a temporary replacement, it is worth attempting to keep the donor site in a region covered by the denture. This protects the palatal wound, which makes more comfortable healing for the patient.

- Care should be taken when suturing the relieving incision. The use of fine suture material (e.g. 6.0/7.0) is advisable as this is less likely to lead to scarring.

- Loading of the implant and soft tissue should be avoided as much as possible during the initial healing phase.

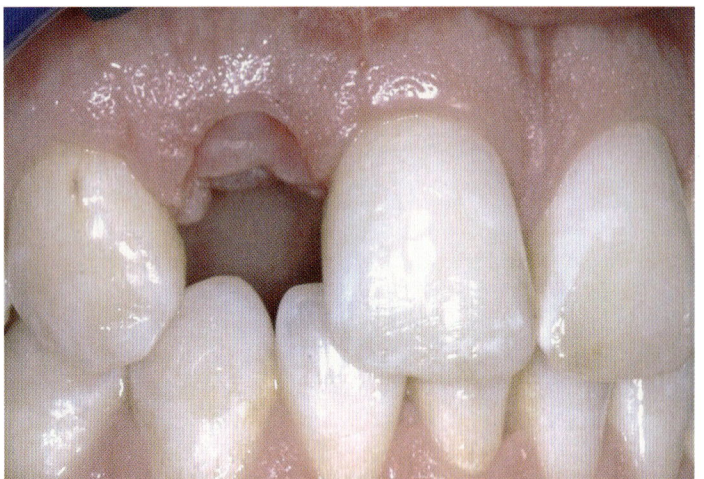

Fig. C5.3.9 Appearance of the soft tissue prior to implant exposure indicates that the buccal defect has been successfully corrected. The provisional restoration has been used to contour the soft tissue.

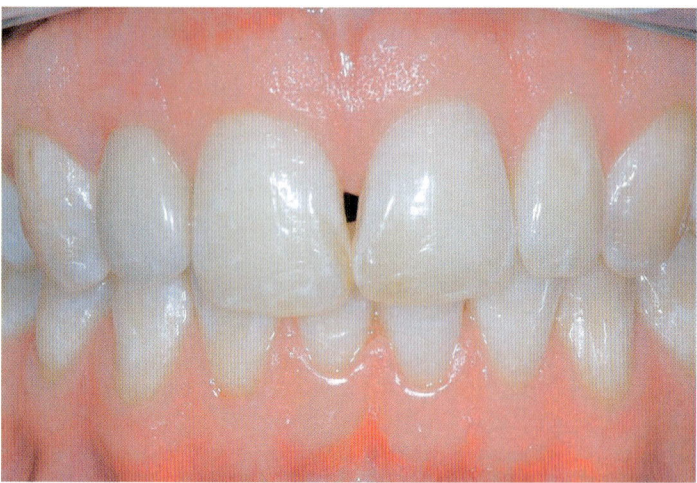

Fig. C5.3.10 The view of the final restoration showing healthy peri-implant mucosa that matches the adjacent tissue in colour and consistency with no evidence of plaque induced inflammation. The emergence profile of the implant-supported crown is satisfactory and the crown mimics the esthetic characteristics of the natural teeth.

KEY CLINICAL TECHNIQUES

- Provisional restorations can be effectively used to mould the soft tissue over the edentulous ridge. Composite resin or acrylic can be added to the temporary replacements after the initial healing.

- If the flap design, as in this case, is such that it involves the interdental papillae, some tissue shrinkage may be observed during the initial healing phase. However, if the periodontal attachment apparatus is intact, the papillae will bounce back to their previous position.

- In a single tooth situation the attachment levels on the adjacent teeth determine papilla height.

Seminal literature

Cohen ES. Atlas of cosmetic and reconstructive periodontal surgery. Hamilton, ON: BC Decker Inc.; 2007.

A detailed and well-illustrated book with thorough descriptions of various surgical techniques. The sections including pedicle flap design are particularly useful.

Dibart S, Karima M. Practical periodontal plastic surgery. Aimes, IA: Blackwell Publishing, 2006.

Periodontal plastic surgery is described well and includes detailed accounts of techniques, required instruments and surgical tips.

Lindhe J, Lang NP, Karring T, editors. Clinical periodontology and implant dentistry, vol. 1. Basic concepts. Oxford: Blackwell Munksgaard; 2008.

Lang NP, Lindhe J, Karring T, editors. Clinical periodontology and implant dentistry, vol. 2. Clinical concepts. Oxford: Blackwell Munksgaard; 2008.

A very comprehensive text on periodontal therapy with extensive scientific data to support an evidence-based approach to periodontal treatment. Familiar to all postgraduate dentists and a great reference book.

REFERENCES

1. The American Academy of Periodontology. Glossary of periodontal terms. 4th ed. Chicago, IL: The American Academy of Periodontology; 2001.

2. Becker W, Ochsenbein C, Tibbetts L, Becker BE. Alveolar bone anatomic profiles as measured from dry skulls. Clinical ramifications. J Clin Periodontol 1997;24(10):727–31.

3. Baker DL, Seymour GJ. The possible pathogenesis of gingival recession. A histological study of induced recession in the rat. J Clin Periodontol 1976;3(4):208–19.

4. Miller PD. A classification of marginal tissue recession. Int J Periodontics Restorative Dent 1985;5(2):9–13.

5. Miller PD. Root coverage using a free soft tissue graft following citric acid application, part 1. Technique. Int J Periodontics Restorative Dent 1982;2(1):65–70.

6. Langer B, Langer L. Subepithelial connective tissue graft technique for tooth coverage. J Periodontol 1985;56(12):715–20.

7. Harris RJ. The connective tissue and partial thickness double pedicle graft. A predictable method of obtaining root coverage. J Periodontol 1992;63(5):477–86.

8. Zucchelli G, Amore C, Sforza NM, et al. Bilaminar techniques for the treatment of recession type defects. A comparative clinical study. J Clin Periodontol 2003;30(10):862–70.

9. Wennström JL, Zucchelli G. Increased gingival dimensions. A significant factor for successful outcome of root coverage procedures? A 2-year prospective clinical study. J Clin Periodontol 1996;23(8):770–7.

10. Cairo F, Pagliaro U, Nieri MJ. Treatment of gingival recession with coronally advanced flap procedures: a systematic review. J Clin Periodontol 2008;35(Suppl. 8):136–62.

11. Zucchelli G, De Sanctis M. Long-term outcome following treatment of multiple Miller class I and II recession defects in esthetic areas of the mouth. J Periodontol 2005;76(12): 2286–92.

12. McGuire MK, Nunn M. Evaluation of human recession defects treated with coronally advanced flaps and either enamel matrix derivative or connective tissue. Part 1: Comparison of clinical parameters. J Periodontol 2003;74(8):1110–25.

13. Berglundh T, Lindhe J, Ericsson I, et al. The soft tissue barrier at implants and teeth. Clin Oral Implants Res 1991;2(2):81–90.

14. Abrahamsson I, Berglundh T, Wennstrom J, Lindhe J. The peri-implant hard and soft tissues at different implant systems. A comparative study in the dog. Clin Oral Implants Res 1996; 7(3):212–19.

15. Berglundh T, Lindhe J, Jonsson K, Ericsson I. The topography of the vascular systems in the periodontal and peri-implant tissues dog. J Clin Periodontol 1994;21(3):189–93.

REFERENCES

16. Araújo MG, Lindhe J. Dimensional ridge alterations following tooth extraction. An experimental study in the dog. J Clin Periodontol 2005;32(2):212–18.

17. Palacci P. Papilla regeneration technique. In: Palacci P, Ericsson I, Engstrand P, Rangert B, editors. Optimal implant positioning & soft tissue management for the branemark system. Chicago, IL: Quintessence Pub. Co.; 1995. p. 59–70.

18. Shahidi P, Jacobson Z, Dibart S, et al. Efficacy of a new papilla generation technique in implant dentistry: a preliminary study. Int J Oral Maxillofac Implants 2008;23(5):926–34.

19. Tarnow DP, Magner AW, Fletcher P. The effect of the distance from the contact point to the crest of bone on the presence or absence of the interproximal dental papilla. J Periodontol 1992;63(12):995–6.

20. Choquet V, Hermans M, Adriaenssens P, et al. Clinical and radiographic evaluation of the papilla level adjacent to single-tooth dental implants. A retrospective study in the maxillary anterior region. J Periodontol 2001;72(10):1364–71.

21. Palmer RM, Farkondeh N, Palmer PJ, Wilson RF. Astra Tech single-tooth implants: an audit of patient satisfaction and soft tissue form. J Clin Periodontol 2007;34:633–8.

22. Grossi SG, Zambon JJ, Ho AW. Assessment of risk for periodontal disease. I. Risk indicators for attachment loss. J Periodontol 1994;65(3):260–7.

23. Grossi SG, Genco RJ, Machtei EE. Assessment of risk for periodontal disease. II. Risk indicators for alveolar bone loss. J Periodontol 1995;66(1):23–9.

24. Bergström J, Floderus-Myrhed B. Co-twin control study of the relationship between smoking and periodontal disease factors. Community Dent Oral Epidemiol 1983;11(2):113–16.

25. Nitzan D, Mamlider A, Levin L, Schwartz-Arad D. Impact of smoking on marginal bone loss. Int J Oral Maxillofac Implants 2005;20(4):605–9.

26. Martins AG, Andia DC, Sallum AW, et al. Smoking may affect root coverage outcome. A prospective clinical study in humans. J Periodontol 2004;75(4):586–91.

27. Lai HC, Zhang ZY, Wang F, et al. Evaluation of soft-tissue alteration around implant-supported single-tooth restoration in the anterior maxilla: the pink esthetic score. Clin Oral Implants Res 2008;19(6):560–4.

28. Harris RJ. The connective tissue with partial thickness double pedicle graft: the results of 100 consecutively treated defects. J Periodontol 1994;65(5):448–61.

29. Pasquinelli KL. The histology of new attachment utilizing a thick autogenous soft tissue graft in an area of deep recession: a case report. Int J Periodontics Restorative Dent 1995;15(3):248–57.

30. Zucchelli G, De Sanctis M. Treatment of multiple recession-type defects in patients with esthetic demands. J Periodontol 2000;71(9):1506–14.

31. Da Silva RC, Joly JC, De Lima AF, Tatakis DN. Root coverage using the coronally positioned flap with or without a subepithelial connective tissue graft. J Periodontol 2004;75(3):413–19.

32. Del Pizzo M, Zucchelli G, Modica F, et al. Coronally advanced flap with or without enamel matrix derivative for root coverage: a 2-year study. J Clin Periodontol 2005;32(11):1181–7.

33. Hürzeler MB, Weng D. A single-incision technique to harvest subepithelial connective tissue grafts from the palate. Int J Periodontics Restorative Dent 1999;19(3):279–87.

CHAPTER 6

Space Management

ANABELLA OQUENDO, STEVEN DAVID

Introduction 152
Clinical considerations 153
Esthetic parameters. 158
The orthodontic role 161
Crowding treatment planning 163
Diastema treatment planning 165
Clinical case 6.1: crowding 171
Clinical case 6.2: clinical procedures for
diastema closure. 176
Acknowledgement 179

INTRODUCTION

Patients who present with excessive intra-arch space, diastemata (Fig. 6.1), or insufficient intra-arch space, crowding (Fig. 6.2), can, in almost all cases, benefit from orthodontic therapy. Orthodontic therapy represents the traditional, predictable means of achieving tooth movement to address esthetic and functional problems presented by excessive or insufficient arch space.[1]

However, orthodontic's inability to produce esthetic results quickly enough to satisfy patient desires and the need to retain the results achieved have inspired the use of tooth preparation and restorative dentistry to manage spatially compromised cases.

Restorative space management (RSM) is defined as the use of tooth preparation techniques and restorative dentistry to manage spatially compromised cases (Box 6.1). It requires the selective and strategic removal of tooth structure and its replacement with either direct or indirect cosmetic restorative materials. At the same time, RSM requires that the quantity of tooth structure removed be

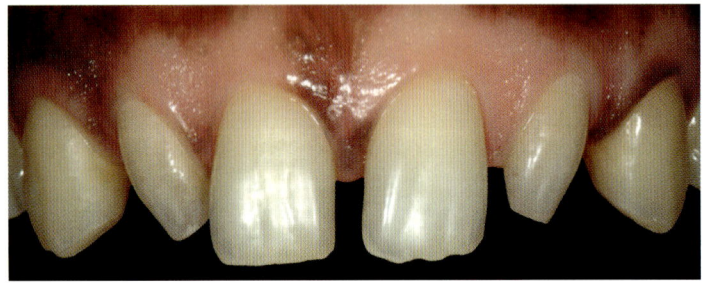

Fig. 6.1 Excessive spaces (diastema).

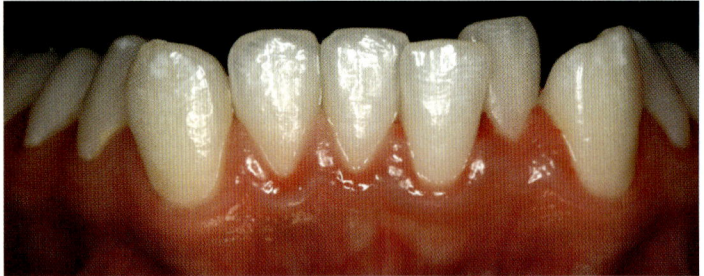

Fig. 6.2 Insufficient space (crowding).

BOX 6.1

Clinical considerations for RSM of spatially compromised cases:

- Do the teeth require restoration?
- Can the occlusion be managed with restorative dentistry?
- Is the existing periodontal architecture healthy and will it esthetically enhance the treatment outcome?
- Will the structural stability of the tooth be compromised?

Spear FM. The esthetic correction of anterior dental mal-alignment conventional vs. instant (restorative) orthodontics. J Calif Dent Assoc 2004;32(2):133–141.

predetermined and defined, with limitations established to avoid subsequent problems associated with over-aggressive removal of healthy tooth structure.[2] Additive techniques are much preferred to subtractive techniques. For the latter, considerable discussion of the alternatives is essential to obtain consent. Patients can only consent to tooth reduction if they fully understand and appreciate the alternatives, likely scenarios and risks.

Unlike traditional orthodontic therapy, which can correct space, tooth alignment and occlusal issues, the benefits of RSM include the improvement of tooth shape and dimension, the elimination of tooth discolourations and the treatment of initial and recurrent caries. The result can be improved tooth proportion, colour and overall intra-oral health.

The goals of RSM therapy are to determine a new, more pleasing esthetic and restorative arch form, and then to create the proper tooth size and proportion within that new arch form. At the same time an environment for excellent gingival health must be maintained or created and the patient should be left with a stable and functional occlusion. The final result should be one that is harmonious and pleasing to both the professional and the patient. To achieve these goals and clinical success the contemporary principles of smile design must be applied and an appropriate treatment sequence followed.[3]

CLINICAL CONSIDERATIONS

RSM as a standalone therapy has, rightly or wrongly, been accused of overuse. Establishing the goals of the completed treatment (in terms of esthetics, periodontal health, occlusion and long-term stability) must guide the decision making process as to whether conventional orthodontics is the most appropriate treatment, and what limitations there might be on treatment outcomes if orthodontics is not employed.

THE NEED FOR RESTORATION

If there is a restoration that needs to be replaced, poor tooth size, shape or proportion, or tooth colour problems, then orthodontics will have to provide some other significant advantage to the case outcome in order to justify its use as the primary course of treatment. On the other hand, if the teeth do not require restorative treatment other than bleaching or selective recontouring then there are compelling reasons for conventional orthodontics and leaving the teeth uncut and unrestored.[4]

As good as our current techniques and materials are, there is no evidence that even the most perfect of restorations will survive a lifetime. In fact, nothing gets close. The most successful dental restoration is the gold crown with 50% survival of around 17 years. Everything else has a shorter survival span and while a crown may survive, the underlying tooth could fail. Patients are sometimes not made aware of the truth about restoration failure and without the facts they often opt for ceramic veneers, but once given the data 2 out of 3 (in a study of 146 patients each with 10 veneers) opted for a noninvasive therapy. This is especially relevant when dealing with young individuals as the expediency of the quick fix must be weighed against the long-term consequences of preparing teeth that would not otherwise require restoration.

Teeth that will remain inherently unattractive after orthodontic treatment is completed will challenge the treatment planning process to determine whether an acceptable result can be achieved by restoration alone, or whether it is necessary to use both orthodontics and restorative dentistry to create the desired esthetic outcome.[4]

Restorative treatment options for correcting spatially compromised cases include esthetic contouring, bonding, porcelain laminates and crowns. The underlying condition of the dentition is a factor in determining which restorative option is best. Teeth without any restorations or caries should be treated as conservatively as possible. If only minor modifications to tooth contours are required to achieve the desired esthetic result then contouring and bonding provides the least invasive treatment. Caries in the teeth to be treated may require that more extensive restorations be considered, such as porcelain laminates or crowns. The size and location of the caries may dictate the design of these restorations.[5]

Occlusal stability:

1. Regardless of the esthetics achieved, whether through orthodontics, RSM or a combination of both, the occlusion must be stable.[6]

2. Varying occlusal patterns can be found in spatially compromised dentitions and treatment of a malocclusion can present a challenge due to the associated spatial discrepancies. In order to achieve a more predictable esthetic and functional result, an occlusal analysis should be included in the treatment planning process and the best option, orthodontics, restorative dentistry or a combination of both modalities, clearly identified.[7] While restorative dentistry can often solve the esthetic problems of anterior teeth, it frequently cannot correct occlusal relationships.

The pretreatment occlusion as compared to the anticipated post-treatment occlusion must be considered. The goal is to create a stable physiological occlusion that can exist healthily regardless of the pre-existing malocclusion.[2] Minor to moderate discrepancies in tooth position and alignment are generally receptive to RSM and slight to moderate disharmony in rotation and tipping are also considered practical candidates. However, moderate to severe intra-arch discrepancies are not appropriate for RSM, and treatment of severe discrepancies of the facial and dentofacial midlines and bodily displaced or transposed teeth is contraindicated due to the limited esthetic improvement that can be achieved when compared to the need for extensive dental mutilation.[2]

PERIODONTAL ARCHITECTURE

The appearance of the teeth and gums must act in concert to provide a balanced and harmonious smile. A defect in the surrounding pink tissue cannot be compensated by the quality of the dental restoration and vice versa.[8] In the past decade, there has been a remarkable upswing in interdisciplinary collaboration among dentist, orthodontist and periodontist in smile enhancement.[9] Chapter 5 covers pink esthetics in more detail.

As a rule, variations in gingival margin height are due to differences in bone level or sulcus depth between teeth in the same patient;[4] however, it is possible that the bone levels vary not because of bony recession but because of differences in tooth eruption. An example would be two overlapped central incisors, one to the lingual and one to the facial aspect. The tooth to the lingual aspect will always exhibit more wear than the one to the facial aspect. As it wears, it will erupt, bringing the bone in a coronal direction and resulting in a coronally placed gingival margin (Fig. 6.3).[4]

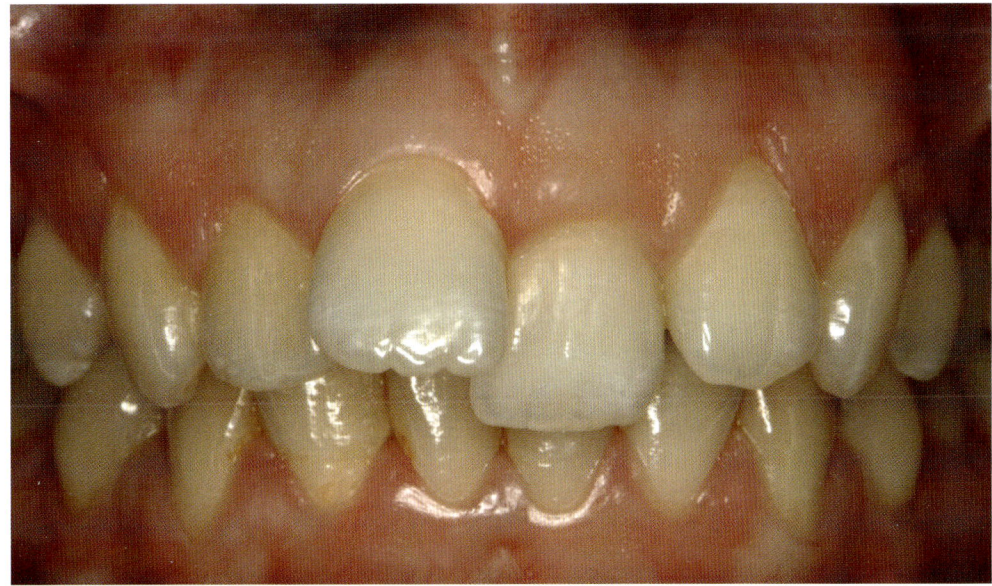

Fig. 6.3 Lingually positioned tooth number 9 presents a more coronal gingival margin when compared to buccally positioned tooth number 8.

Another possible cause of aberrations in gingival margin height is variation in sulcus depth between the central incisors, despite correct bone levels. The tooth with the shallower sulcus will have a more apically positioned gingival margin than the one with a deeper sulcus. This variation in sulcus depth is common in cases of anterior tooth malposition. The more labially inclined teeth have a thinner gingiva and a shallow sulcus. The more lingually placed teeth have a thicker gingiva and a deeper sulcus (Fig. 6.3).[4]

Periodontal surgery can alter gingival margins and it is much easier to remove soft tissue or bone than to create it. If the most apical free gingival margin level is determined to be appropriate, it is possible to use either gingivectomy or osseous surgery to apically position the gingival margin heights of the other teeth to this position. However, if this process would create excessively long and thin-appearing teeth, then a new problem has been created. Although connective tissue grafting is predictable and effective for covering exposed root surfaces, it is far less predictable for moving tissue coronally to cover enamel or ceramic on labially positioned teeth. Therefore, in cases that have a high smile line and the most apically positioned free gingival margin is unacceptable, orthodontics to reposition the teeth and tissue is the most predictable solution.[4] Coronally positioned gingival margins and deep sulci, which are the result of lingually positioned teeth, can be corrected by tooth repositioning. The gingiva will thin to a normal thickness and sulcus depth will move to a normal level. Similarly, a tooth in labial version with slightly apical thin tissue and a shallow sulcus can be correctly positioned causing the gingiva to thicken and the sulcus to assume a normal depth.

Laser or electrosurgery can be used to sculpt the free gingival margins to ideal levels during cosmetic restorative procedures. The modifications can result in a far more pleasing esthetic effect. However, the practitioner must identify the cause of the gingival aberration prior to selecting the mode of treatment for the gingival levels. If the problem is one of bony levels, then either osseous flap surgery or transmucosal laser recontouring is necessary to provide biological health and tissue stability. It is biologically acceptable to correct by sculpting an excessive sulcus depth that exists due to a lingually positioned tooth. Unfortunately a significant amount of tissue regrowth may occur since the tooth is in lingual version. Orthodontic repositioning of the tooth can also alleviate this problem.[4]

The papilla levels are at least as critical to the overall esthetics of anterior teeth as are the levels of the free gingival margins. Papillae that are positioned too far apically result in either an open gingival embrasure (black triangle) or the development of an excessively long contact and rectangular looking teeth. This is a risk associated with enamel stripping that is common in aligner treatments. See

Chapter 7 for discussion on aligner therapies. Three factors come into play in establishing papilla levels: underlying bone level; the patient's biological width; and the gingival embrasure and contact area. The patient's biological width is relatively constant, and bone level, embrasure form and contact area can vary dramatically with tooth eruption. A significant esthetic challenge for the restorative dentist is created by this variance. In general, unless a patient has had wear or excessive overjet and secondary eruption, the interproximal bone is rarely positioned too far coronally. Additionally, unless the patient has had periodontal disease, the interproximal bone is rarely positioned too far apically. Thus, in most patients who present for cosmetic procedures, variations in papilla level are related to embrasure form and contact area. Interestingly, excessively large embrasures, as in diastemata, can result in papillae that are positioned apically. Excessively small embrasures, as in overlapped or rotated teeth, can also result in papillae that are positioned apically.[4] If the most apically positioned papilla would result in the need for an excessively long contact area and unpleasing coronal form, then, in order to achieve a truly esthetic result, orthodontics is the only solution. Currently there are few reliable periodontal procedures that can increase the height of interproximal bone and none that can predictably grow interproximal soft tissue. However, overlapped teeth can be aligned, interproximal bone and soft tissue moved coronally, and the entirety of the esthetic result of diastemata closure can be enhanced with orthodontic treatment.[4]

DENTOGINGIVAL STRUCTURAL COMPROMISES

Restorative correction of a malalignment frequently requires aggressive tooth preparation. Near amputation of the existing coronal form is often required of a labially positioned tooth to bring it into line. To avoid an excessively thick incisal edge, a lingually positioned tooth needs significant lingual tooth preparation. Rotated teeth may require a combination of significant labial and lingual reduction on mesial and distal aspects to accomplish the desired alignment. It is an interesting challenge to determine how much tooth preparation is acceptable in a treatment plan. There are no clear-cut guidelines indicating that a particular degree of reduction will result in a successful result. Nevertheless, it does seem prudent to consider the patient's age and current dental condition when determining appropriate reduction.[4] As the pulpal chamber size decreases with age, this parameter is influenced by the individual characteristics of each case and the age of the patient.[1]

The parameters for RSM are defined by the dimensions and structures of the teeth and the surrounding periodontium within the dental arches. There are limits to the amount of tooth structure that can be removed before pulpal and periodontal violation results. Excessive tooth removal to accomplish the goals of therapy may require mutilation of the remaining tooth structure. The biological and structural outcomes will be compromised from three essential aspects: endodontic stability regarding questionable pulpal health and long-term prognosis of root canal treatment; structural stability of the remaining tooth structure to support the restoration and/or occlusal scheme; and periodontal stability impacted by resultant changes in restorative tooth morphology. Proximal contours that impede proper oral hygiene and encourage food impaction and plaque retention are one example of a compromised outcome of overly aggressive tooth reduction.[1] If the desired contour requires a tooth preparation that exposes the pulp or amputates the pulp and coronal tooth structure, strong consideration must be given to treating the situation with orthodontics. Additionally, negative gingival and interdental papilla architecture cannot be remediated through RSM treatment.[1]

KEY POINT SUMMARY

In many countries, cutting into dentine and devitalizing pulp tissue for esthetic reasons is frowned upon.

A pure RSM esthetic correction must also take into account the risk of adversely affecting the biology of the periodontium. The potential exists for significant alterations in emergence profile when correcting restoratively a rotated or lingually positioned tooth. The impact on gingival health must be considered in these cases. Restorative alignment of severely overlapped teeth also has the potential to have a negative impact on the periodontium as the contacts and supporting bone has moved apically as the overlap developed. The risk of chronic periodontal inflammation increases due to the violation of biological width as a consequence of the required aggressive tooth preparation and the subsequent restoration. In fact, when the teeth are overlapped, the very act of separating the contact with a bur creates a high likelihood that the preparation margin will be placed in the attachment.[4]

ESTHETIC PARAMETERS

The use of RSM to treat spatially compromised cases demands that several esthetic factors be considered.[10] The elements that make up facial composition must be evaluated. Frontal and lateral examination of the subject, including analysis of the position of the eyes, nose, chin and lips, is required for identification of the reference points and lines that are indispensable to performing RSM. Analysis of these features is made using horizontal and vertical reference lines, which allow correlation of the patient's face with the dentition.[11,12]

The dentolabial analysis is essential for evaluating the correct ratio between teeth and lips during the various phases of speaking and smiling. Maxillary incisor tooth display, with the lips at rest, is a major parameter in justifying incisal edge lengthening.[13,14] Appropriate vertical tooth position, incisal edge position and vertical gingival margin control are as important as correcting horizontal and buccolingual deficiencies in achieving an ideal result when treating spatially compromised cases.[3] Many of the procedural choices that the clinician will make to provide a suitable restoration are significantly affected by the correct incisal edge position.[13] This is also covered in detail in Chapters 2 and 3. The key parameter is the determination of the portion of the maxillary teeth that is visible with the lips at rest.[14]

The smile line analysis evaluates the exposure of the anterior teeth and the display of the gingival margins while smiling.[15] In patients with high smile lines, the esthetic considerations for periodontal surgery are as important as those for teeth. In cases where discrepancies in the soft tissues interfere with the proposed tooth proportion, the gingival tissues can be altered via periodontal surgery to accomplish an ideal architecture.[3]

Measurement of the teeth, through micro-esthetic dental analysis, is the primary building block within the framework of a smile. Anterior tooth display in the finished case must be consistent with the principles of proportion in order to be considered a success.[16] When proper tooth proportions are violated, as may happen in RSM therapy, the restored teeth look 'wrong'.[10] The ideal width of the maxillary central incisor should be approximately 80% of its length (Fig. 6.4). A higher width to height ratio means a squarer tooth, and a lower ratio indicates a longer, more rectangular appearance.[9] For greater detail refer to Chapter 1, Esthetic Diagnosis on the proper use of the Esthetic Evaluation Form.

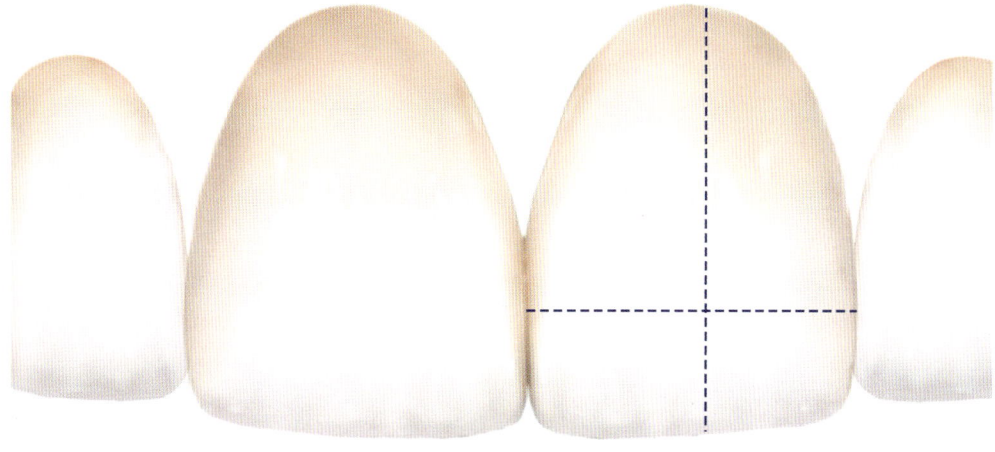

75% to 85%

Fig. 6.4 A pleasant width to length proportion for a maxillary central incisor is 75–85%.

In patients with diastemata, inappropriately small natural anterior teeth or normal teeth with an excessively large arch form are the primary causes of this condition. For each of these causes, the treatment is very different. The patient with diastemata owing to small teeth is usually best treated with restorative dentistry, regardless of whether orthodontics is also performed.[4] At the other end of the spectrum are patients with severely overlapped and crowded teeth. As one might expect, this condition occurs either because of inappropriately large anterior teeth or normally sized teeth within an excessively small arch form. The esthetic concern, in both diastemata and crowding cases, is the appearance of the teeth if they are restored in their current position.

There are several articles discussing the use of the 'golden proportion'[17] when planning treatment for patients with malalignment. Although this may be a useful tool for doing a wax-up or setup, it can fall short of creating ideal esthetics in patients with diastemata or crowding. Only the relationship between the teeth widths is considered within the golden proportion. As logical as this may seem, there is strong evidence that some anterior teeth, particularly the maxillary central incisors, carry more weight than others in the assessment of esthetic outcomes.[4] The maxillary lateral incisors, however, can have large variations in their width and still be judged esthetically pleasing as long as they are symmetrical. More pleasing esthetic results can be created by designing central incisors with ideal proportions and allowing the laterals to be wider or narrower than the golden proportion would require. Proportionate central incisors create the illusion of a pleasing smile, whereas mis-sized lateral incisors are rarely noticed as long as they are symmetrical to each other.[4]

Chu[18] describes yet another way to relate the width of teeth within the esthetic zone and proposes that the width of the maxillary lateral incisor should be approximately 2 mm less than the central incisor and that the canine should be 1 mm less than the central incisor (Fig. 6.5).

The methods available to compensate esthetically for anatomical crowns that are excessively wide include: restorative lengthening of the crown incisally, increasing the clinical crown length apically with periodontal surgery, using restorative optical illusions that make a wide tooth appear narrow or any combination of these methods (Box 6.2).[10] When compensating esthetically for teeth with excessively long clinical crowns, the width may be increased, the incisal edge may be shortened if the lip line and phonetics permit or the location of the gingival margins may be altered to a more coronal position through orthodontic extrusion or additive periodontal surgery. Again, restorative optical illusions or any combination of the aforementioned techniques may be employed to make a long tooth appear wider (Box 6.3).

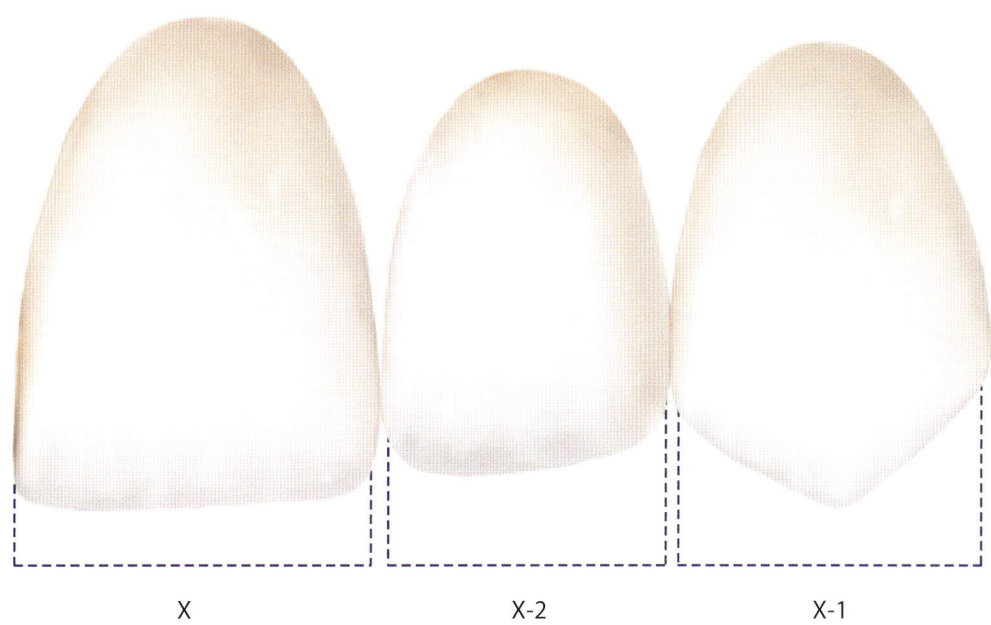

Fig. 6.5 The width of the maxillary lateral incisor is approximately 2 mm less than the central incisor and the width of the canine is approximately 1 mm less than the central incisor.

BOX 6.2	
	To compensate esthetically for crowns which are excessively wide:
	• Lengthen the clinical crown incisally with a restoration
	• Lengthen the clinical crown apically with the use of periodontal surgery
	• Move the mesial and distal line angles towards the midline of the tooth to create the illusion of a narrower tooth
	• Use a combination of the above techniques
	Dlugokinski M, Frazier K, Goldstein R. Restorative treatment of diastema. In: Goldstein R, Haywood V. Esthetics in dentistry, vol. 2: Esthetic problems of individual teeth, missing teeth, malocclusion, special populations. Ontario, Canada: BC Decker, 2001:703–731.

THE ORTHODONTIC ROLE

Most patients can benefit functionally and esthetically from orthodontic therapy. This is particularly true in patients who present with a smile affected by a crowded dentition. The periodontal restorative and cosmetic benefits of orthodontic therapy have been well documented. Additionally, interest in orthodontic therapy among the adult patient population has been stimulated by techniques developed and based upon the introduction of new materials. Removable

> **BOX 6.3**
>
> The methods available to compensate for excessively long clinical crowns include:
>
> - Restoratively widening the crown
> - Shortening the incisal edge if the lip line and phonetics permit
> - Repositioning the gingival margins coronally through orthodontic intrusion or additive periodontal surgery
> - Creating restorative optical illusions
> - Using a combination of the above techniques
>
> ---
>
> Oquendo A, Brea L, David S. Diastema: correction of excessive spaces in the esthetic zone. Dent Clin North Am 2011;55(2):265–281.

resin-based orthodontic aligners, temperature sensitive/activated archwires and ceramic brackets, to mention a few, have been introduced into the orthodontic armamentarium. Streamlined treatment times and minimal lifestyle-impacting orthodontic therapies have stimulated acceptance of orthodontics by adults. Despite these advances in orthodontic treatment, patient acceptance is still not universal. Orthodontic's inability to produce quick results and the need to retain the results of successful orthodontic therapy have inspired the use of tooth preparation and restorative dentistry to manage spatially compromised cases and eliminate the potential for relapse.[1]

The dentist should educate and motivate the patient to accept orthodontic therapy when the spatially compromised case is best treated by that modality. No restorative material is equal to healthy tooth structure and, regardless of the time taken, skill employed or material used, a restoration cannot duplicate the beauty of the natural dentition. Due to the periodic repairs or remaking of the restored dentition over the patient's lifetime, there is also considerable financial savings for those who choose orthodontics over restorative dentistry.[10]

When orthodontic therapy itself is not feasible, an integrated orthodontic–restorative approach may enhance the esthetic result while preserving tooth structure.[19] Undoubtedly, any type of esthetic restoration will look its best when the patient's teeth are aligned at their ideal position within the dental arch. Indeed, the orthodontist's goal may be to 'set up' the case for the restorative dentist. For example, in some diastema cases the mesiodistal width of the teeth may not permit complete space closure and the best course of action might be positioning the teeth for veneers that will close the spaces. The approach is best decided by the restorative dentist with the aid of the diagnostic wax-ups.[2] Orthodontics is generally the first consideration when the patient presents with crowded teeth. If a patient is unable to accept comprehensive orthodontic procedures, the general practitioner must determine whether the patient can be treated with minor tooth movement, restoration, extraction or a combination of these procedures.[5]

In certain situations, orthodontic–periodontic–restorative procedures may be necessary.[20] The ideal goal is to find a conservative and biologically sound treatment plan for every clinical situation. In order to achieve this goal, the participation of several dental disciplines is frequently required[2] and a clear understanding of the various roles in developing and executing the treatment plan is essential.[21]

CROWDING TREATMENT PLANNING

Tooth crowding can pose an intellectual and technical challenge, since both mesiodistal and buccolingual discrepancies must be addressed.[1] A thorough evaluation of the patient will establish the basis for potential treatment options. Minor corrections of crowded teeth can be achieved with conservative treatments such as esthetic contouring, disking combined with minor tooth movement, and bonding. When corrections that are more substantial are required then porcelain laminates and crowns become the treatment of choice.[5]

Restoration of proper tooth proportions and establishment of a stable physiological occlusion are the objectives of RSM therapy in a case with insufficient space. In these cases, the clinician must assess where the necessary space can be gained to accomplish the treatment objectives through the reduction of existing tooth substance rather than orthodontically shifting the teeth.[1] Space is frequently gained by preparing the teeth in ways that require removal from the mesial aspect and addition to the distal aspect (Fig. 6.6A–C). Moderate crowding can often be successfully treated using this technique.

An average of 1.0–1.5 mm of total reduction per tooth can be comfortably obtained due to the interproximal contours of teeth and the anatomy of available enamel.[22] When multiplied by the number of teeth involved, the frequent result is adequate space to realign the crowded dentition.[1] The amount of tooth reduction required can be determined using digital software, e.g. 'Spacewise' on an imported occlusal photograph and using the calibration tool.

Buccolingual changes in tooth position can be associated with discrepancies in gingival architecture, such as midfacial tissue height, papilla height or papilla shape. These problems will require adjunctive periodontal therapy or orthodontic correction depending on the severity of the discrepancy. Elective endodontics may be required in extreme borderline cases to correct the functional and esthetic deficiencies.

CROWDING TREATMENT PLANNING

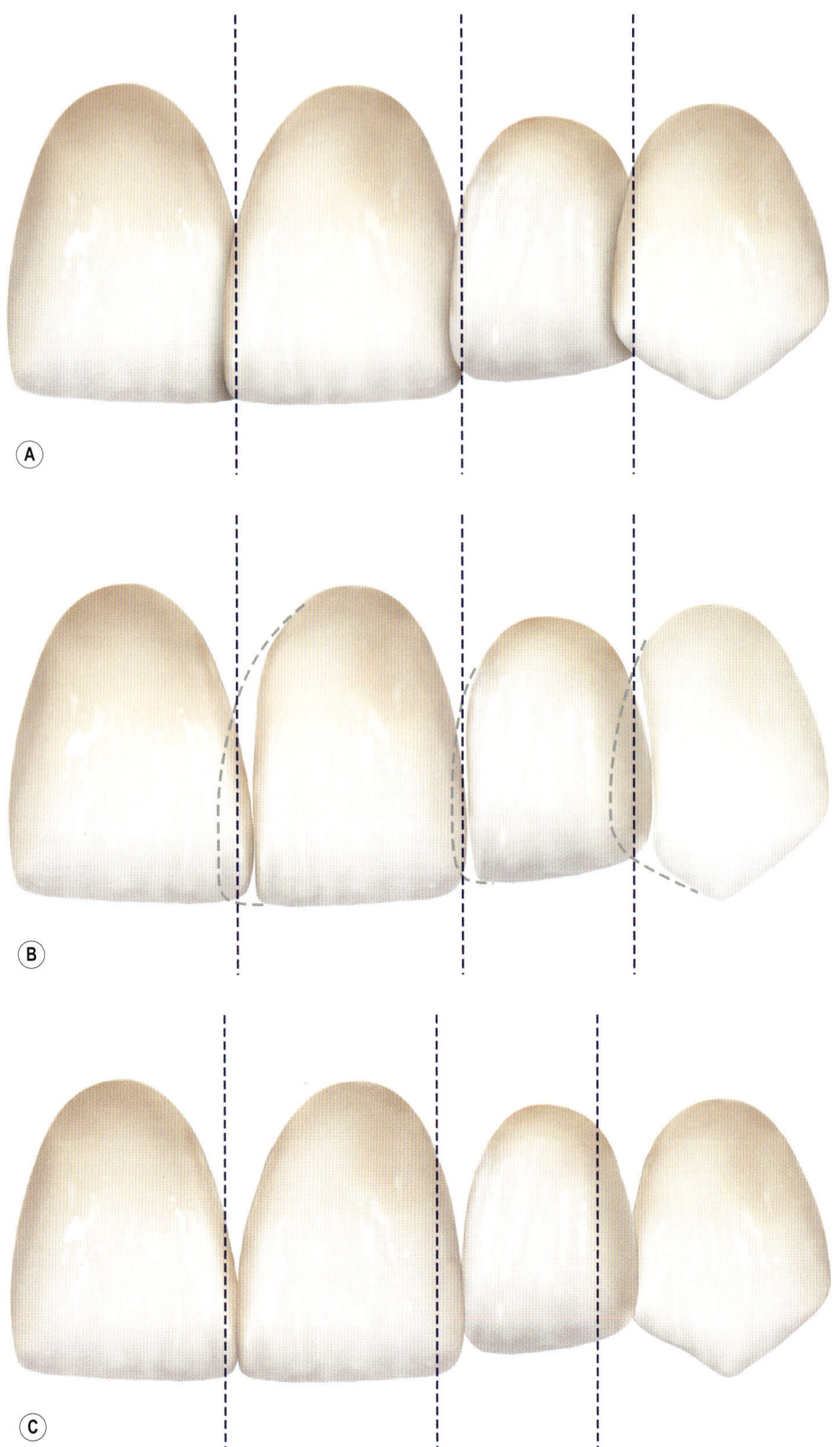

Fig. 6.6A–C Some crowding cases may require restorative space management involving the removal of mesial tooth structure and the addition of restorative material to the distal surface.

Lingually locked teeth that are to be restored with porcelain laminates offer the advantage of requiring little or no tooth preparation on the facial surface. The lost tooth volume will be filled with the porcelain restoration. The critical area is the incisal edge which, if not correctly prepared, will result in a thick surface with improper occlusion, poor esthetics often due to increased chroma and reduced translucency, and compromised masticatory function. To ensure correct final anatomy, the incisal edge of the prepared tooth should be trimmed to a new preparation line that facilitates the application of a properly proportioned veneer with a true incisal edge.[2] Teeth positioned far buccally require particularly careful planning, as these will have large amounts of tooth structure removed. As the facial surface is reduced the incisal edge will disappear.[2]

The diagnostic wax-up is the key and it will identify to what degree corrective contours must be made to idealize a crowded dentition. Both the addition of wax to deficient areas of the dentition and the removal of stone will be required to achieve the desired esthetic results.[5] Through this process, arch space deficiencies can be worked out and the specifically needed modifications to each tooth can be identified.[5]

A preparation guide made from the wax-up should be used so that adequate, but not excessive, tooth reduction can be accomplished. The waxed incisal length and position of the facial surface can then be replicated in the final case. A matrix for temporization can also be fabricated using the same materials and technique, and will accurately duplicate the subtleties of the diagnostic wax-up. With proper embrasure form and gingival contours accurately duplicated in the provisional restorations, chairside adjustment will be significantly reduced.[5]

DIASTEMA TREATMENT PLANNING

Typically, the presence of small teeth indicates the need for restorations to treat diastemata cases. However, additional therapies may be needed to achieve optimal esthetics. Tooth repositioning may be necessary to tweak the space distribution prior to restoration and periodontal surgery may be required to provide additional clinical crown length to accommodate the newly increased tooth width. To provide appropriate proportionality, teeth not directly affected by a diastema may need to be included in the restorative treatment.[10]

Direct adhesive composite may represent an excellent treatment alternative.[10] Due to its ability to save time, money and tooth structure, composite resin is a popular choice for many patients.[10] Additionally, the direct composite technique provides the ability to modify the restorations during the course of orthodontic treatment.

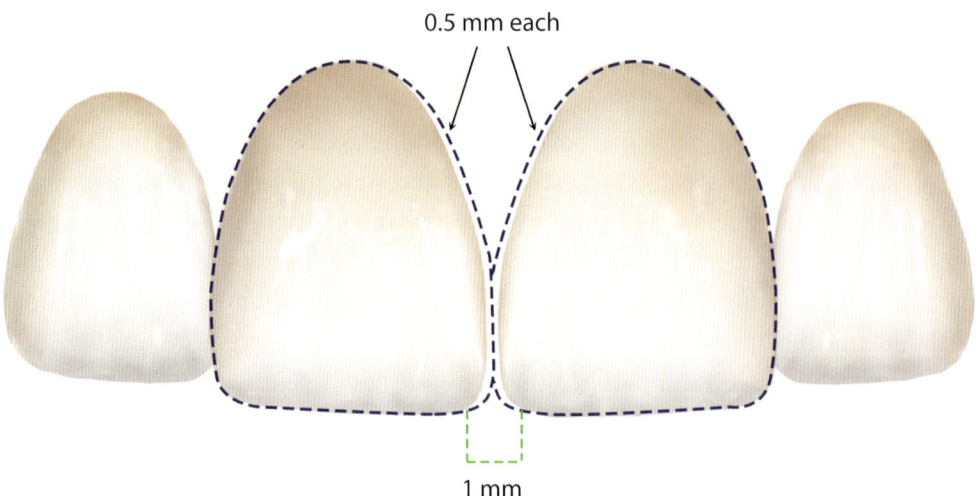

Fig. 6.7 Patients with gaps equal to or less than 1 mm, and with teeth of near ideal proportions, can be managed by adding approximately 0.5 mm to each tooth.

Diastema closure is one of the most common indications for porcelain laminate veneers.[23] Due to the 2-dimensionality of diastema cases, the proximal surfaces are commonly involved while the labial and lingual surfaces rarely need much, if any, preparation. Most attention should be given to the facial view in closing the diastema while maintaining natural tooth proportions.[2]

In the case of a midline diastema, the build-up should be equal for both teeth. If the case presents with a gap of less than 1 mm then the maximum amount to be added to each tooth will be 0.5 mm (Fig. 6.7). Therefore, if the teeth are within acceptable proportions then tooth proportion will not be negatively affected by an addition of 0.5 mm to the width. If the addition does present a visual problem then anatomical characterization techniques can be used on the facial surface to mask the problem. The teeth can be made to appear thinner through controlling the reflection of light, for example, by playing with the distance between the mesiolabial and distolabial line angles. Rounding the disto-incisal corners of the teeth and increasing the incisal embrasure will have similar illusionary effects. These techniques will help make the apparent proportions of the newly reshaped teeth consistent with proportions commonly found in smiles that are considered to be esthetically pleasing.[2]

When treating a diastema case involving spaces that are larger, i.e. 1–3 mm, achieving esthetic tooth proportions becomes an issue. While these cases can be treated restoratively, advanced treatment planning is required and precautionary measures must be considered. The length of the teeth will almost certainly need to be increased in order to maintain desirable proportions.[2] Length can be altered either apically through a periodontal approach or incisally with

SPACE MANAGEMENT

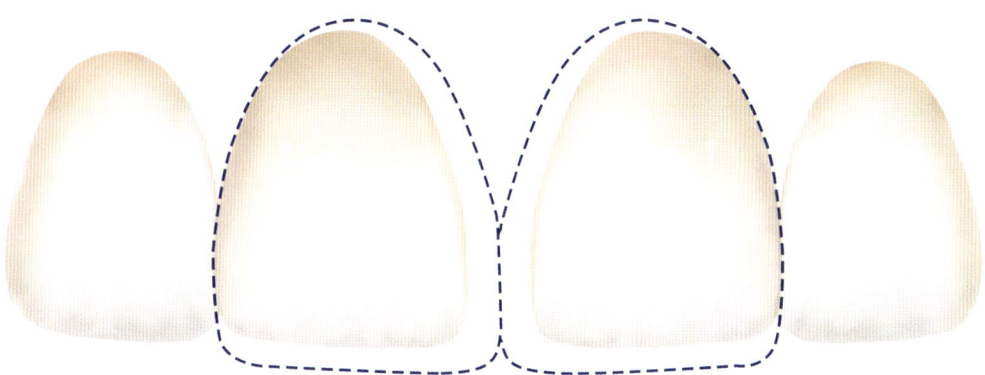

Fig. 6.8 Short clinical crowns may be lengthened apically by means of a periodontal procedure, incisally with restorations, or by a combination of both techniques.

restorations. The incisal edge position, which is the primary esthetic parameter, will be affected by the latter approach. Occlusal and other esthetic considerations may not permit sufficient incisal lengthening to maintain the desired width to length ratio. A combination of apical and incisal lengthening may be appropriate for these situations (Fig. 6.8).[2] The basic three positions of the lips – rest, half smile and full smile – must also be observed. Based upon the treatment option selected, the laboratory can wax the desired changes on the diagnostic models. A mock-up obtained from the wax-up and seated over the unprepared teeth is the preferred method of visualizing the final outcome and the location of appropriate interproximal contacts may also be finalized using this technique.[23]

Leaving tooth length unaltered, both incisally and gingivally, implies that the apparent width to length ratio is favourable. 'Distalizing the defect' is the alternative technique used to close the diastema under these circumstances. When employing this technique, the distal portion of each tooth is reduced by half the size of the more mesial diastema. The amount removed is then restoratively added to the mesial surface of the same tooth (Fig. 6.9A,B). When treating centrals, this technique assumes that the midline is in the proper position and need not be altered. In order to close all of the spaces, the process is continued with the laterals, canines and premolars as necessary. As the distal portion of the canine is not seen from a facial aspect, due to its position, its widening usually cannot be visually distinguished. This illusion as applied to proportion management is quite useful in treatment planning and case management.[23] Although conservative dentistry is a worthy goal in itself, attempting to close a diastema by treating only two teeth in this type of case will almost always result in an esthetic failure.[10]

Tooth preparation is another issue in dealing with diastema closure. On the diastema side, the papilla has an undesirable, blunt shape. In order to have a

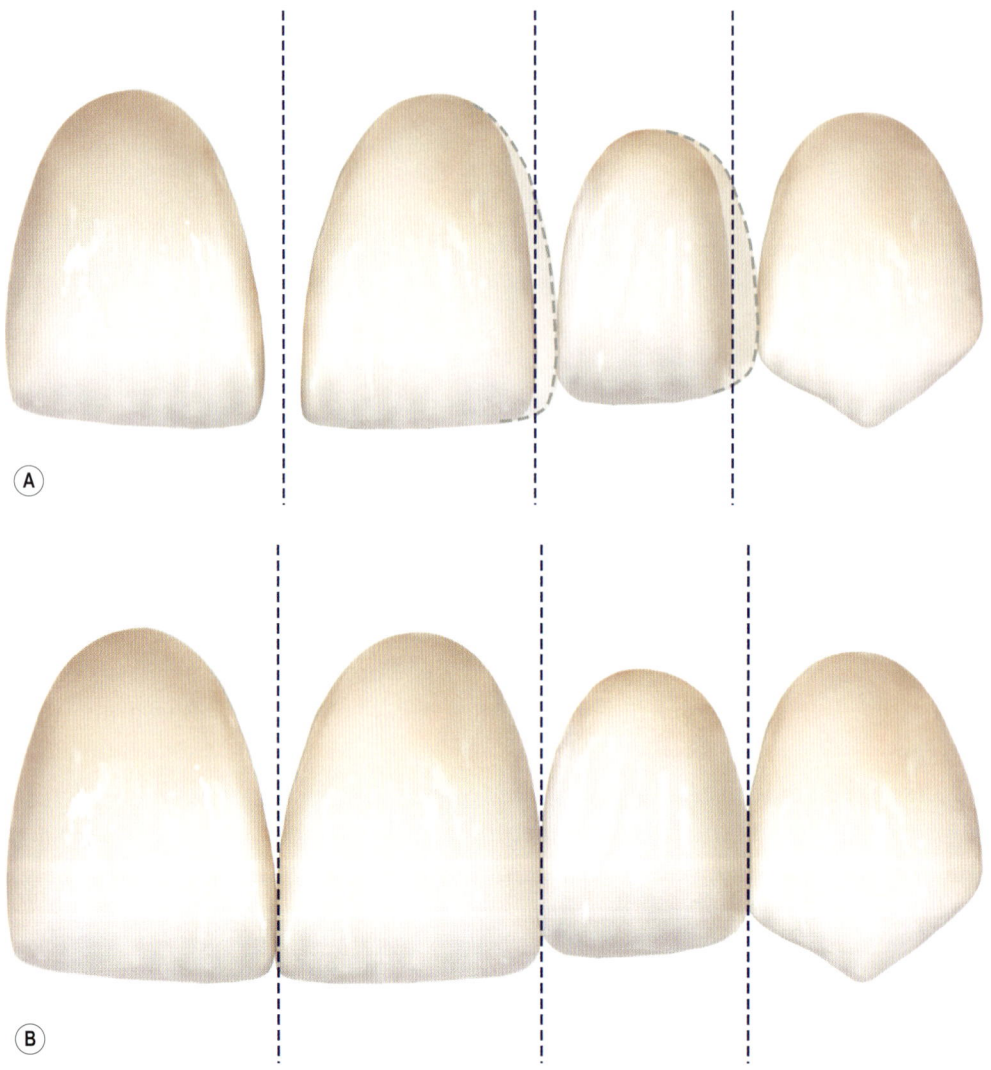

Fig. 6.9A,B When maintaining existing incisal edge position, gingival margin location and tooth proportion during a diastema closure, at least four teeth must be treated to 'distalize the problem'. Restorations are added to the mesial edge while the distal surfaces are narrowed.

crisp, clear triangular-shaped papillae, the tissue has to be gently pushed from each side and reshaped incisally. Locating the interproximal preparation subgingivally permits a slight overcontouring of the emergence profile of the area and allows for a gentle reshaping pressure on the papilla (Fig. 6.10A,B).[2] Overcontouring can be accomplished by dropping the preparation subgingivally from the facial third nearest the diastema. The laboratory technician can then establish a progressive emergence profile for the extension of the restoration into the interproximal contact area.[23] To produce an ideal tooth form for closing the gingival embrasure and maintaining optimal gingival health, and ensure that

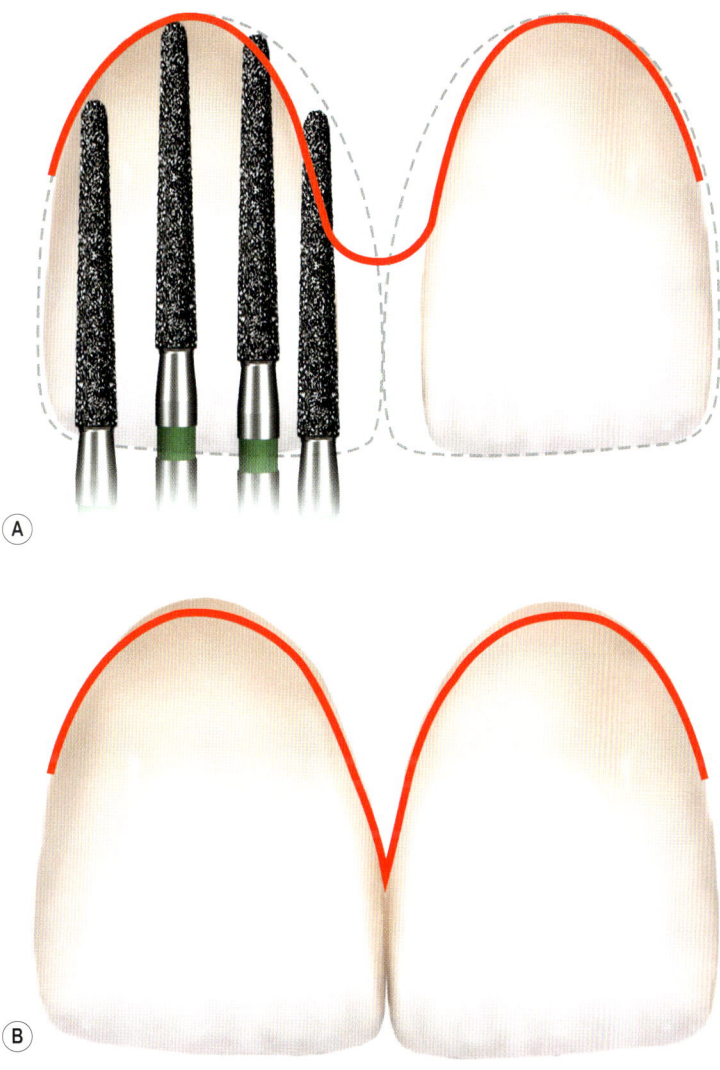

Fig. 6.10A,B To produce a triangular-shaped papilla on the diastema side, the gingival preparation is placed subgingivally to allow overcontouring of the emergence profile of the restoration and gentle pushing of the papilla.

the area can be easily flossed, the subgingival preparation is extended towards the palate to include the col area. Care should be taken not to create undercuts while creating this design.[23]

The most apical position of the labial free gingival margin of each tooth is referred to as the zenith point, which is a major esthetic factor. If zenith points are left unchanged, they will be located too far distally after the diastema closure. The unwanted result will be teeth that appear to be tilted mesially. Periodontal surgery is needed to shift the zenith points mesially and overcome this result (Fig. 6.11A,B).[2]

DIASTEMA TREATMENT PLANNING

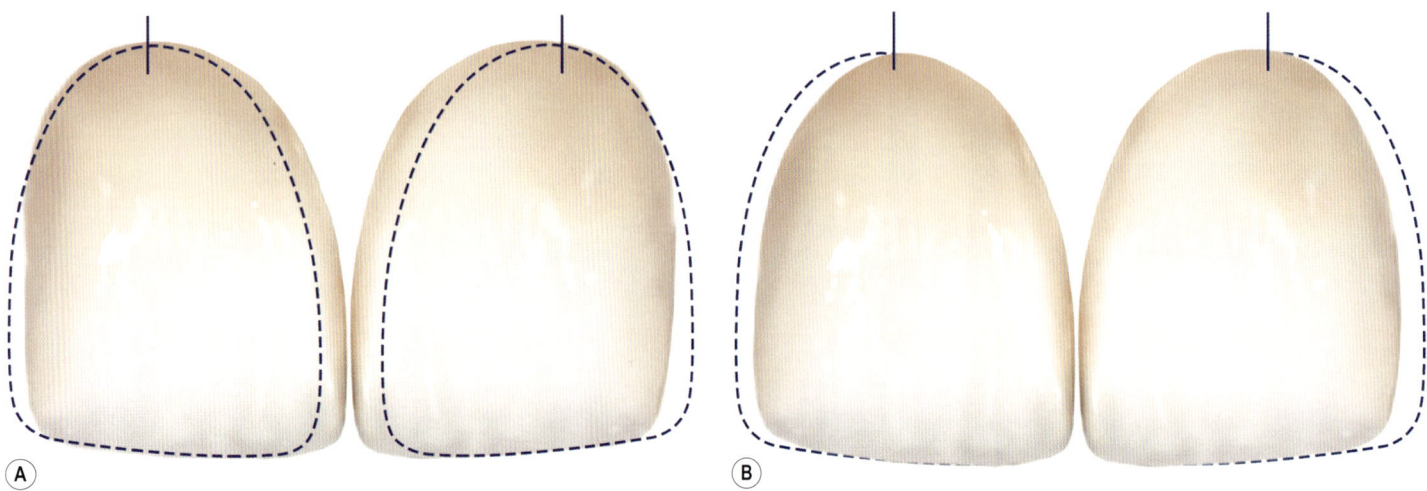

Fig. 6.11A,B Unaltered zenith points will be located too far distally after the diastema closure. The result will be teeth that appear tilted to the mesial. This problem may be avoided by relocating the zenith point with a periodontal procedure or by recontouring the gingival trough in the provisional restorations.

Crowns are only indicated when the teeth included in the treatment plan are very broken down and require support. Similarly, while the bond strength of composite to dentine has increased over time, enamel still remains the optimal tooth structure to retain bonded restorations. Teeth that do not have a sufficient amount of enamel for bonding procedures should be restored with full coverage restorations.[10]

PATIENTS' FAQS

Q. I do not like the idea of having my teeth ground.

A. The necessary space to accomplish the treatment objectives by RSM is gained through the reduction of existing tooth substance rather than shifting the teeth orthodontically.

Q. How much reduction of my teeth is needed?

A. The shade, shape and position of the tooth will determine the amount of reduction we need in order to achieve the desired result.

Q. Why are you recommending orthodontic movements in my case rather than restoration?

A. No restorative material is equal to healthy tooth structure and (regardless of the time taken, skill employed, or material used) a restoration cannot duplicate the beauty of the natural dentition.

KEY POINT SUMMARY

Nowadays many clinicians believe that there are no, or few, indications for crowning teeth due to the amount of further destruction needed. Adhesive dentistry has enabled broken down teeth to be built up without further tissue removal. Partial coverage restorations that preserve tooth tissue are preferred.

CLINICAL CASE 6.1: CROWDING

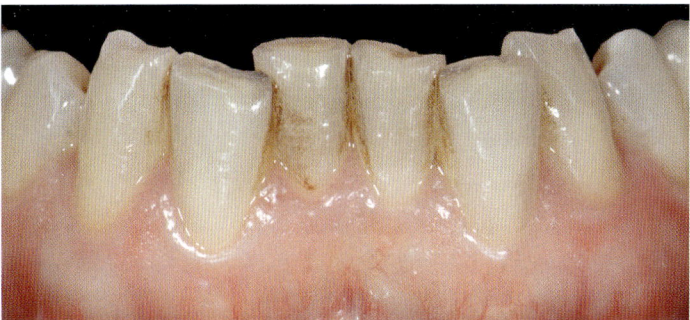

Fig. C6.1.1 A 50-year-old female patient presented with moderate to severe misalignment of teeth numbers 22 through to 27. Although the patient was informed that the ideal treatment in her case was orthodontic therapy, she chose an immediate correction with porcelain laminate veneers. While teeth numbers 23 and 26 were positioned facially, teeth numbers 24, 25 and 27 were lingually retroclined and created an uneven, overlapping appearance.

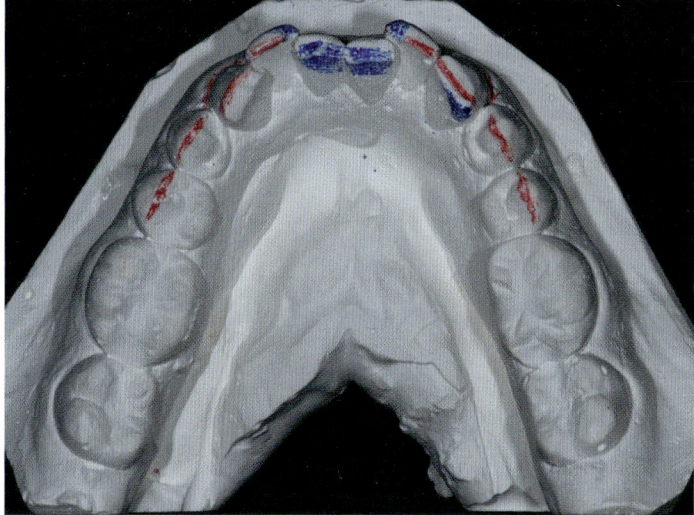

Fig. C6.1.2 The mandibular arch was evaluated with the goal of achieving proper incisal contours. Intra-oral impressions and stone casts were made. Areas that required reduction were marked in blue and red lines were drawn on the incisal edges to indicate the ideal restored arch form.

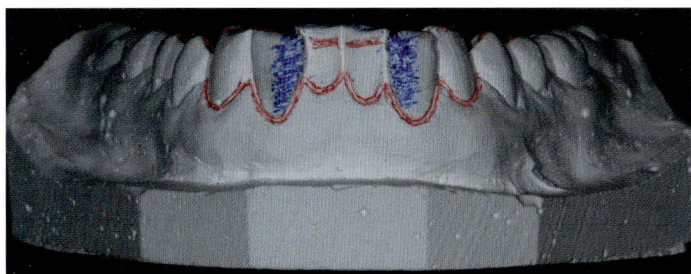

Fig. C6.1.3 The mesiodistal overlaps were marked with blue vertical lines to ensure proper reduction and to allow subsequent expansion of the restored dental arch. The free gingival tissue height was also marked to ensure development of the correct gingival architecture. Creating a natural looking gingival architecture is one of the most significant problems in treating the crowded case type. The facially positioned teeth present a thin alveolar crest with relatively thin gingival tissue that is generally positioned apically. In this case it was easier and more predictable to move the soft tissues apically rather than to attempt to bring the teeth coronally. Conversely, if the teeth were positioned lingually it would be common to find coronally overgrown gingival tissue and a distorted gingival symmetry. A simple gingivectomy will suffice to achieve the correct gingival form in the majority of these cases.[1]

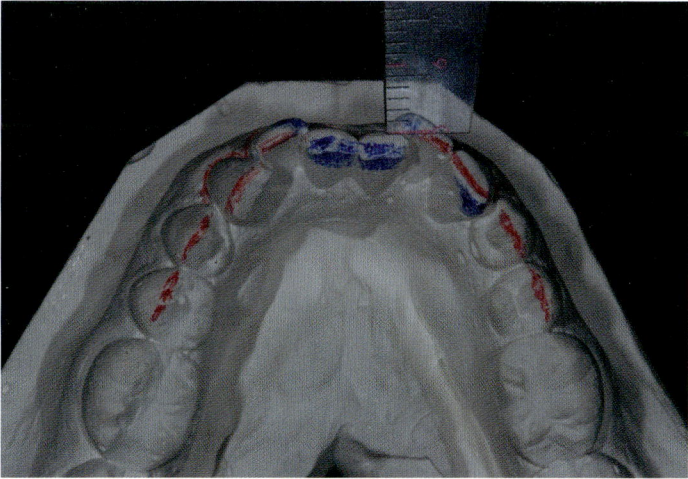

Fig. C6.1.4 A buccolingual overlap of approximately 2 mm was evident between incisal edges as was a mesiodistal overlap of less than 2 mm. To create a space sufficient to shift the lingually positioned tooth facially, the mesial and distal interproximal areas of the labially positioned tooth were removed.[1,7]

CLINICAL CASE 6.1: CROWDING

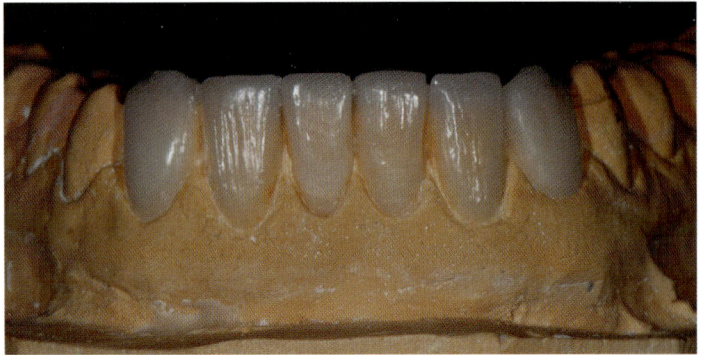

Fig. C6.1.5 Deciding where to place the facial surface was a critical decision in developing a pleasing and functional arch form. A functional wax-up was created to ensure maximum patient satisfaction and to allow the desired outcome to be realized.[4] The wax-up was also used to fabricate the preparation guides.[1] Although not done for this patient, visualization of the anticipated tooth form and final result can be accomplished by using the preparation guides to fabricate a preoperative intra-oral mock-up.

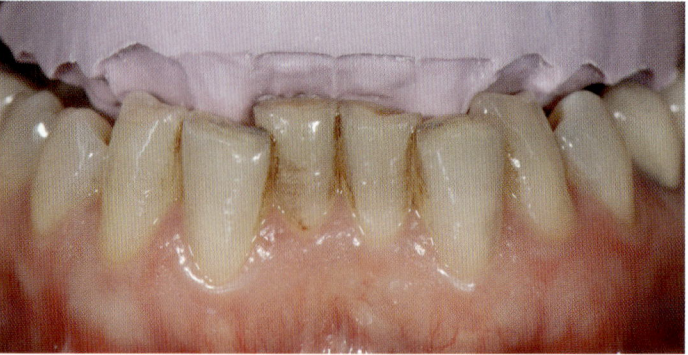

Fig. C6.1.6 Incisal and buccal preparation guides were fabricated from the wax-up using condensation silicone putty. The preparation guides were tried over the teeth and the areas interfering with the full seating of the guides were identified as needing reduction.

KEY CLINICAL TECHNIQUES

Preparation guides should be used during tooth reductions to:

- Avoid excessive tooth reduction.
- Ensure that the location and amount of reduction is appropriate.
- Indicate the correct final positions of the teeth.
- Help in visualizing the final dimensions of each tooth.

KEY CLINICAL TECHNIQUES

The diagnostic wax-up:

- Serves as a blueprint for the subsequent interdisciplinary treatment.
- Helps the patient, dentist and technician visualize the final outcomes of treatment.
- Helps to indicate the desired improvements in proportion, shape and position of the teeth.
- Is used to fabricate the preparation guides.

CHAPTER 6
SPACE MANAGEMENT

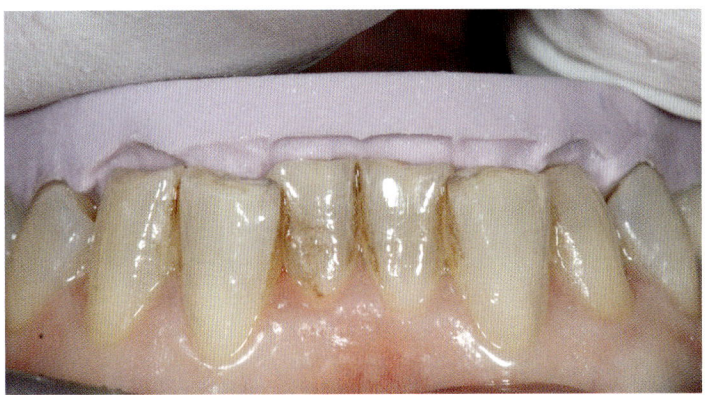

Fig. C6.1.7 Esthetic recontouring, in this case used for the removal of tooth areas interfering with the passive seating of the preparation guides, was performed. Proper seating of the guide is a critical step in gathering the correct information for the subsequent preparations.

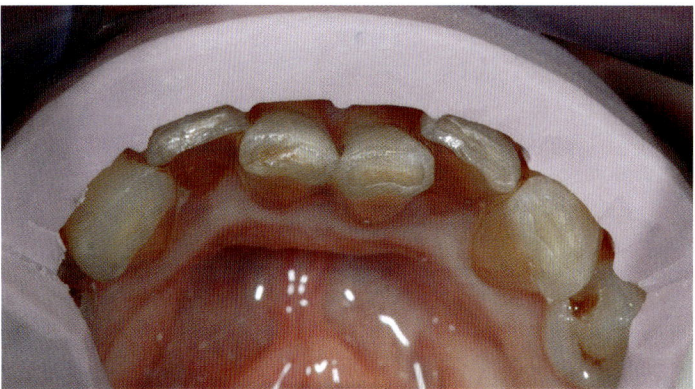

Fig. C6.1.8 The same procedure was followed for the buccal index. Proper seating of the preparation guide was achieved through removal of protruding areas. The buccal guide was used as a reference during tooth reduction and preparation. This guide was also used to indicate the correct final positions and to help with visualizing the final dimensions of each tooth.

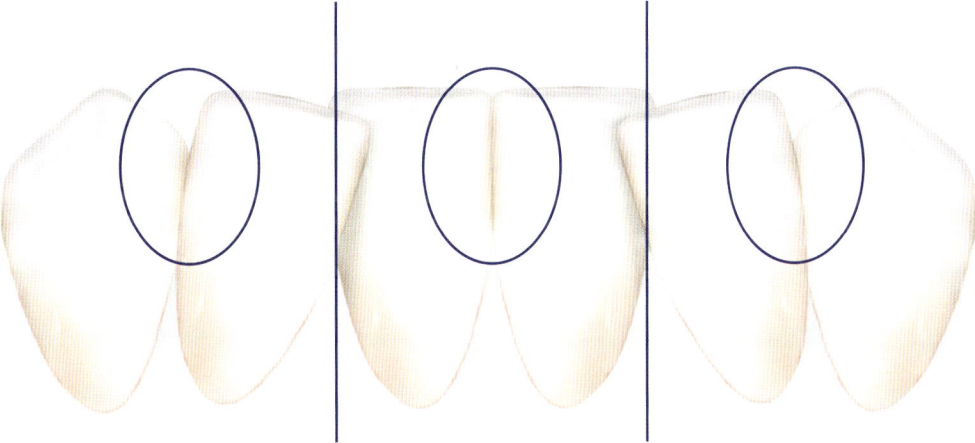

Fig. C6.1.9 In cases with overlapped teeth, the contact areas must be opened during tooth preparation to permit the technician to re-establish the new shape, position, proportion and interproximal contact relationship. In the case presented here, the contact between the central incisors, as well as between laterals and canines, was correct and there was no need to break the contacts. Ideally, the contacts should be preserved whenever possible.

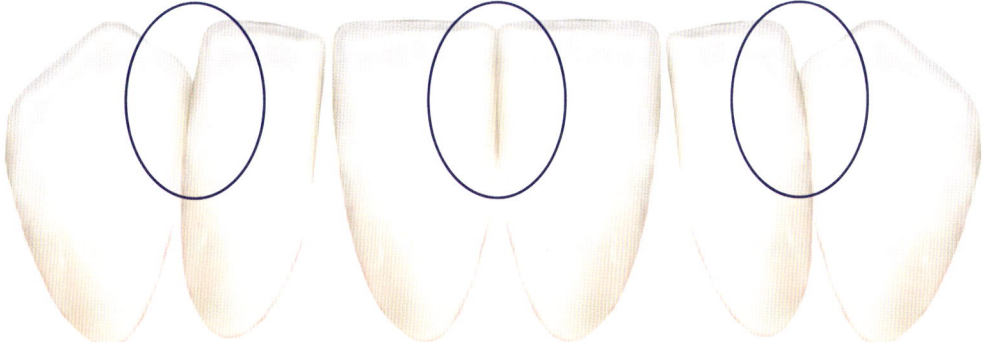

Fig. C6.1.10 Due to the mesiodistal and buccolingual overlaps between the centrals and laterals, the contacts were opened to create enough room to accommodate the restorations.

CLINICAL CASE 6.1: CROWDING

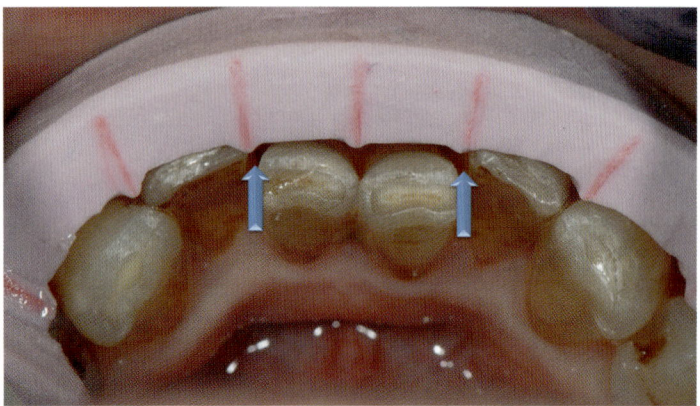

Fig. C6.1.11 Using a very fine diamond bur, the contact areas were opened from their base to the incisal edge. Pencil lines were drawn on the index to indicate the proper spatial relationship as well as the width of teeth on the incisal edge.

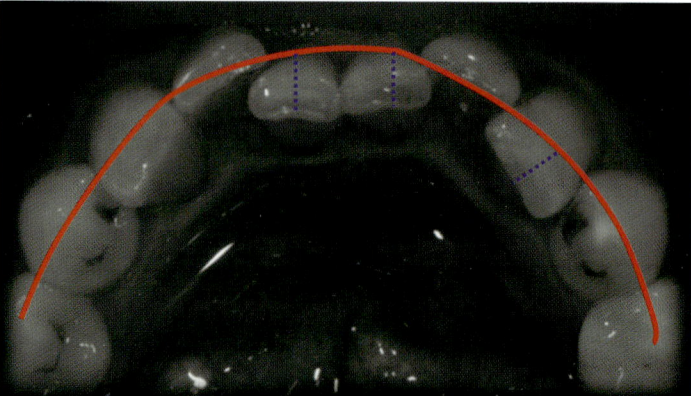

Fig. C6.1.12 The relationship between the final arch form and the proper thickness of the incisal edges is one of the keys to success when preparing crowding cases. Leaving too thick an incisal edge for the lingually positioned teeth is a common mistake in RSM therapy for crowding cases. Not adequately preparing the lingual surface of the lingually positioned teeth is the usual cause of this problem. In this case, the red line represents the corrected restorative arch form. The blue lines represent the excessive and inappropriate thickness of the lingually positioned teeth if the proper lingual reduction is not performed.

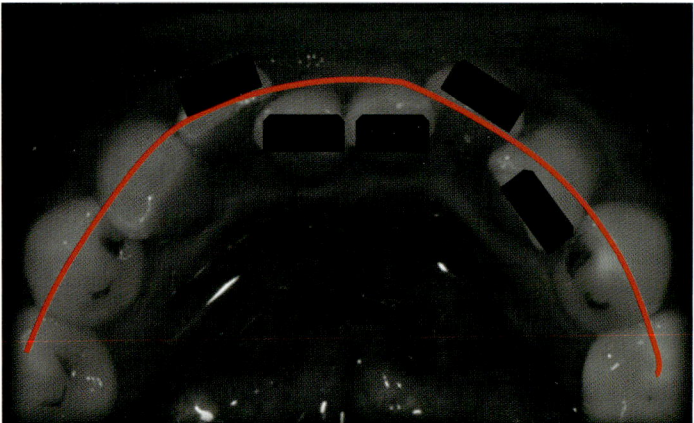

Fig. C6.1.13 To align crowded cases with restorations, such as veneers, selected teeth must be reduced more than in cases presenting without crowding. In the present case, teeth 24, 25 and 27 required minimal preparation on the facial surfaces to ensure that lost labial volume is filled by the porcelain laminate veneer. The incisal edges were trimmed lingually to prevent the development of excess thickness. Teeth numbers 23 and 26, due to their labial positioning, required more reduction labially to bring them within the ideal arch position. Unmodified tooth number 22 was aligned within the proposed arch form and will do well with a classical veneer preparation. Black areas indicate the reduction needed to accomplish the goals.

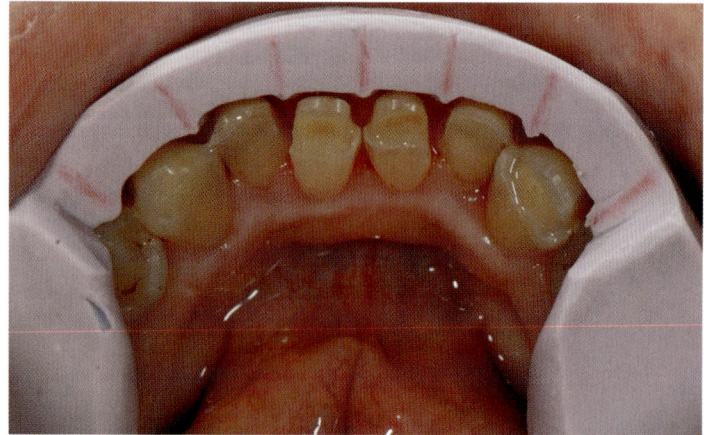

Fig. C6.1.14 Clinical view of the reduction providing enough space for the technician to build porcelain and to achieve the esthetic goals. Notice the lingual reduction to numbers 24, 25 and 27.

SPACE MANAGEMENT

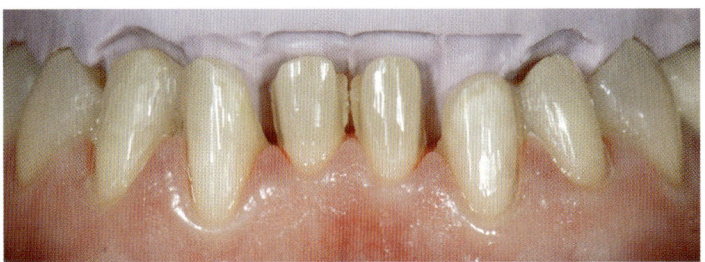

Fig. C6.1.15 Again the finished preparations were checked with the preparation guides to ensure that the location and amount of reduction was appropriate.

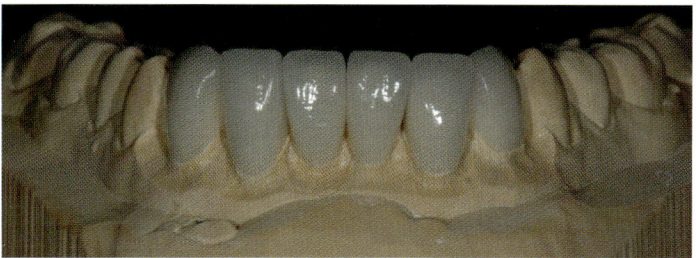

Fig. C6.1.16 An impression of the completed preparations was made and sent to the laboratory for fabrication of the final case. The incisal index was used in the laboratory to allow the technician to develop an optimal ceramic build-up. The restorations were fired and characterized as necessary, and when finished were returned for cementation.

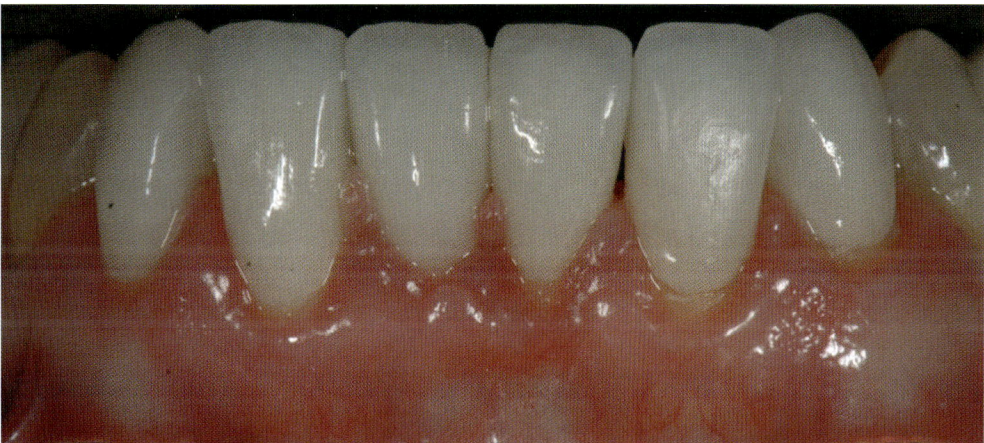

Fig. C6.1.17 The definitive restorations were cemented using a bonding agent and resin cement.[1] Shown here is a final case immediately after insertion.

KEY CLINICAL TECHNIQUES

The teeth can be made to appear thinner through controlling the reflection of light by:

- Bringing the mesiolabial and distolabial line angles closer together.
- Rounding the disto-incisal corners of the teeth and increasing the incisal embrasure.

CLINICAL CASE 6.2: CLINICAL PROCEDURES FOR DIASTEMA CLOSURE

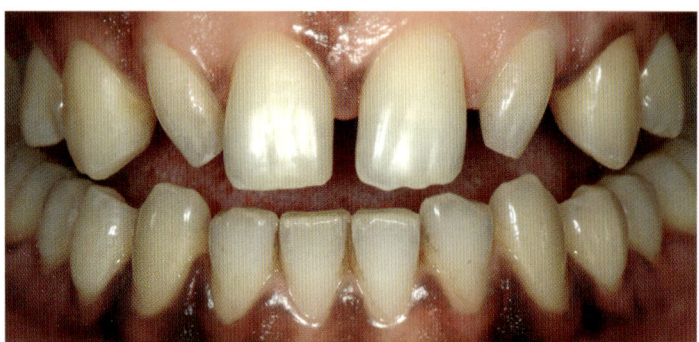

Fig. C6.2.1 The patient presented with a chief complaint of spaces between her teeth. An esthetic evaluation was performed leading to a diagnosis of diastemata associated with peg laterals and poor tooth proportions. Corrections were appropriate to restore esthetics and establish a stable occlusion. RSM was determined to be the best approach for space closure and for addressing the patient's complaints.

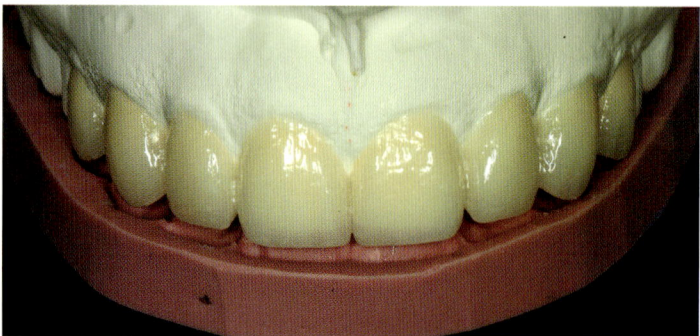

Fig. C6.2.2 The diagnostic wax-up created for this patient served as a blueprint for the subsequent interdisciplinary treatment and helped the patient, dentist and technician visualize the final outcome of treatment. The wax-up indicated the desired improvements in the proportion, shape, and position of the teeth.[18] Preparation guides were fabricated from the wax-up and dictated the amount and location of tooth reduction needed during the preparation to achieve the desired goals.

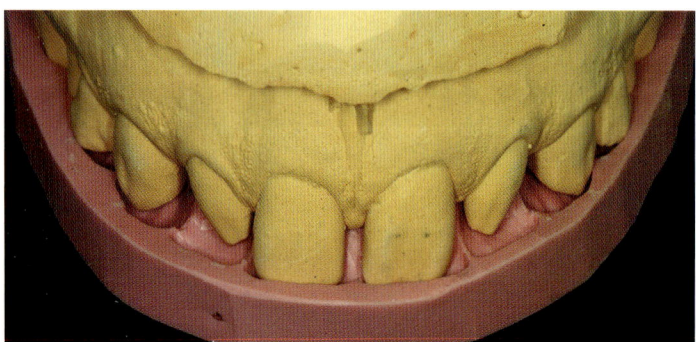

Fig. C6.2.3 By trying the guides in the mouth, the case will be determined to be additive, subtractive or both additive and subtractive. This case was mostly additive, which meant tooth reduction was minimal. The preparation guides dictate the amount and location of any needed tooth reduction.

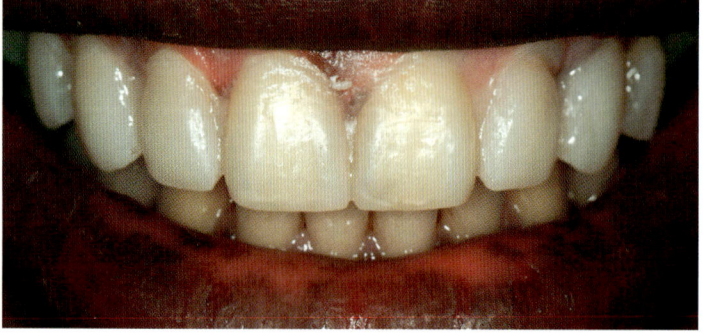

Fig. C6.2.4 A bis-acrylic mock-up was fabricated intra-orally with the help of a transparent silicone impression made from the wax-up. The facial, oral and tooth proportions, the incisal edge position, the occlusal parameters, speech and smile were evaluated. The mock-up is an effective and valuable procedure that is used to produce a very close replica of the definitive restoration. This procedure provides a comfortable communication tool between dentist and patient and allows the artistic creation of a smile to take place through a trial-and-error designing process. The goal is visualization of a result that leads to case acceptance by the patient and convinces the dentist that the maximum potential can be achieved with the planned restorations.[23]

KEY CLINICAL TECHNIQUES

The mock-up is an effective and valuable procedure that:

- Evaluates the facial, oral and tooth proportion parameters.
- Evaluates incisal edge position, occlusion, speech and smile.
- Produces a very close replica of the definitive restoration.
- Provides a comfortable communication tool between dentist and patient.
- Allows the artistic creation of a smile to take place through a trial-and-error design process.

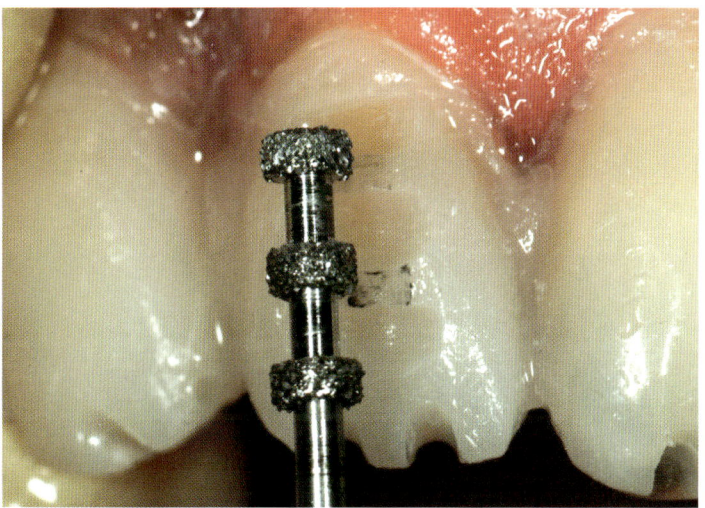

Fig. C6.2.5 The preparations began with depth cutters and the mock-up in place. The depth cutters have a great value for controlling the amount of tooth structure removed. The preparations were completed to permit a consistent thickness of porcelain to be developed by the technician. This approach allows maximum conservation of enamel and strength in the porcelain veneers.

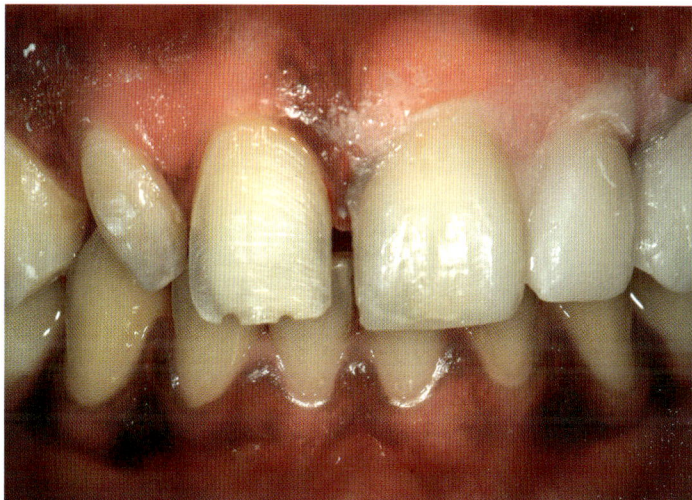

Fig. C6.2.6 The tooth surfaces were reduced using a round-ended diamond bur following the convexity of the tooth. The mock-up was cut back until the demarcation lines were removed, indicating that the essential depth was achieved. Sufficient reduction of the preparations was verified by placing the silicone index over the teeth. Final impressions of the prepared case were made and sent to the laboratory with the wax-up, guides and clinical photographs of the mock-up.

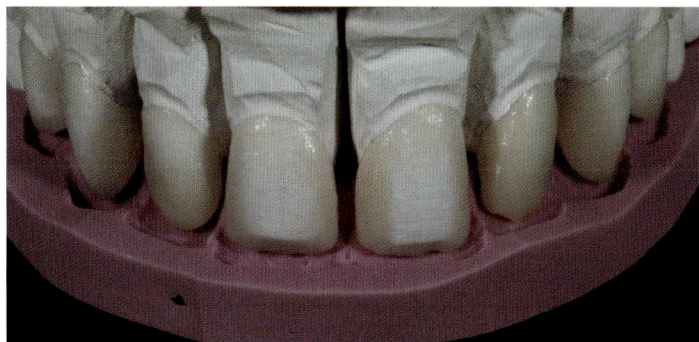

Fig. C6.2.7 The porcelain restorations were initiated in the laboratory using the guides made from the wax-up.

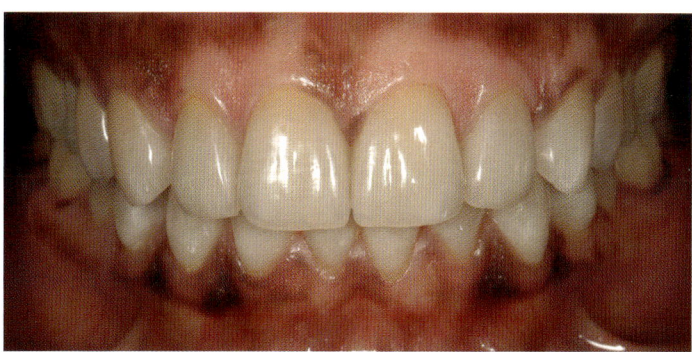

Fig. C6.2.8 The completed restorations were placed using a two-step bonding agent (total etch) and a light-cured resin cement.[3]

CLINICAL CASE 6.2: CLINICAL PROCEDURES FOR DIASTEMA CLOSURE

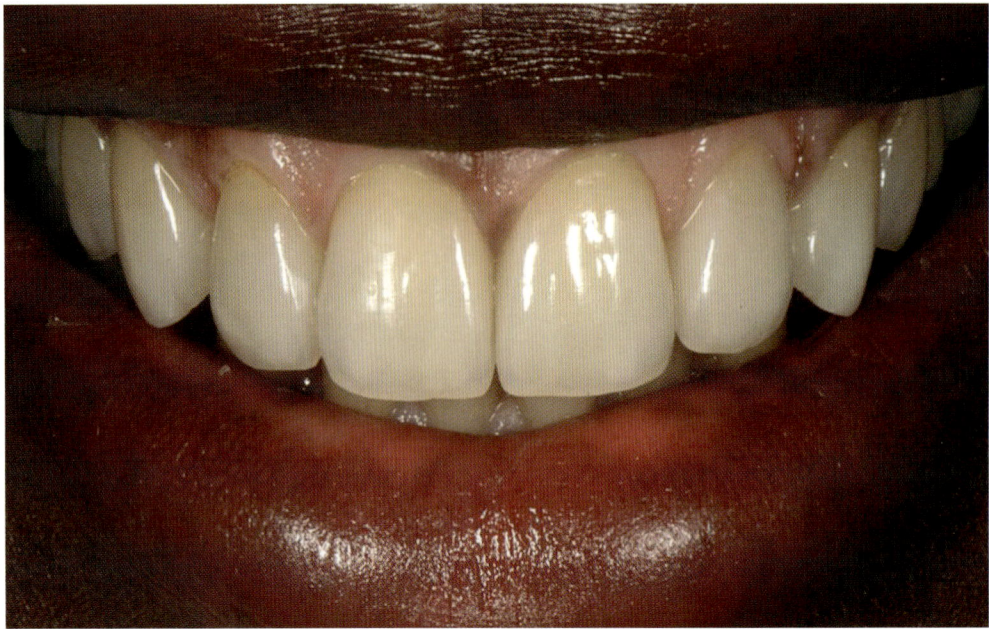

Fig. C6.2.9 Final result after the esthetic rehabilitation.

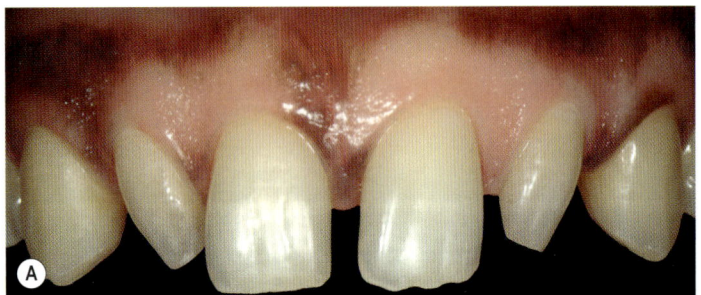 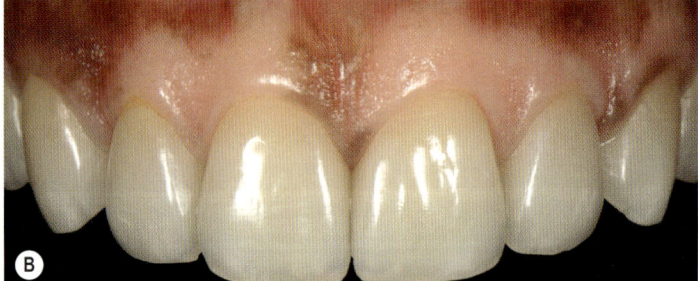

Fig. C6.2.10 Maxillary views (A) before and (B) after case completion.

ESSENTIALS

RSM can be a predictable treatment for many esthetic and functional dental problems.[1]

The ideal patient for RSM should meet the following requirements:

- Needs tooth restoration regardless of whether orthodontic treatment is performed.
- Has an ideal occlusion without any orthodontic treatment.
- Has free gingival margin and papilla levels that are manageable without orthodontic treatment.
- Requires tooth preparations that will not structurally or biologically compromise the teeth.

Even after careful case selection many patients will be found to meet these requirements and are good candidates for nonorthodontic esthetic correction.[4]

An understanding of RSM theory and techniques enables the clinician and laboratory technician to adopt a biologically and functionally sound approach to the management of esthetic improvement for patients with spatially compromised teeth. Used, when necessary, in conjunction with orthodontic therapy and employing contemporary restorative materials, predictable, accurate and natural appearing esthetic results can be achieved.[2]

ACKNOWLEDGEMENT

The authors thank Dr Stephen Chu for providing the diastema clinical case presented in this chapter.

Seminal literature

Brea L, Oquendo A, David S. Dental crowding: the restorative approach. Dent Clin North Am 2011;55(2):301–10.

Crowded dentition is commonly found in the esthetic zone. Many forms of therapy can be used to treat the overlap of teeth caused by insufficient space within the dental arch. A careful analysis of patients with dental crowding is necessary to determine the most appropriate treatment of each individual case. Clinical considerations, advantages, disadvantages and alternative treatment modalities for crowding dentition are discussed in this article and a clinical case is presented to illustrate the application of these techniques.

Gurel G, Chu S, Kim J. Restorative space management. In: Tarnow D, Chu S, Kim J, editors. Aesthetic restorative dentistry principles and practice. Mahwah, NJ: Quintessence; 2008. p. 405–25.

In attempting to provide a restorative solution for cases that have been compromised by spatial considerations, clinicians have traditionally opted for an orthodontic approach that does not provide optimal esthetics due to changes in tooth morphology, specifically tooth size and shape as a result of dental deterioration. This article presents the clinical considerations that must be addressed when providing a prosthetic restoration for spatially compromised cases.

Oquendo A, Brea L, David S. Diastema: correction of excessive spaces in the esthetic zone. Dent Clin North Am 2011;55(2):265–81.

The presence of diastemata is a common feature found in the anterior dentition. Many forms of therapy can be used for diastema closure and advanced planning allows the most appropriate treatment to be determined for each individual case. Clinical considerations, advantages, disadvantages and alternative treatment modalities for diastema closure are discussed in this article and a clinical case is presented to illustrate the application of these techniques.

REFERENCES

1. Kim J, Chu S, Gürel G, Cisneros G. Restorative space management: treatment planning and clinical considerations for insufficient space. Pract Proced Aesthet Dent 2005;17(1):19–25.

2. Gurel G, Chu S, Kim J. Restorative space management. In: Tarnow D, Chu S, Kim J, editors. Aesthetic restorative dentistry principles and practice. Mahwah, NJ: Quintessence; 2008. p. 405–25.

3. Oquendo A, Brea L, David S. Diastema: correction of excessive spaces in the esthetic zone. Dent Clin North Am 2011;55(2):265–81.

4. Spear FM. The esthetic correction of anterior dental mal-alignment: conventional vs. instant (restorative) orthodontics. J Calif Dent Assoc 2004;32(2):133–41.

REFERENCES

5. Sheen G, Goldstein R, Hackman S. Restorative treatment of crowded teeth. In: Goldstein R, Haywood V, editors. Esthetics in dentistry, vol. 2. Esthetic problems of individual teeth, missing teeth, malocclusion, special populations. Ontario, Canada: BC Decker; 2001. p. 733–52.

6. Dawson P. Requirements for occlusal stability. In: Dawson P, editor. Functional occlusion from TMJ to smile design. Missouri: Mosby; 2007. p. 345–8.

7. Brea L, Oquendo A, David S. Dental crowding: the restorative approach. Dent Clin North Am 2011;55(2):301–10.

8. Chu S, Tarnow D, Bloom M. Diagnosis, etiology. In: Tarnow D, Chu S, Kim J, editors. Aesthetic restorative dentistry principles and practice. Mahwah, NJ: Montage Media. 2008. p. 1–25.

9. Sarver DM. Principles of cosmetic dentistry in orthodontics, part 1. Shape and proportionality of anterior teeth. Am J Orthod Dentofacial Orthop 2004;126(6):749–53.

10. Dlugokinski M, Frazier K, Goldstein R. Restorative treatment of diastema. In: Goldstein R, Haywood V, editors. Esthetics in dentistry, vol. 2. Esthetic problems of individual teeth, missing teeth, malocclusion, special populations. Ontario, Canada: BC Decker; 2001. p. 703–31.

11. Fradeani M, Corrado M. Facial analysis. In: Fradeani M, editor. Esthetic rehabilitation in fixed prosthodontics. Carol Stream, Illinois: Quintessence Pub. Co.; 2004. p. 35–62.

12. Levine JB. Esthetic diagnosis. In: Current concepts in cosmetic dentistry. Chicago: Quintessence; 1994. p. 9–17.

13. Fradeani M. Dentolabial analysis. In: Fradeani M, editor. Esthetic rehabilitation in fixed prosthodontics. Carol Stream, IL: Quintessence Pub. Co.; 2004. p. 63–116.

14. Vig RG, Brundo GC. The kinetics of anterior tooth display. J Prosthet Dent 1978;39(5):502–4.

15. Tjan A, Miller G. Some esthetic factors in a smile. J Prosthet Dent 1984;51(1):24–8.

16. Chu SJ. Range and mean distribution frequency of individual tooth width of the maxillary anterior dentition. Pract Proced Aesthet Dent 2007;19(4):209–15.

17. Lombardi RE. The principles of visual perception and their clinical application to denture esthetics. J Prosthet Dent 1973;29:358–82.

18. Chu SJ. Range and mean distribution frequency of individual tooth width of the maxillary anterior dentition. Pract Proced Aesthet Dent 2007;19(4):209–15.

19. Furuse AY, Herkrath FJ, Franco EJ, Benetti AR, Mondelli J. Multidisciplinary management of anterior diastemata: clinical procedures. Pract Proced Aesthet Dent 2007;19(3):185–91.

20. Beasley WK, Maskeroni AJ, Moon MG, et al. The orthodontic and restorative treatment of a large diastema: a case report. Gen Dent 2004;52(1):37–41.

21. Spear FM, Kokich VG, Mathews DP. Interdisciplinary management of anterior esthetics. J Am Dent Assoc 2006;137(2):160–9.

22. Ferrari M, Patroni S, Balleri P. Measurement of enamel thickness in relation to reduction for etched laminate veneers. Int J Periodontics Restorative Dent 1992;12(5):407–13.

23. Gurel G. Porcelain laminate veneers for diastema closure. In: Gurel G, editor. The science and art of PLV. Chicago: Quintessence; 2003. p. 19–58, 369–92.

CHAPTER 7

Clear Aligner Therapy

FRANK CELENZA

Overview.	184
Comparison of fixed and removable appliances	185
Getting started.	186
Aligner uniqueness	187
Other aligner advantages.	187
Aligner evolution	188
Clinical application	189
Clinical cases	202
Acknowledgement	212

Orthodontics is a key treatment option and adjunct in esthetic dentistry. It is the natural, noninvasive way to re-align teeth. Re-aligning teeth with an air turbine must always be seen as more damaging, irreversible and less acceptable. Fortunately aligners are now widely available and popular, offering high patient acceptability in many cases. However, there are limitations.

Orthodontic care, particularly for adults in the permanent or even late transitional dentition stage, has undergone a dramatic shift in acceptability and awareness, largely due to the invention and acceptance of clear aligner therapy. The combination of computer-generated virtual treatment and sequential appliance manufacture has provided a means by which tooth movement can be planned and executed in a manner that is far more acceptable than conventional fixed or removable appliances. Consequently, there has been a noticeable rise in the implementation of orthodontic care and the breadth of age range than was previously the norm. Either as a means unto itself, or in many pre-restorative situations, the appreciation and utilization of orthodontic treatment is becoming more commonplace. However, with this trend in mind, a few caveats still remain, and will remain, in the opinion of the author.

OVERVIEW

Of paramount importance is the understanding that clear aligner therapy represents a removable appliance technique, and although vastly superior to any previous removable appliance (more on that shortly), it is still just that: an appliance technique. Other appliances exist and can be substituted for a myriad of orthodontic situations; this technique merely represents a new appliance choice. Consequently, it is the firm assertion of this author that a fundamental understanding of orthodontics, particularly diagnosis and treatment planning, remains essential to the successful implementation of this treatment. The notion that sending the requisite records and allowing the manufacturer, or a computer, to plan and sequence the case by merely approving their rendition will surely lead to less than ideal results, possible complications and the question of who is responsible for the orthodontic treatment. Was the general practitioner practising orthodontics? Was a suitably trained orthodontist involved at any stage? Although theoretically acceptable in simple cases, in orthodontics a trained and experienced eye is often essential to distinguish difficult situations.

Orthodontic treatment by its very nature requires a thorough understanding of and appreciation for the physiology of tooth movement and treatment goals as well as compromises. In addition, an appreciation of appropriate retention strategies and retainer design is of great importance, again pointing to the understanding that this is merely another appliance, not a magical change in the way teeth will respond and stabilize. Orthodontic treatment can be associated with unintended, unanticipated and untoward side effects, and aligner therapy cannot be relied upon to eliminate these deterrents. Operator experience and expertise remains an important and essential ingredient for successful implementation, which computer generated suggestions cannot and likely will not ever provide a substitute for. Further, it is this author's opinion and experience that effective retention planning and design is often more challenging and important in adults than the actual treatment phase.

This chapter is intended to provide an overview of the technique and to display an assortment of cases, selected solely from the author's experience with aligner therapy, ranging from simple to complex in order to demonstrate the technique of clear aligner therapy. Lastly, a direction of interdisciplinary inclusion that forecasts a promising and sophisticated potential for the future application of this technique is suggested. This chapter is not, however, intended as a training manual.

COMPARISON OF FIXED AND REMOVABLE APPLIANCES

Fixed appliance therapy is still the gold standard but aligners win on patient acceptance. Further, advances in the technique and material science continue to improve and broaden the application. However, aligner therapy is to be viewed as treatment using a new appliance, which means the principles and fundamentals of orthodontics still apply.

Whereas there have been and exist many variations and competitors to the main manufacturer and supplier of the original aligner technique, namely Invisalign, many of them have come and gone. Invisalign remains the leader and the originator in this field and consequently this chapter is devoted in its content to infer the use of Invisalign in describing and discussing aligner therapy in general, as the author's experience with that product far outstrips any other. However, there are other popular similar systems in use throughout the world and the reader may be able to assess these, reach their own conclusions and treat patients accordingly based on the techniques described in this chapter, which relate to the original version, i.e. Invisalign.

Examples of aligner systems in use:

- Invisalign
- Clear Correct
- Essix
- Tru-Tain.

GETTING STARTED

The orthodontic treatment of patients with this technique involves the submission of patient records, which comprise impressions (be they digital or conventional), clinical photographs and X-ray images. From these records, computer simulations of the actual treatment are derived and delivered via computer for the operator to modify, sequence and approve. Once that approval is gained, the manufacturing process of the actual sequential aligners commences. There are some interesting aspects of this process that warrant consideration.

It is worth considering a unique aspect of the manufacturing challenge that aligner therapy demands. Normally, in manufacturing, the goal is to systematize production to allow for constant repetition and the elimination of any variation in the process, thereby maximizing the efficiency. The goal is to produce as many identical items as possible. However, in the case of orthodontic aligner production, not only is every individual unique but each individual aligner for that patient is also unique. Consequently, aligner manufacturing necessitates the exact opposite of conventional manufacturing in that no two items being produced are ever the same!

Aligner therapy, by definition, involves the use of a removable appliance. However, there are significant features of this style of removable appliance that lead to the realization that aligners are a significantly superior form of removable appliance, and, as a result, many of the limitations of conventional removable appliances do not necessarily apply. For instance, it has long been held that the main difference between fixed and removable appliances lies in what they can accomplish. More specifically, removable appliances can only effect tipping type movements on teeth. Bodily movements, such as large space closures or translations, have historically required fixed appliance utilization to achieve properly paralleled tooth roots. This is because of the nature of construction of traditional removable appliances, which is most frequently from acrylic and wire. They apply force to a tooth (or teeth) by minimal or single point contact. The movement that results is a function of the relationship of these contact points to the centre of rotation of the tooth. Since the force is applied at the coronal aspect of the tooth, or some distance from the centre of rotation, it results in a tipping moment upon the tooth. Fixed appliances work similarly by applying a force at the coronal level but they also feature an archwire that precisely fits the slot of a bracket that is attached to the tooth and acts as a track or guide for the movement, thereby controlling the moment of force (which is defined as a force application some distance from the centre of rotation or resistance). Other subtleties to the application of the force and the fit of the archwire, as well as various bends and compensatory details that will allow the tooth to move in a bodily fashion, are also utilized but are beyond the scope of this chapter. Suffice it to say that historically the ability to effect a bodily movement has been the main difference between fixed and removable appliances, with respect to attainable outcomes.

ALIGNER UNIQUENESS

Aligner therapy, however, by the nature of its features and construction is an exception to this dictate. Still technically a removable appliance, aligners are, however, manufactured in such a way that they do not apply single or limited contact to the tooth surface, in fact they are intimately and accurately moulded to the entire tooth crown. By careful evaluation of the desired movements and then by detailed translation of those movements into the computer rendition, 'virtual gables' and other combined computer–orthodontic terminology can be inserted into the prescription and the resulting configuration of the aligner results in very sophisticated and accurate tooth movement or tracking. Again, however, the degree of accuracy and sophistication of these movements is largely a function of the prescriber's ability to treatment plan and forecast the outcome, as well as familiarity with this technique and an ability to communicate details in the prescription.

OTHER ALIGNER ADVANTAGES

Aligner therapy also realizes other advantages over conventional orthodontic treatment, some of which are logistic in nature. For example, fewer visits as well as fewer emergency repairs (for debonded brackets or extruding archwires) rank high among the advantages. Less frequent visits and a longer interval between regular visits is attractive to many patients, with 6–8 weeks becoming the norm as compared to 4–6 weeks. Much less discomfort is reported from patients, as aligners are much less bulky and obtrusive than fixed appliances or conventional removables, especially with regard to the maxillary arch since palatal coverage is no longer needed. Aligners are certainly more hygienic than fixed appliances by virtue of the fact that they are removed for eating and so are not food retentive, and they afford the ability to brush and floss an unencumbered natural dentition before replacing them in the mouth. For the operator, a great feature of aligner treatment is significantly reduced chair time. This is appreciated because the case is designed and manufactured 'up front' and succeeding appointments are for very minor procedures (such as bonding of 'attachments' and 'interproximal reduction') and, more usually, for progress checks and dispensing of subsequent aligners. There is virtually no adjustment or manipulation of the actual appliances, although 'midcourse corrections' and 'refinements' can be accomplished when necessary. Lastly, although the aforementioned advantages are by no means complete, the main advantage of aligner therapy is the very reason patients have flocked to it: they are virtually unnoticeable in public or social settings. Not all cases suit aligners, removable appliances depend on patient compliance, retention is mandatory, teeth with severe undercuts can be unsuitable, etc.

ALIGNER EVOLUTION

When Invisalign was first introduced it was considered by many to be a modality suitable for minimally to moderately involved situations, particularly with regard to crowding or spacing. Many practitioners, perhaps those well aware of their own limitations, continue to utilize it solely for these situations, such as Class I malocclusions. However, with training and experience the ability to apply this technique to more challenging and involved case types will become the norm. Furthermore, as the art and science developed, there have been significant modifications and improvements to the modality that have further expanded its application. It is now safe to say that clear aligner therapy has gained acceptability far beyond what many had originally anticipated, and that orthodontic offices offering clear aligners as their exclusive, if not preferred, appliance design are becoming more commonplace.

Furthermore, the development of 'express' treatment has reduced the laboratory fee for minor cases and put this treatment within reach of many more patients, as well as operators. First introduced as a maximum of 10 sets of aligners (corresponding to 20 weeks of treatment), newer versions have now introduced 'express 5' (10 weeks) for an even greater reduction in laboratory fee.

The perception is that Invisalign is high cost compared with conventional fixed appliance treatment and competitor aligner systems. However, the cost of Invisalign has come down to where most orthodontists can offer it as no additional cost. Operators are also realizing certain efficiencies in utilizing Invisalign and are able to pass these savings on to patients. Additionally, the need to keep a vast orthodontic inventory and armamentarium is obviated with aligner systems.

The introduction of a more detailed and descriptive computer program (labelled G4) has provided the operator with a more sophisticated platform from which to communicate and prescribe intended treatment, and has resulted in better outcomes. An integral part of that development was 'optimized' or more sophisticated 'attachments' that are bonded to the teeth and moulded into the aligners. These attachments provide for greater control of movement and anchor units, in addition to adding retentive components for greater control. 'Power ridges' are features that can now be moulded into the aligners as well, which permit significant and effective torque application to anterior teeth.

The provision for 'precision cuts' and 'button cutouts' has opened the door for providers to include and implement interarch elastics with greater ease. No longer is it necessary to modify each aligner by hand as the auxiliary fasteners can be included in the manufacturing of each set from the outset. Consequently, a wide array of case types of greater sophistication can be accommodated with ease. Class II and III cases can much more effectively be addressed and corrected, and the efficiency of attaching elastics to a very secure aligner to apply force is proving to be considerable (see Clinical Cases, Figs C7.9A,B and C7.10A,B). In addition, dramatic tooth movements can also be achieved. Further, the use of extra-dental sources of anchorage, such as miniscrews, can now be easily accommodated and combined with aligner therapy, opening possibilities for other treatments and outcomes (see Clinical Cases, Figs C7.11A,B and C7.12A–D).

'Invisalign Teen' is a development that allows for the expansion of Invisalign into a whole new patient population, by accommodating some of the features of the late transitional and early permanent dentition into the aligners. Second molar eruption, late vertical detailing movements, anterior torquing and a compliance indicator are examples of this technology.

As the application of aligner therapy continues to expand, new treatment possibilities arise and the utilization of aligner technology and methodology grows. As a new appliance choice, aligner therapy has proven to be viable, effective and even advantageous. Aligner therapy is here to stay.

Invisalign and aligner therapy in general must be viewed as a new appliance choice. It is not a magic wand but a new technology that must be understood in order to be correctly utilized. It offers many significant advantages over conventional appliances but does not rewrite the basic fundamentals of orthodontics. Consequently, relapse and retention issues must be addressed and provided for, with much the same philosophy as with conventional appliances. Aligners can change how you move a tooth, but not how you maintain it. There are now many aligner systems on the market worldwide but this chapter will discuss Invisalign as it is the most comprehensive.

CLINICAL APPLICATION
INITIAL VISIT

Figure 7.1 is a schematic flow chart of the sequence of delivering aligner therapy. The first visit, or consultation appointment, is intended to both examine and diagnose the case and to inform the patient of options. Appropriate records are gathered to facilitate this process. It is also preferable to start the case by

CLINICAL APPLICATION

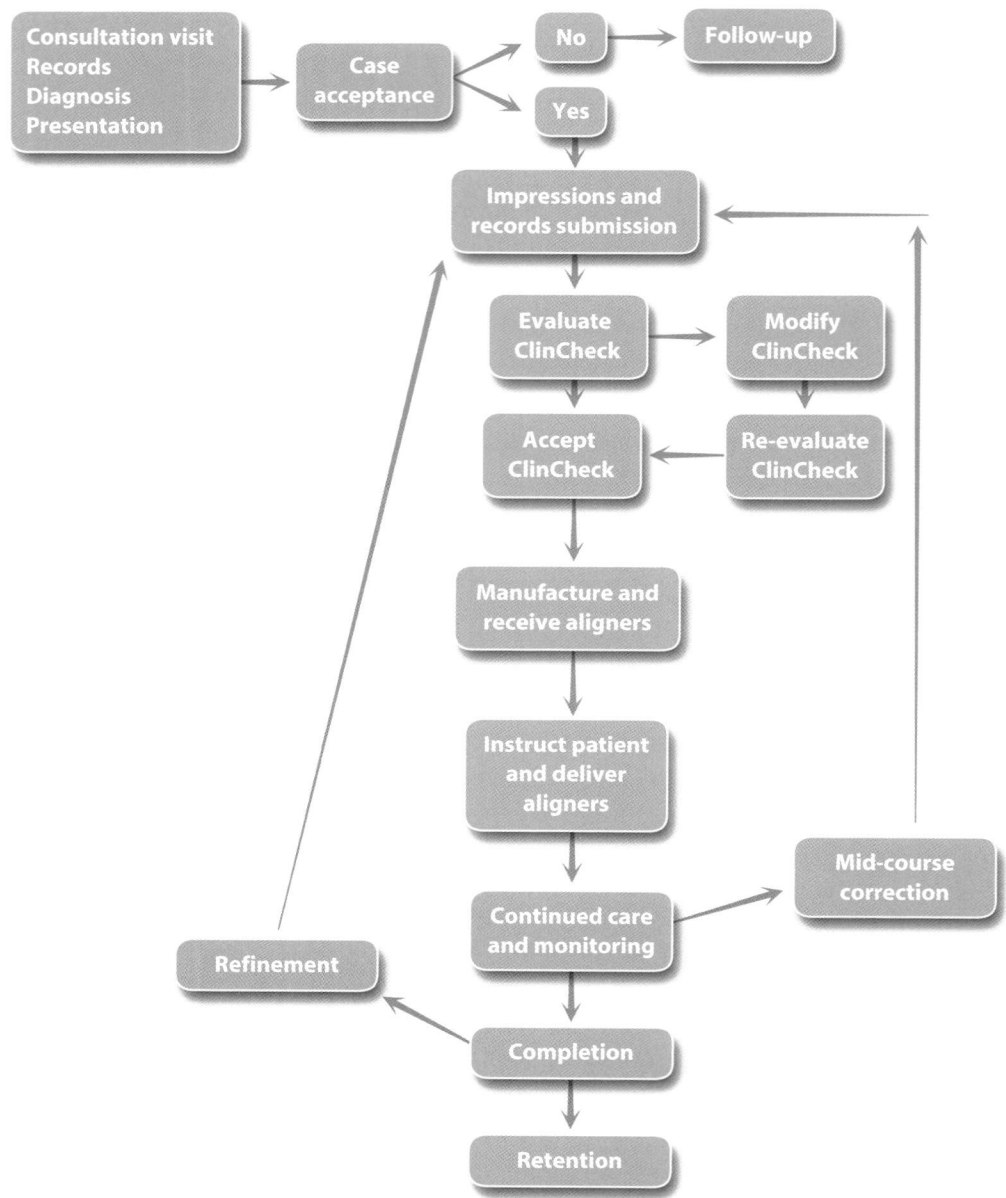

Fig. 7.1 A flow chart for aligner therapy and the decision-making process involved.

submitting the records and prescription soon thereafter. Operators should be experienced and knowledgeable enough to eliminate the need to analyse the records requiring the patient to return for a second consultation appointment to gain that insight. An exception to this strategy might be when ancillary specialists need to be sequenced into the case, such as the need for third molar or any other extractions or preparatory restorative dentistry and periodontal preparation.

PATIENT PREPARATION

With regard to oral preparation, the same guidelines that apply to conventional orthodontics also should be implemented with aligner therapy. Again, this philosophy points to the realization that aligner therapy is merely the choice of a different appliance and an understanding of the dental physiology behind tooth movement still applies. Consequently, the operator needs to diagnose and eliminate all pathology in preparation for the initiation of tooth movement. This may include oral pathology, caries or periodontal disease. These conditions can be treated subsequent to the making of impressions provided that they do not significantly change the oral configuration. For instance, if soft tissue inflammation is observed to be present, the patient can undergo scaling and root planing without causing an adverse effect on the impression. Minor carious lesions conceivably could also be addressed. However, any change to the oral environment that causes a big enough alteration such that aligner fit would be compromised contraindicates impressioning and case submission during this visit. Extraction of permanent teeth for space provision, third molars if erupted and restorations large enough to alter the shape of a tooth are examples of this latter situation. Furthermore, any changes that can be anticipated that might occur during the course of treatment are better addressed at this time, to prevent the need to re-impress and remanufacture the aligners. The patient should be informed that it might be better to complete any treatment that is already in progress before initiating aligner therapy.

As far as periodontal disease is concerned, the same dictates as used for conventional orthodontics apply. To achieve success and prevent damage to the dentition or any untoward periodontal breakdown, a thorough evaluation of the periodontium and its condition beforehand is warranted. Radiographic assessment of the bony topography in conjunction with clinical probing to assess attachment levels and inflammation, as evidenced by bleeding upon gentle probing, is a quick and easy enough determinant. Prior to commencing any form of tooth movement, all soft tissue inflammation should be eliminated. This will ensure that movement without attachment loss can ensue. Procedures such as scaling, root planing, oral hygiene instruction, grafting and open flap debridement can be considered as basic and often necessary to achieve this goal.

ORTHODONTIC RECORDS

Orthodontic records pertinent to the case are imperative; however, traditional plaster study models are not and may well be en route to obsolescence in themselves, owing to the advent of digital model storage as well as the records that

Invisalign will generate, known as 'ClinCheck'. Similarly, digital images have now become nearly imperative, both for clinical photographs and radiographic images. Panoramic or full mouth radiographs are preferable (or at least bitewing type surveys), even though Invisalign no longer requires their submission. Lateral cephalograms have become largely optional in general, but again it is up to the operator's experience and diagnostic acumen to determine the need for one and to know how to evaluate it properly.

Accuracy of fit is an essential aspect of successful aligner therapy. The impressioning of dentitions has undergone several generations of improvement since the introduction of Invisalign and the progression from custom tray fabrication to one-step PVS materials, but the ultimate expression of this has only recently become available and promises to be a big improvement. The manufacturing process of aligners does not actually include the pour of a stone model from the provided impression, but rather results from the digital scan of that impression and subsequent 3-dimensional printing. Consequently, with the elimination of the impressioning step, by virtue of a direct scan of the actual dentition, a significant source of potential error is eliminated. Readily available intra-oral scanners for impressioning have arrived and offer numerous advantages in aligner therapy, in addition to greater accuracy. Figure 7.2 is an image of an office-based intra-oral digital scanner, known as iTero, which is designed to be mobile between operatories. It scans the dentition and produces the image files to be sent out for processing. Early indications are that aligners manufactured from digital scans feature much greater accuracy and fit than those generated from conventional PVS impressions. They also eliminate the need to retake impressions, as the computer simply will not accept an image unless it is accurate. Figure 7.3 is a digital impression of a dentition, produced by an iTero, as it would appear on a computer monitor. This method also saves time because virtual impressions are transferred and shared digitally, not by couriers or mail. Digital impressions are also far less uncomfortable to patients as they no longer need to wait for material to set intra-orally, while trying to stifle gag reflexes. Further, as with any new device or technique, unanticipated modalities and developments will inevitably result and digital impressioning certainly suggests possibilities along those lines. Figure 7.4 is a digital record, or study model that is stored on a computer hard drive, eliminating the need to catalogue and provide physical storage for stone casts.

VIRTUAL TREATMENT

Once a case is diagnosed and treatment is proposed and submitted, the provider is presented with a virtual treatment animation, or ClinCheck, for evaluation.

CHAPTER 7
CLEAR ALIGNER THERAPY

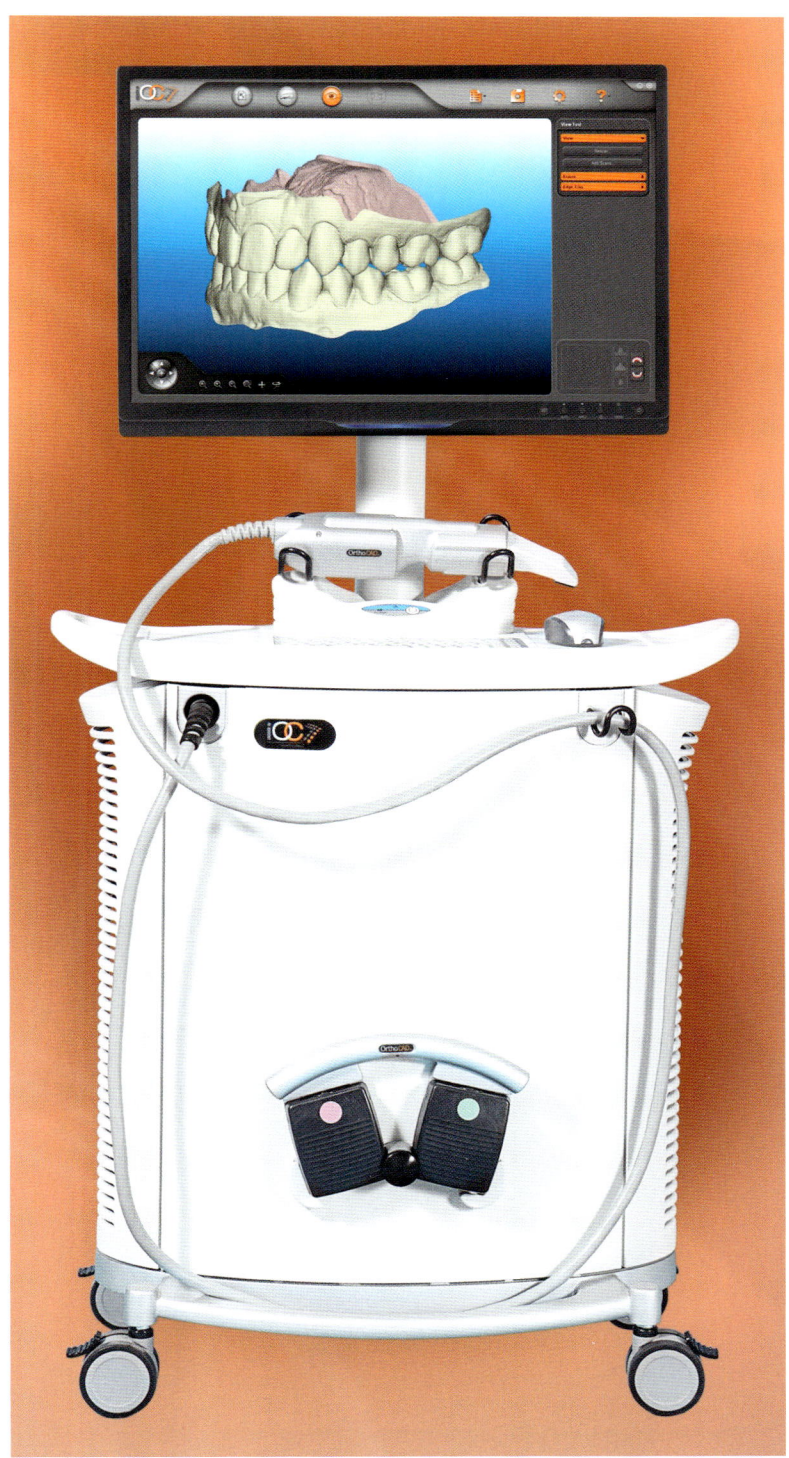

Fig. 7.2 An iTero unit for making digital impressions intra-orally is shown. The unit is self-contained and mobile, with a temporary power supply to allow transport without rebooting. Foot pedals are hanging on the front of the machine, and the intra-oral scanning wand is visible just under the monitor, atop the keyboard.

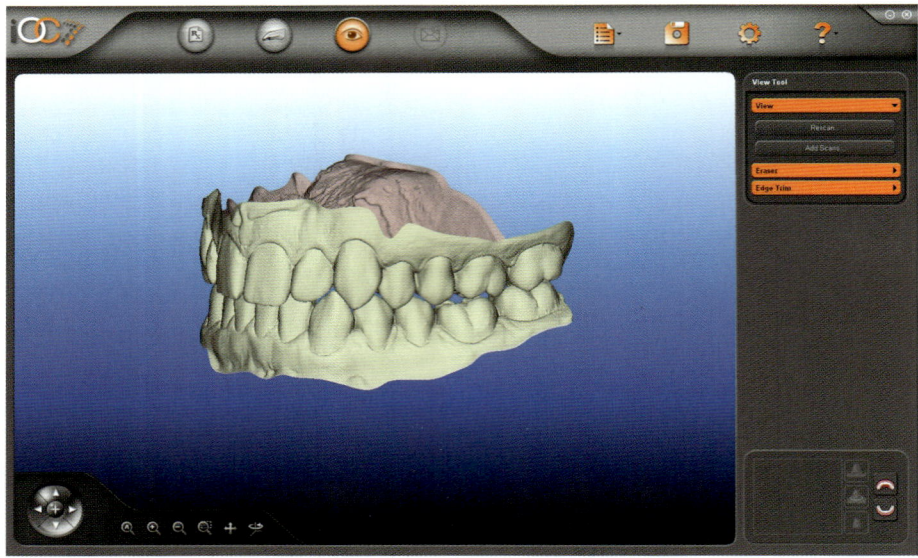

Fig. 7.3   An iRecord sample, or digital scan of a dentition, as produced by an iTero and ready to be sent for treatment planning. This digital image completely replaces a conventional physical impression.

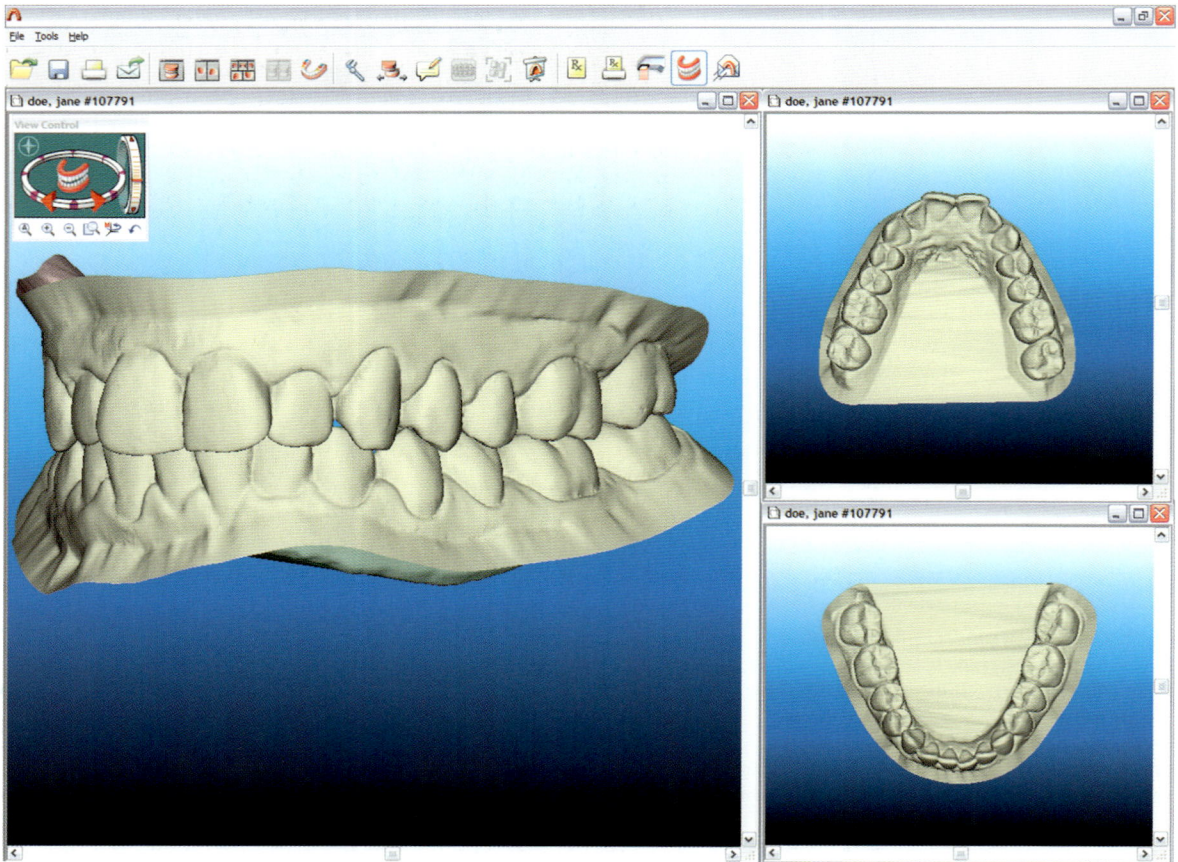

Fig. 7.4   An iRecord or example of a digital cast made from an iTero scan and used in place of conventional study casts for analysis and record storage.

CLEAR ALIGNER THERAPY

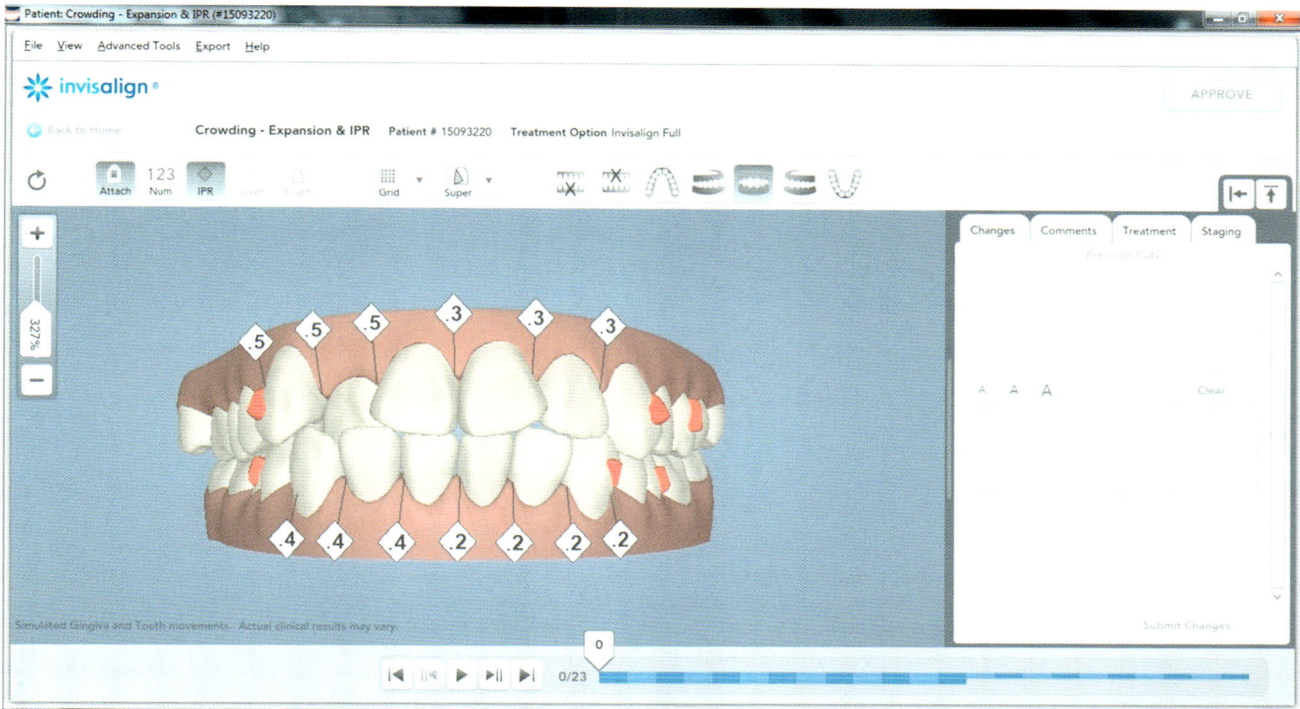

Fig. 7.5 A typical ClinCheck interface. On a computer monitor, the operator has the functionality to manipulate and alter the image and treatment plan at this stage using the various tabs and controls provided. There is also a place to write explanations and requests, allowing the operator to communicate verbally with the laboratory technician. Multiple rounds of detailing are feasible, which can lead to great detail in the treatment plan, until the practitioner clicks to approve the rendition, sending the case into aligner production.

Figure 7.5 is a typical ClinCheck, which the operator can use to manipulate and alter the treatment plan and aligner design. In the static representation presented here the functionality of the ClinCheck is lost, but when displayed on a computer this is a very interactive interface. There are numerous tabs and buttons for analysing the proposed treatment and communicating any changes to the laboratory. The ClinCheck also displays the number of aligners that are to be produced, which can then be translated into treatment time. The ClinCheck is a motion picture of the treatment that can and should also be used as a motivational tool when presented to the patient. At this point in time, the practitioner's input is crucial to the outcome, as the plan can be altered and modified prior to the aligners' production. Selection of attachments (Fig. 7.6) as well as their orientation and configuration is a science unto itself and should be carefully evaluated and designed by the practitioner, who needs to be proficient at understanding their design and purpose. The auxiliaries must be properly selected and included at this time. Items such as 'precision cuts' for the use of elastics and 'button cutouts' for the use of bondable attachments to the teeth

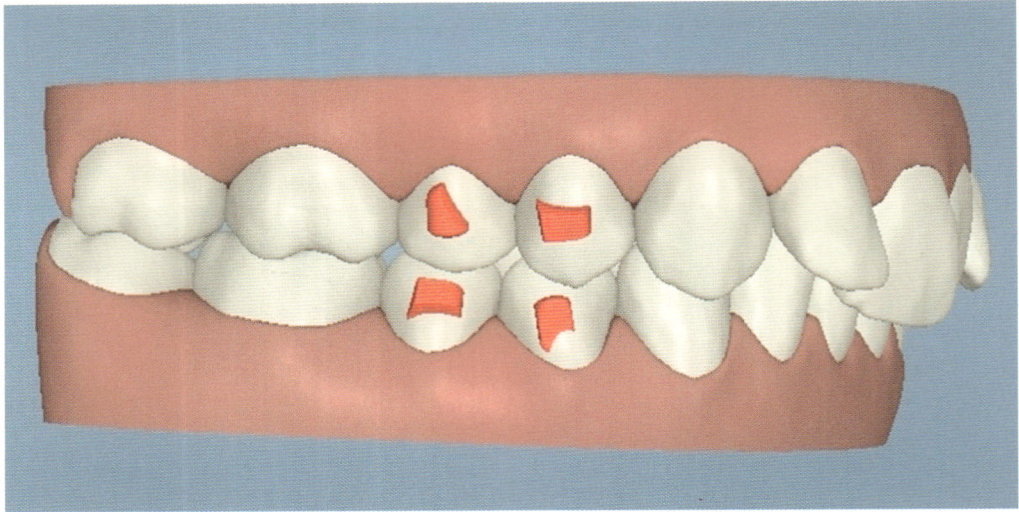

Fig. 7.6 A typical example of how 'attachments' appear on a ClinCheck. Shown in red, the attachments are actually bonded to the teeth using typical tooth-coloured composites, and moulded using precise templates that are provided with the aligners. The shape, location, size and orientation of these attachments are crucial to the outcome, and a thorough understanding of their design and use is important to the success of aligner therapy.

are also included at this stage. Figure C7.8 (see Clinical Cases) illustrates the combined use of bondable auxiliaries in conjunction with suitably relieved aligners. Further, the practitioner needs to assess the feasibility of the actual case and its movements and time frame, to prevent an overly ambitious or clinically unachievable result from being designed. Again, only a suitably experienced operator can best evaluate these parameters. Relying upon the technician's judgement to design the case is at best risky, and certainly irresponsible. When the practitioner is satisfied with the proposed treatment, the ClinCheck is accepted and the case goes into production.

APPLIANCE DELIVERY

Upon receiving the aligners, of which the entire set is delivered to the practitioner's office, the next step is to appoint the patient for delivery. At that appointment, instructions for use and demonstration of insertion and removal is important. Some practitioners prefer to delay the placement of the bonded attachments for an aligner or two, to allow the patient to become accustomed to using them first. IPR, or interproximal reduction, is performed as specified by the practitioner and according to clinical preferences. From this point on, aligners are changed every 2 weeks and appointment intervals are set as is customary for the practitioner, usually every 6 or 8 weeks (corresponding to 3 or 4 sets of aligners, respectively).

KEY CLINICAL TECHNIQUES

Tips on the placement of attachments:

- Patients should be shown what attachments are, and what they will look like and feel like, preferably on a model or in photographs, before their treatment commences. In this way, there is no disappointment when they are placed.

- Some patients are overwhelmed at the start of aligner therapy and need to be 'phased in' to treatment. For this reason, it is often beneficial to delay the placement of attachments after the initial delivery of the first aligner set.

- The author recommends that the placement of attachments is accomplished at the delivery of the third aligner set. In this way, the patient has had the experience of placing and removing two sets before the added retention of attachments is realized, and they are more adept at utilizing them.

CASE PROGRESS

During the ensuing visits, aligner fit is to be evaluated. The main indication that the system is working effectively is the fit of the aligners. Teeth that are not 'tracking' properly, or are showing signs of not fitting in the aligner, may need to be addressed. Figure 7.7 illustrates a situation where the upper right cuspid

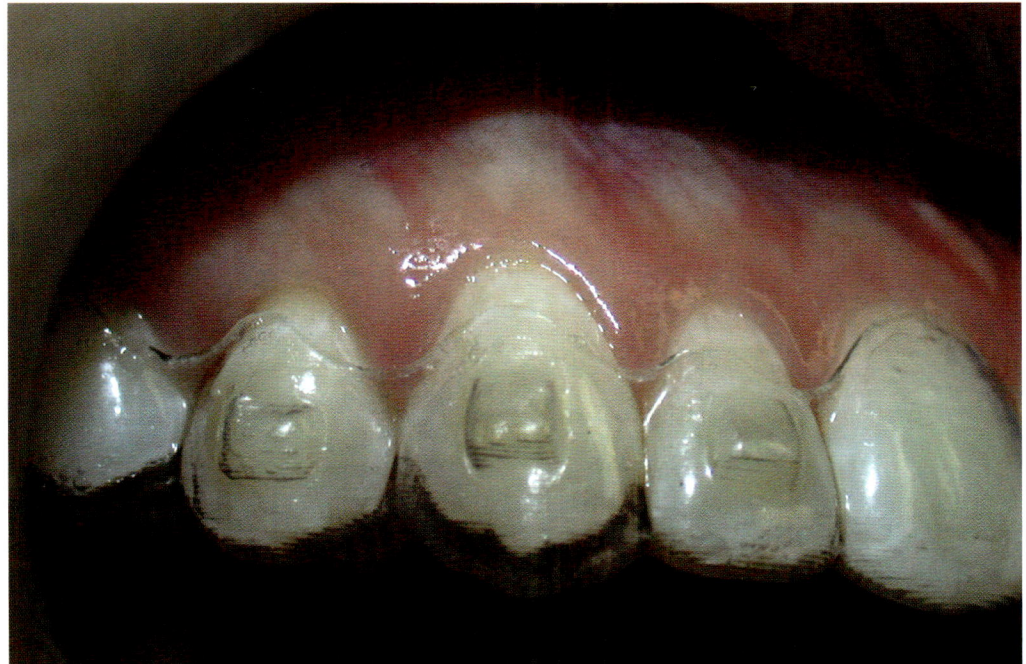

Fig. 7.7   Here is an example of an ill-fitting aligner. The upper right cuspid no longer fits the aligner precisely, and its attachment is no longer engaged to it. An unoccupied portion of the aligner is visible and is not tracking properly. Once the intimate fit of the aligner is lost, it cannot guide the tooth accurately and the result will be compromised. Corrective action such as re-impressioning and remanufacture or utilization of auxiliary means is recommended.

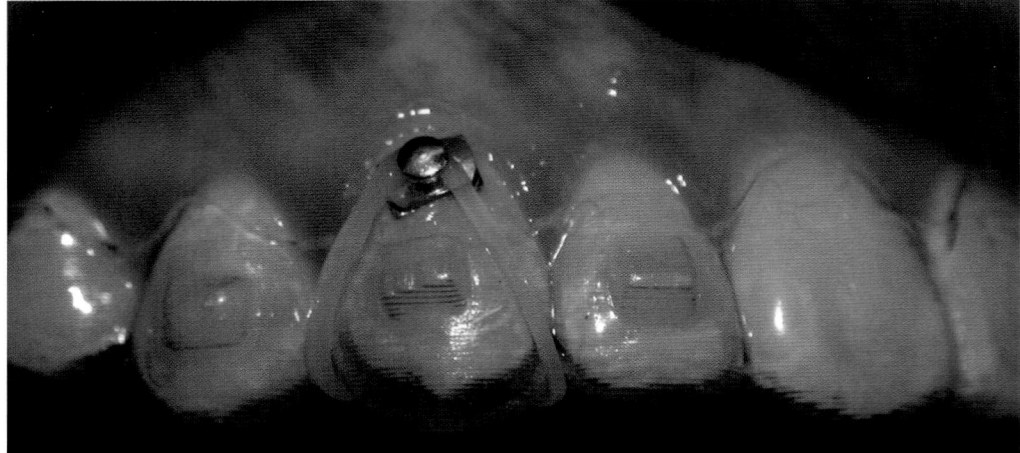

Fig. 7.8 The use of auxiliary means to recapture aligner fit is depicted. Buccal and lingual bonded buttons are placed on the tooth and the patient is instructed to wear an elastic connecting the buttons and over the aligner, in effect erupting the tooth into the aligner. Relief of the aligners to prevent conflict with the buttons must be provided. When the tooth is recaptured by the aligner, the auxiliaries can be removed.

is not properly fitting in the aligner and is an example of improper tracking. The tooth is not following the prescribed movement, and the fit of the aligner has been compromised. In cases of poor compliance or other reasons for less than ideal fit, new impressions may need to be made and a 'mid-course correction' enacted to remanufacture the aligners to recapture a proper fit. This would also entail another course of ClinCheck evaluation and approval. Another choice for the correction of this single tooth is depicted in Figure 7.8. Buccal and lingual bonded buttons are placed on the tooth and the aligners relieved to provide clearance. The patient is instructed to place and wear elastics over the aligner and fastened to the bonded buttons to effect an eruption of the tooth and consequent reinsertion and engagement in the aligner (Fig. 7.9).

CONCLUSION OF ACTIVE TREATMENT

At the end of aligner therapy, the result must be evaluated and the patient's satisfaction addressed. Hopefully, objectives have been achieved, and then suitable retainers can be designed and fabricated. In the event that objectives have not been fully satisfied, then re-impressioning and a course of 'refinement' (with the requisite ClinCheck evaluation and approval) is indicated to manufacture additional sets of aligners, which will allow progress to continue to its endpoint. Refinement is viewed by many orthodontists as a detailing stage, very much part of the procedure and routine, much as with fixed appliances, and by no means an indication of failure.

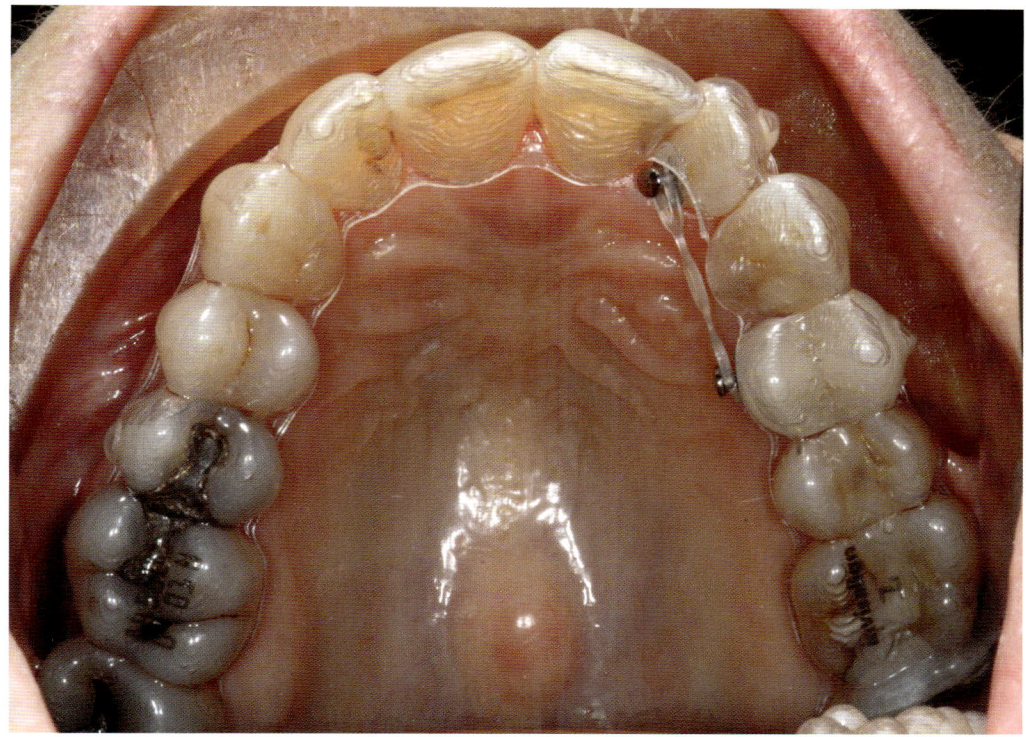

Fig. 7.9 Another use of auxiliaries is illustrated here, in conjunction with aligner therapy. Here a lateral incisor is being de-rotated by a palatal elastic that stretches from a button on the palatal aspect of the lateral to one on the palatal of a bicuspid. Counter rotation of the bicuspid is provided by the aligner and an optimized attachment bonded to its buccal surface. The rotation movement of the lateral is also programmed into the aligner design, and button cutouts are also preprogrammed, obviating the need to modify each aligner set chairside.

CLINICAL TIPS: REFINEMENT

- Refinement, and/or mid-course correction, should be viewed and discussed as a frequent and routine occurrence, not as a failure of treatment or a quick fix for less than ideal results.

- Just as with more traditional fixed appliances, refinement is to be viewed as a final detailing step, a way of achieving some last small details.

- Patients are well served if they are made aware from the beginning that additional aligners are frequently fabricated for this purpose, and they should not fixate on the number of aligners originally forecast because there may be additional aligners made at or near the end.

- Patients should know that the additional sets of aligners are included in their treatment as an integral part of the therapy.

- Patients appreciate the extra step and attention to detail and see it as an added benefit.

CLINICAL APPLICATION

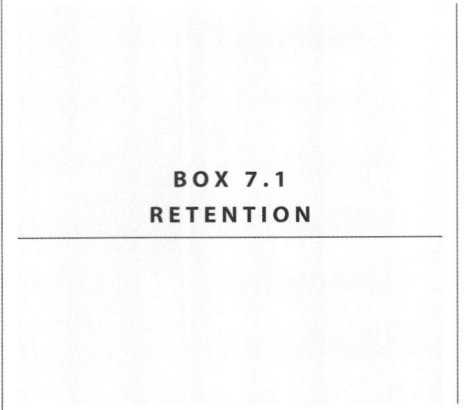

BOX 7.1 RETENTION

- The retention scheme for many patients is frequently more important than the actual treatment. For this reason, it needs to be outlined at the very outset and during the initial consultation.

- Retention suggestions and policy should also be outlined in the patient's written instruction manual.

- The retention scheme can be of either a fixed or a removable variety, and is often a combination thereof.

- The patient should be informed of choices and have a say in what might be best for them.

RETENTION STRATEGIES

Retention (Box 7.1) will be achieved via either fixed or removable means, or a combination thereof. This is a judgement that again is up to the experience and philosophy of the practitioner. Invisalign has various strategies for the use of the removable version. Basically, a more durable duplicate of the last, or any specific aligner, is produced and a new impression is not even required. Replacements are similarly easy to order, as are aligners. Frequently, bonded lingual retainers are deemed preferable, and examples are shown in the Clinical Cases that follow (see p. 202).

Post-treatment considerations:

- Patients with retainers should be seen on a regular and ongoing basis.

- Patients are asked to bring any removable retainers with them to appointments for inspection and evaluation.

- Retention patients should be advised that removable retainers do have a life expectancy and need to be replaced, ideally every 3–4 months, depending upon how much they are worn.

- Discolouration, staining, poor cleaning and care will also affect their longevity.

- Retainer replacement can and should be priced reasonably so that patients are properly served and the provider is adequately compensated.

ESSENTIALS: CLEAR ALIGNER THERAPY

- Clinician understanding of orthodontic fundamentals.
- A thorough and sound understanding of aligner modalities and intricacies.
- Healthy dentition and periodontium that is free of inflammation.
- A compliant and motivated patient.
- Accurate and pertinent records, especially impressions and preferably digital ones.
- A sound scheme for retention post-treatment is often more important than the actual treatment.

PATIENTS' FAQS

Q. How long will this treatment take?

A. Of course, the provider's experience is important in making an accurate estimate of treatment time, but a traditional rule of thumb with conventional appliances can also apply as a guideline here: 1 mm/month. If the clinician can assess the amount of movement required, this can be used as a rough guide. A few other classes of estimate can be considered, e.g. simple cases: 4–6 months, moderate cases: 9–12 months and advanced cases: 1.5+ years.

Q. How much will this treatment cost?

A. Of course, this will depend upon the office policy, but the provider is advised to be well versed, and have colleagues well versed, on office policy in this regard. Further, it is frequently advisable to defer all monetary discussions to the treatment coordinator who can outline terms and office policy for the patient at the appropriate time.

Q. Will I need to have teeth extracted?

A. The answer to this question requires that the provider carefully examines and properly diagnoses the case. In borderline situations the clinician can defer that judgement pending a more careful analysis of records, or even the acquisition of such records. Further, some cases can be treated by 'virtual diagnosis' philosophy, in which treatment is initiated and the extraction decision postponed, but the patient should know and expect that this judgement is forthcoming. However, an experienced clinician should be able to provide a definitive answer to this question, in the vast majority of cases, at the initial examination and based on his or her treatment philosophy.

Q. Aren't I too old for orthodontics?

A. This is a common misconception for many. In fact, age is not the limiting factor to successful orthodontics. Patients should be comforted and reassured that the limitation on orthodontics is not their age but rather their health, more specifically the health of their dentition and oral cavity. In this way, a discussion of preparatory procedures to render their oral cavity healthy, and maintain it that way, is introduced.

Q. Will the result be permanent?

A. The result will be lasting if the clinician's guidelines are carefully followed, but nothing is permanent. In this way, the importance of a sound retention scheme is introduced and the patient is informed of this from the very outset. As previously stated, the design and implementation of a sound and effective retention strategy can be more important than the actual treatment, and is essential to patient satisfaction.

CLINICAL CASES

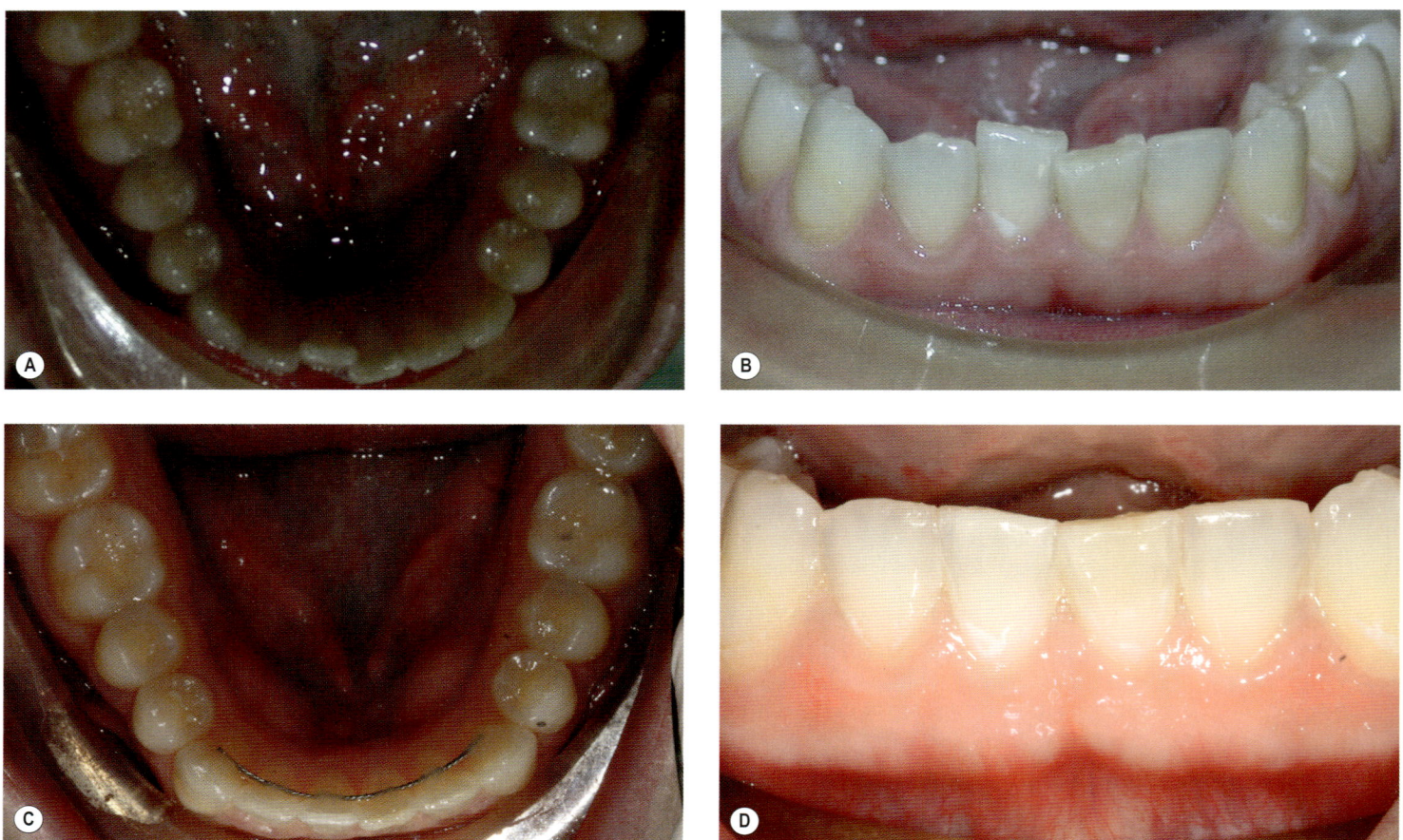

Fig. C7.1A–D   Pre- and post-treatment photographs of a mandibular arch that was diagnosed as minimal anterior crowding. In this case, 2 mm of arch length was needed to align the incisors, and this was gained by some interproximal reduction and aligned with the Invisalign system. Post-treatment, an extracoronal lingual bonded splint was evident as a fixed retainer (C). Active treatment took 5 months.

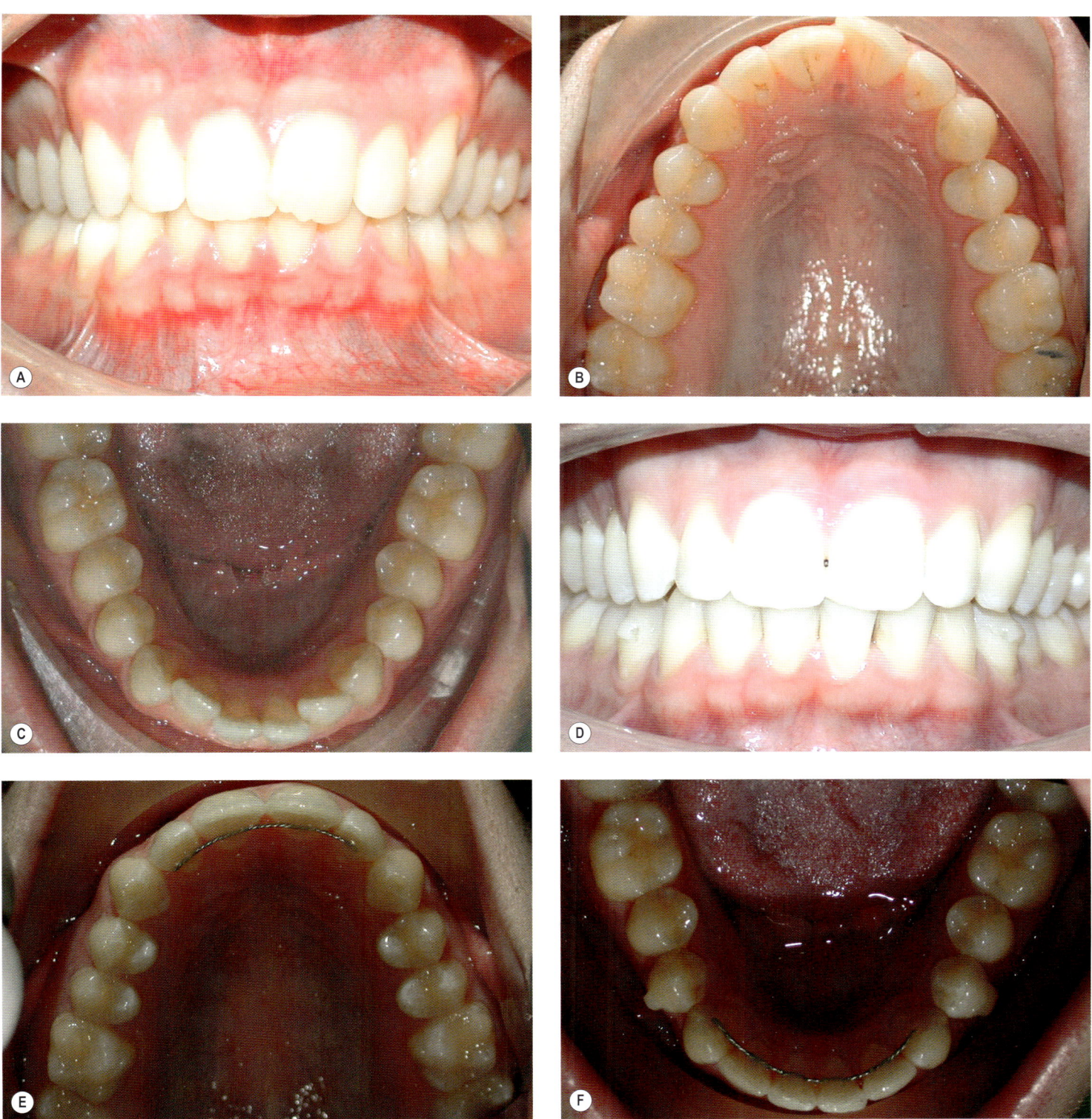

Fig. C7.2A–F (A–C) Pretreatment views of a bimaxillary Class I moderately crowded dentition. Alignment was achieved by a combination of interproximal reduction and lateral expansion using Invisalign. (D–F) Post-treatment result. Retention was achieved using extracoronal bonded lingual anterior splints (E,F). Active treatment took 7 months.

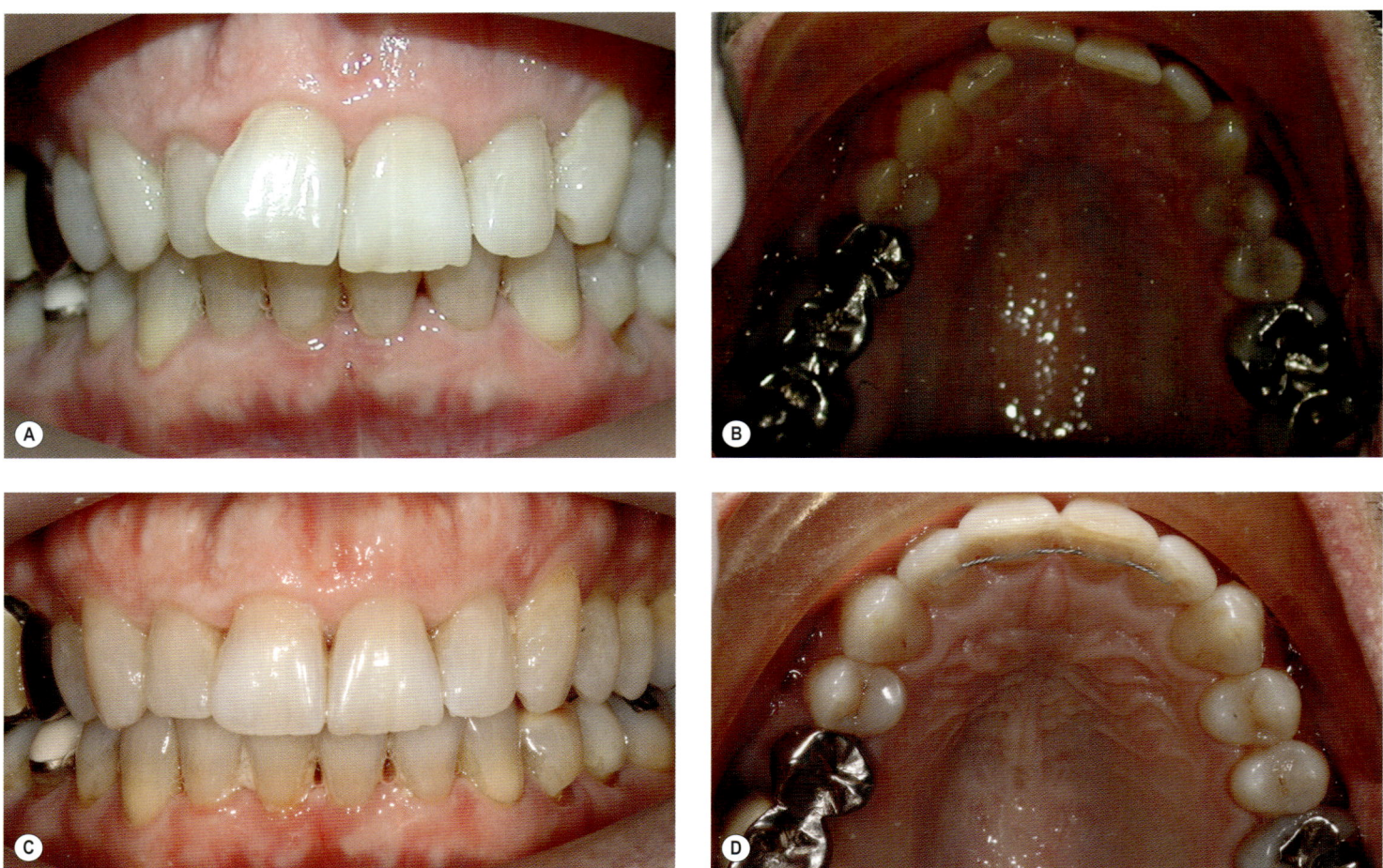

Fig. C7.3A–D A moderate–severely crowded maxillary arch characterized by incisal overlap. Alignment was achieved by a combination of lateral expansion and proclination. Retention was by extracoronal fixed lingual splint (D). Active treatment took 9 months.

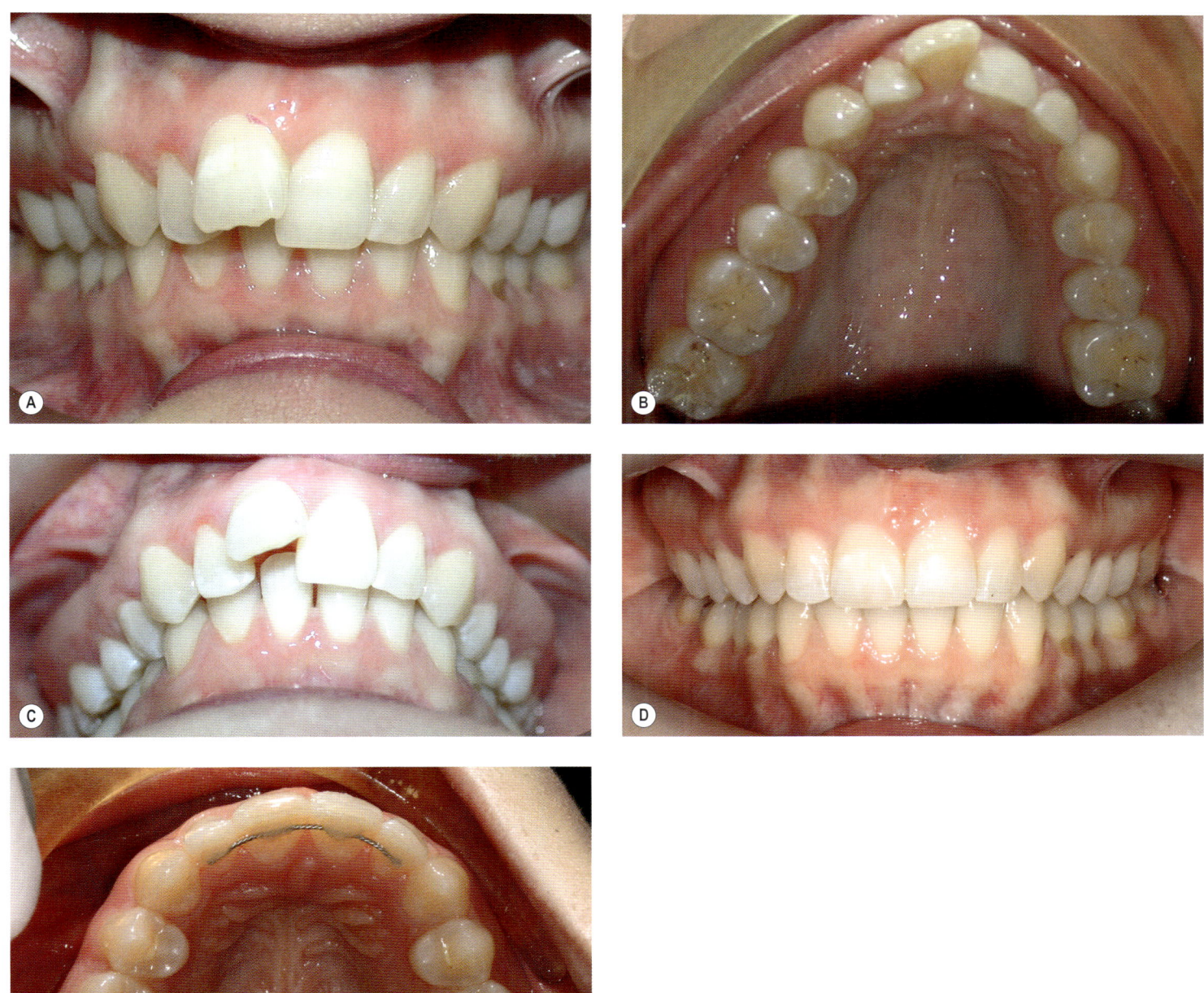

Fig. C7.4A–E (A–C) Pretreatment of a Class II severely crowded maxilla with a labially ectopic upper right central incisor and arch constriction. Alignment was achieved through Invisalign therapy programmed for arch expansion and anterior proclination. (D,E) Post-treatment result and a fixed lingual retainer. Active treatment time was 1 year.

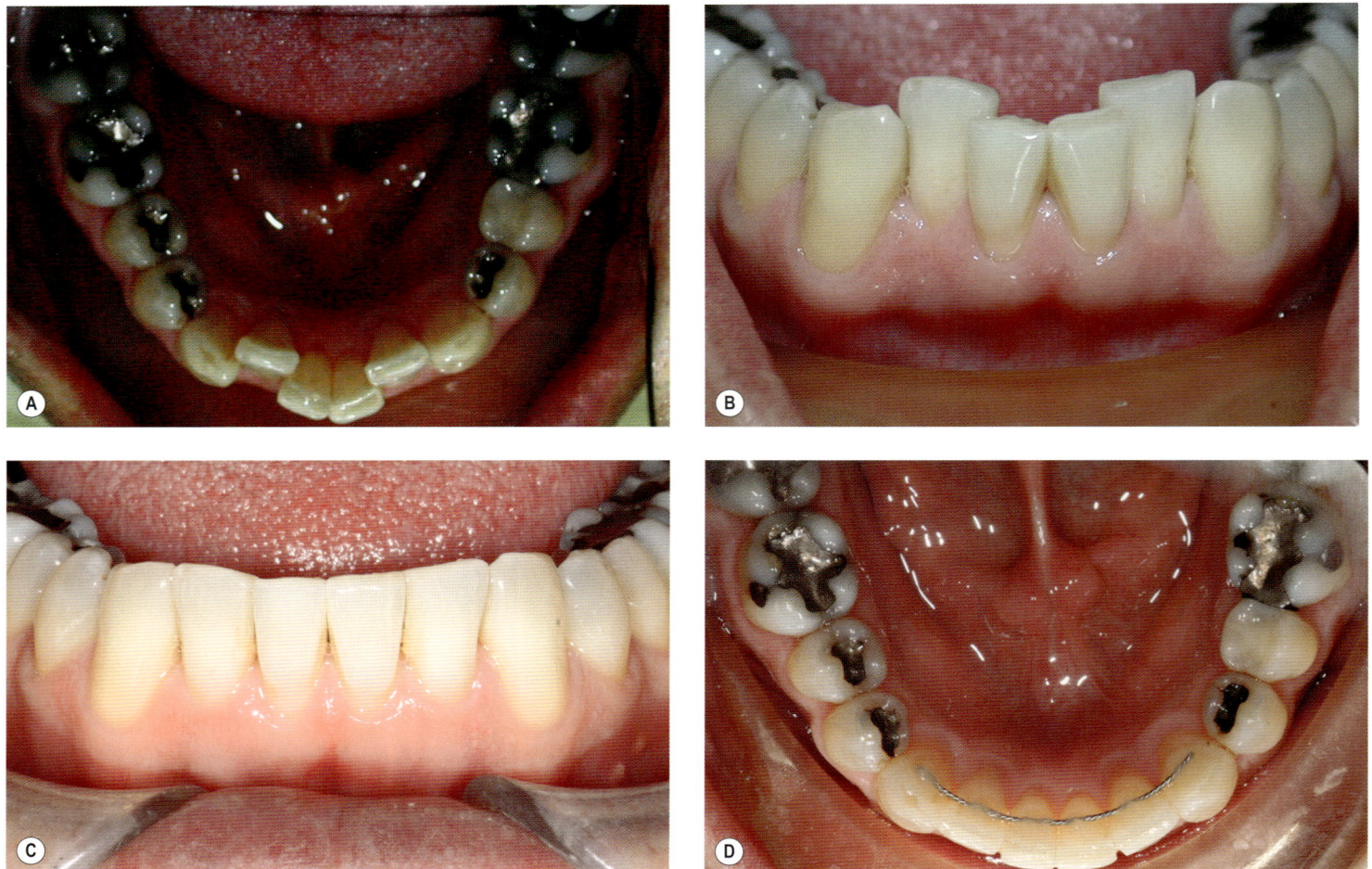

Fig. C7.5A–D This case shows severe mandibular anterior crowding characterized by lingual displacement of the lateral incisors. Alignment was achieved over 9 months of Invisalign therapy including a combination of interproximal reduction and anterior proclination. Retention was accomplished with a fixed lingual splint (D).

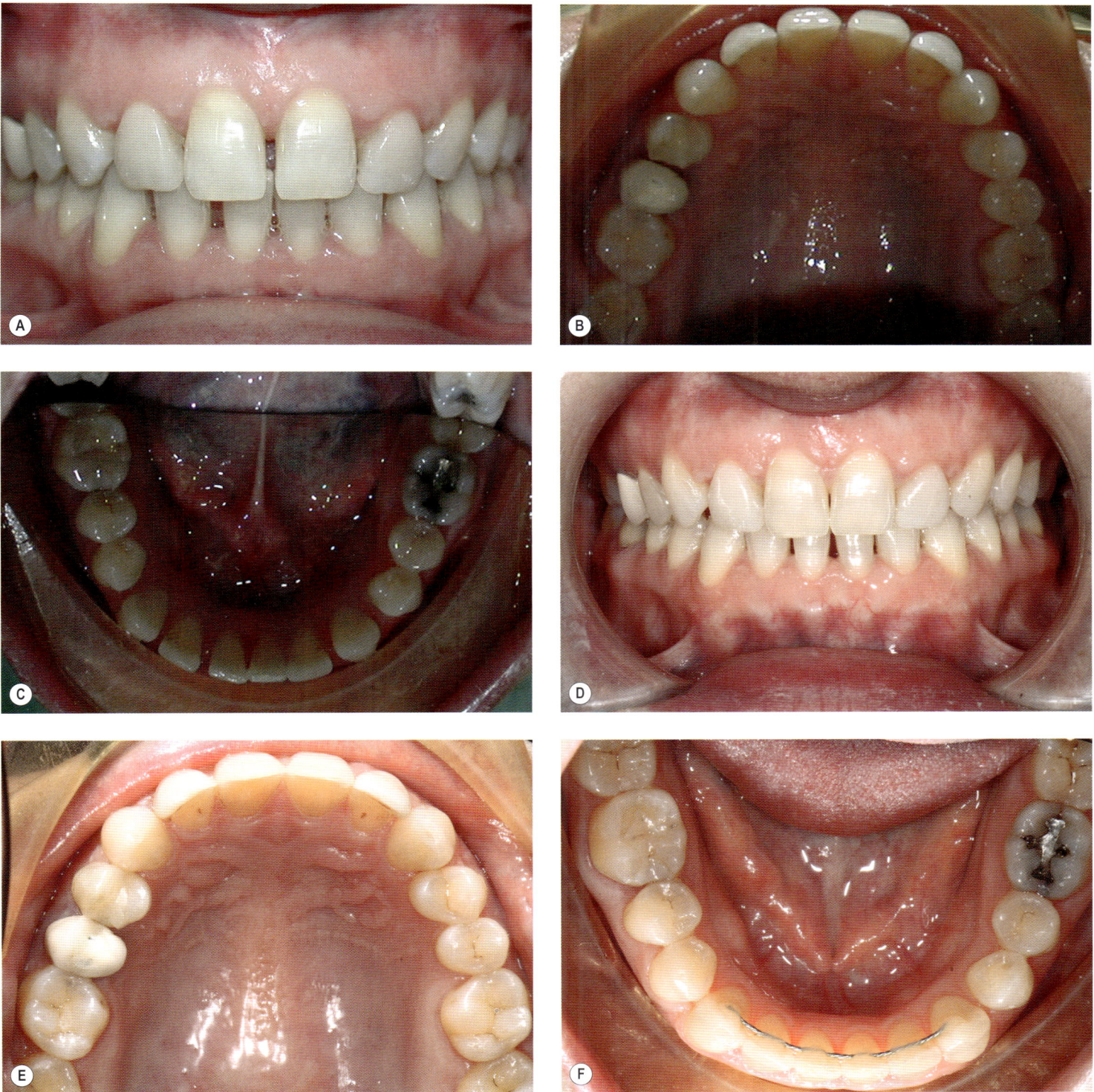

Fig. C7.6A–F (A–C) A Class I moderate spacing case. Spaces were closed over a 9-month period using a bimaxillary Invisalign appliance programmed for retraction. In cases like this, if there is minimal dental overjet, the mandibular movement must precede the maxillary to provide space. (D–F) Post-treatment result. Retention was achieved in this case by a combination of Invisalign retainer in the maxilla (removable) and a fixed lingual for the mandibular arch.

CLINICAL CASES

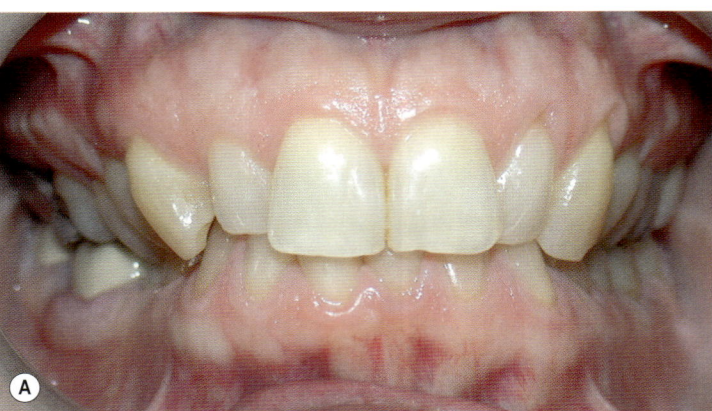 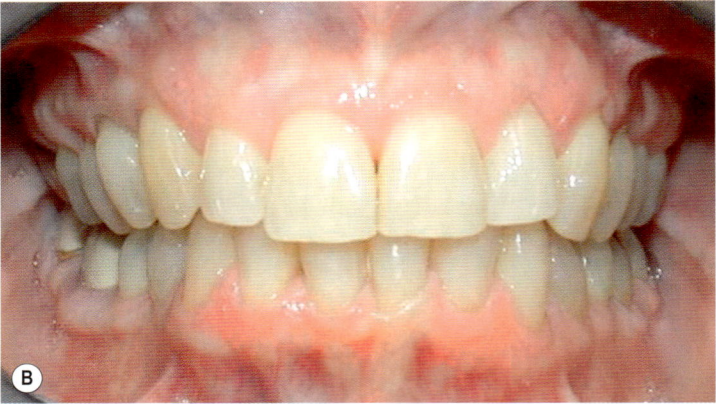

Fig. C7.7A,B   This case is severely crowded Class I dentition characterized by bimaxillary transverse constriction. Evident in the preclinical photo is extreme axial inclination of the bicuspid region. Correction would require lateral expansion and necessitates dual arch treatment. The post treatment photo is one year later. Much more of the dentition is visible and a broader smile is the result. In a case involving posterior lateral expansion, such as this, retention must extend to the posterior regions to prevent transverse relapse, and is accomplished in this case with removable retainers.

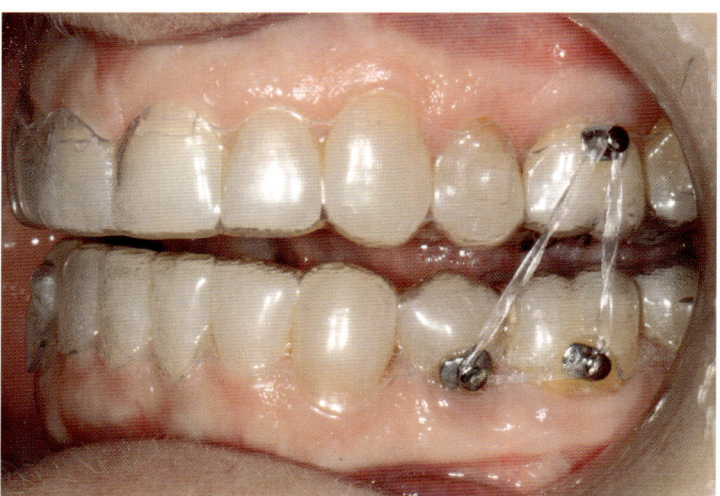

Fig. C7.8   This case shows the use of auxiliaries in conjunction with Invisalign aligners. Bonded buttons were used for the purpose of attaching triangulated intermaxillary elastic to erupt the left side molars and close a lateral open bite. The aligners were prefabricated with button cutouts to provide clearance for the bonded auxiliaries.

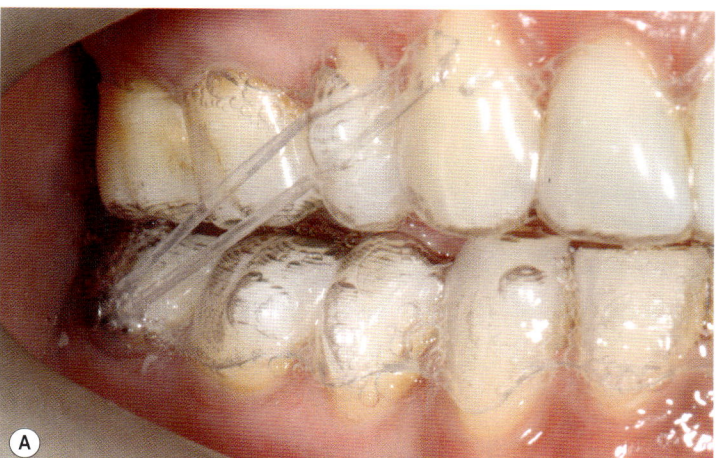
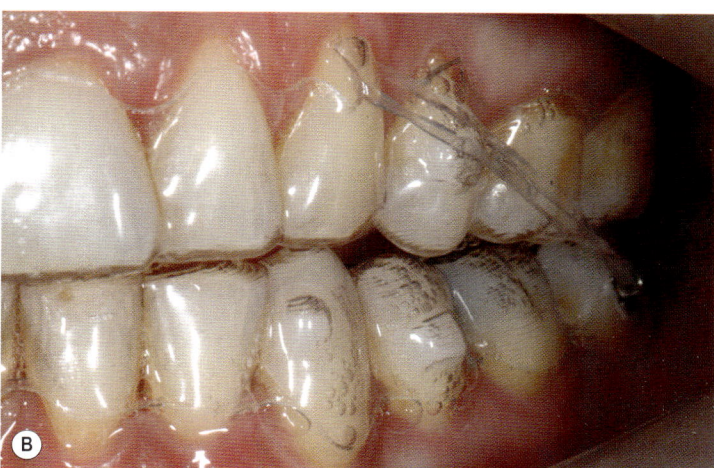

Fig. C7.9A,B A case illustrating Invisalign aligners prefabricated for provision of Class II elastics. The maxillary aligner features a 'precision cut' over the cuspids into which an interarch Class II elastic was hooked directly. There is also a mandibular 'button cutout' to provide clearance for a bonded auxiliary button to the lower molar to which the elastic was also hooked.

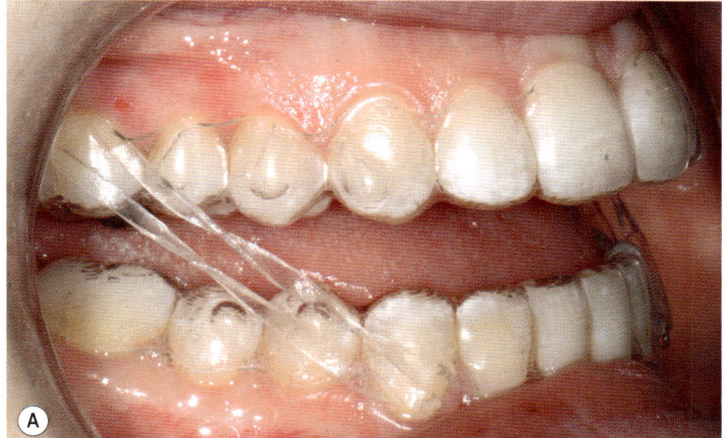
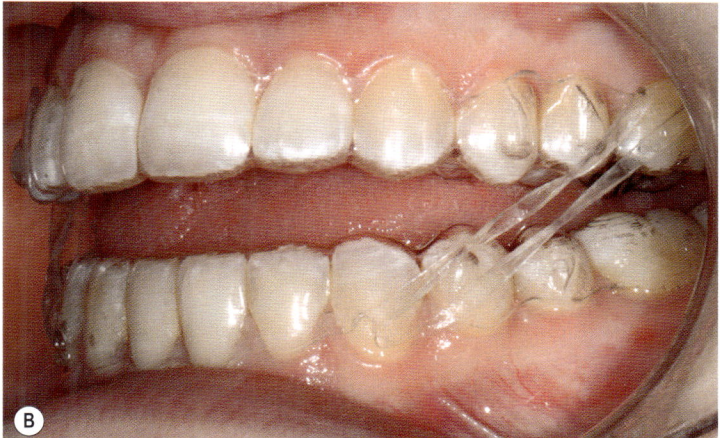

Fig. C7.10A,B This case illustrates the use of Invisalign to correct a Class III situation. Here the aligners were preprogrammed with 'precision cuts' to the maxillary molars and mandibular cuspids to facilitate the use of intermaxillary Class III elastics.

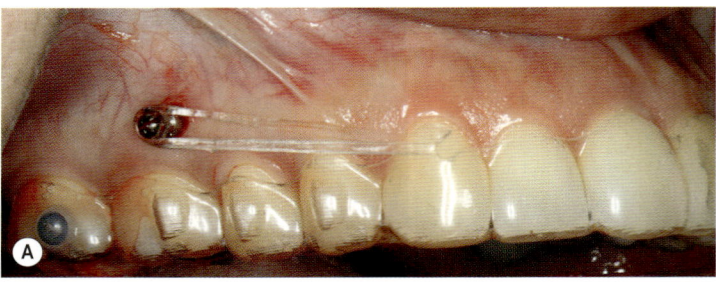
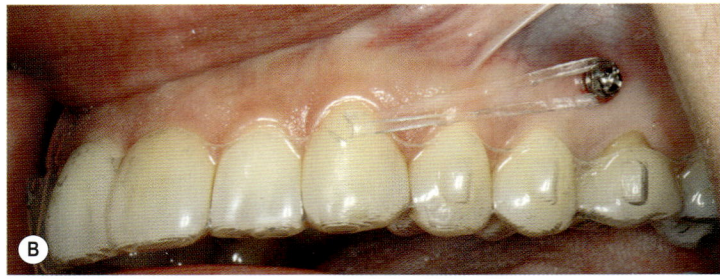

Fig. C7.11A,B The use of an orthodontic miniscrew, or temporary anchor device, for the purpose of securing a Class I elastomeric in conjunction with Invisalign therapy is shown. Full arch retraction can be effected in this way. The aligners were programmed with 'precision cuts' on the maxillary cuspids to allow the elastic to be fastened by the patient each time the aligner is placed. In this way, the elastomeric provides the necessary force and the aligners provide the guidance.

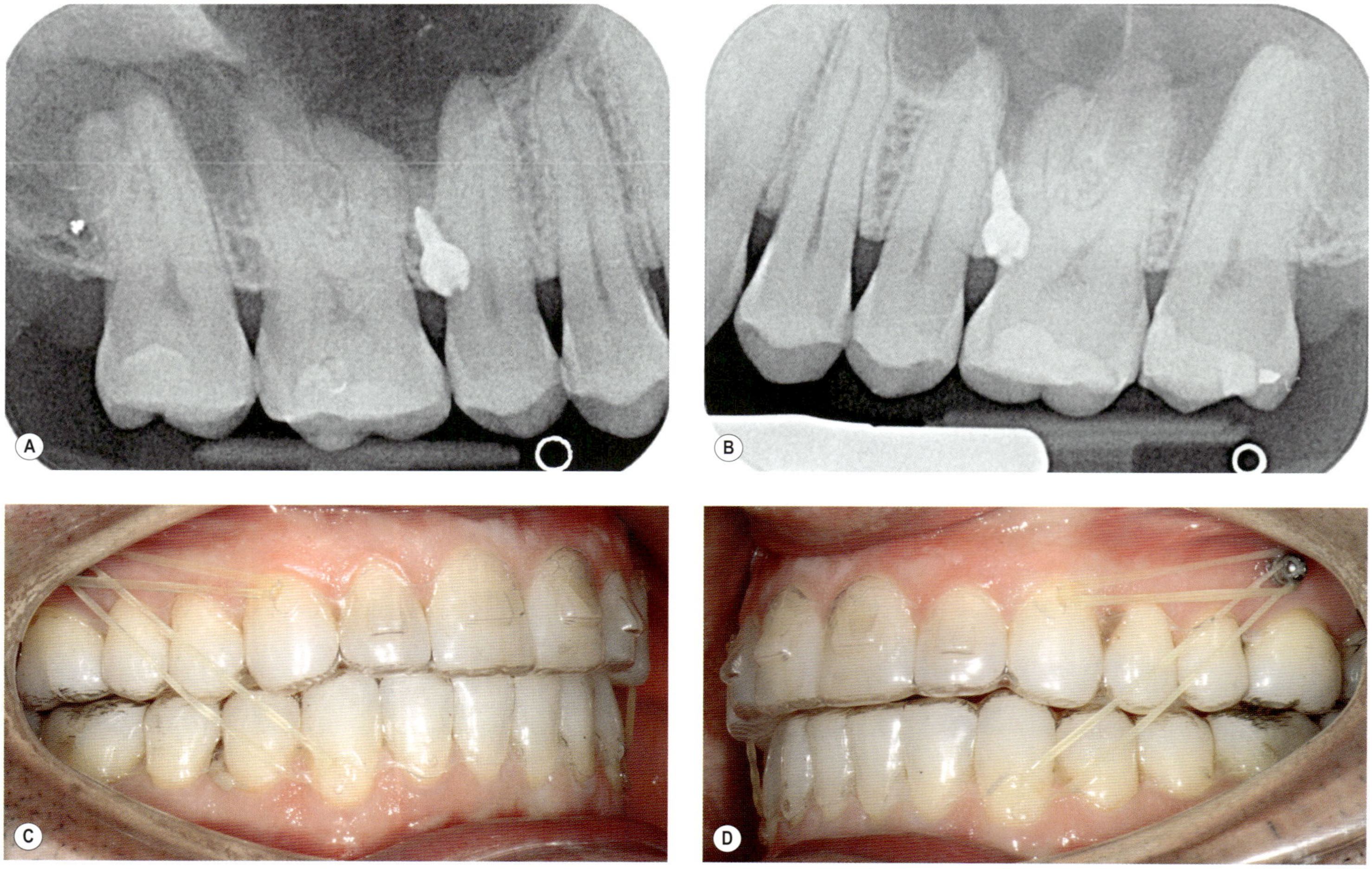

Fig. C7.12A–D Images showing the use of bilateral maxillary temporary anchor devices or miniscrews for bimaxillary anterior retraction. (A,B) Radiographs depicting the inter-radicular placement of miniscrews. (C,D) Class I and Class III elastics placed from the miniscrews to 'precision cuts' that were prefabricated in the aligners for fastening. The combination of miniscrews and elastics provide the necessary force and the aligners guide the movement. Once their function is completed, the temporary anchor devices are easily removed.

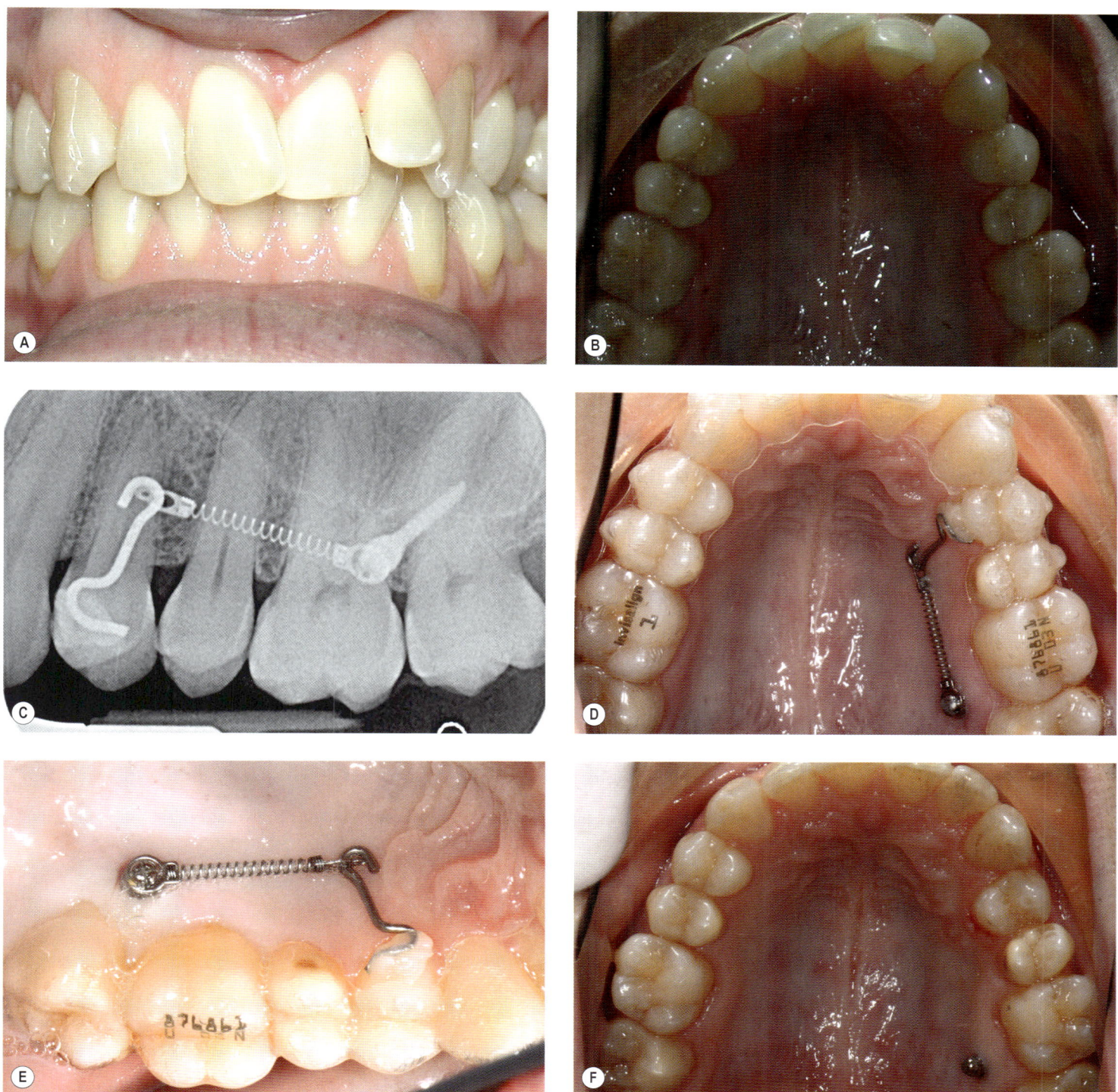

Fig. C7.13A–F This case shows a very simple and elegant way to utilize aligner therapy to achieve unilateral distal driving. A unilateral Class II division 2 case (or a subdivision) is shown and is characterized by a left-side Class II occlusion and corresponding labially locked upper left lateral incisor (A,B). (C) An Illustration of the force system, which comprises a palatally placed inter-radicular temporary anchor device and a bonded power arm to the bicuspid. A nickel titanium coil spring links the two. The power arm permits the application of force down the root surface, at or even apical to the tooth's centre of rotation. In this way, bodily movements can very efficiently be achieved. (D,E) Clinical intra-oral views illustrating how streamlined this force system is. Also visible in these photographs is the aligner, which was programmed to provide guidance for the movement. (F) A view after 10 months of therapy, with ideal arch alignment having been achieved. The power arm has been debonded and the miniscrew will subsequently be removed.

ACKNOWLEDGEMENT

The author would like to acknowledge and thank Mr Robert Maughn of Align-Technology for his assistance in the preparation of this manuscript and for providing some of the nonclinical images.

Further reading

Bollen AM, Huang G, King G, et al. Activation time and material stiffness of sequential removable orthodontic appliances. Part I: Ability to complete treatment. Am J Orthod Dentofacial Orthop 2003;124(5):496–501.

Boyd R, Miller R, Vlastic V. The Invisalign system in adult orthodontics: mild crowding and space closure cases. J Clin Orthod 2000;34(4):203–12.

Boyd R, Nelson G. Three-dimensional diagnosis and orthodontic treatment of complex malocclusions with the Invisalign appliance. Semin Orthod 2001;7(4):274–93.

Chisari J, McGorray S, Nair M, Wheeler T. Variables affecting orthodontic tooth movement with clear aligners. Am J Orthod Dentofacial Orthop 2014;146(Suppl. 4):S82–91.

Djue G, Shelton C, Maganzini AL. Outcome assessment of Invisalign and traditional orthodontic treatment compared with the American Board of Orthodontics Objective Grading System. Am J Orthod Dentofacial Orthop 2005;128(3):293–8.

Joffe L. Invisalign: early experiences. J Orthod 2003;30(4):348–52.

Kuncio D, Maganzini A, Shelton C, Freeman K. Invisalign and traditional orthodontic treatment postretention outcomes compared using the American Board of Orthodontics Objective Grading System. Angle Orthod 2007;77(5):864–9.

Lagravere M, Flores-Mir C. The treatment effects of Invisalign orthodontic appliances: a systematic review. J Am Dent Assoc 2005;136(12):1724–9.

Maganzini A. Outcome assessment of Invisalign and traditional orthodontic treatment and subsequent commentaries. Am J Orthod Dentofacial Orthop 2006;129(4):456.

Miller R, Duong T, Derackhsharn M. Lower incisor extraction treatment with the Invisalign system. J Clin Orthod 2002;36(2):95–102.

Phan X, Ling P. Clinical limitations of Invisalign. J Can Dent Assoc 2007;73(3):263–6.

Vlaskalic V, Boyd R. Orthodontic treatment of a mildly crowded malocclusion using the Invisalign system. Aust Orthod J 2001;17(1):41–6.

Womack W, Ahn J, Ammari Z, Castillo A. A new approach to correction of crowding. Am J Orthod Dentofacial Orthoped 2002;122(3):310–16.

Wong B. Invisalign A to Z. Am J Orthod Dentofacial Orthop 2002;121(5):540–1.

CHAPTER 8

Anterior Bonded Restorations

JONATHAN B. LEVINE, SIVAN FINKEL, ADRIAN JURIM

Introduction/History	**216**
Armamentarium for veneer preparation	**217**
Guidelines for veneer preparation	**220**
Step-by-step veneer preparation	**221**
Considerations for shade selection	**232**
The APT preparation technique	**235**
Retraction and impressioning	**236**
Provisionalization	**238**
Considerations for anterior mandibular veneers	**243**
Considerations for posterior veneers	**243**
Restoration of fractured and carious teeth with porcelain laminate veneers	**245**
Material selection	**246**
Insertion and finishing	**248**
Continuous care	**255**
Clinical case 8.1	**259**
Clinical case 8.2	**261**
Clinical case 8.3	**264**

INTRODUCTION/HISTORY

Our goal is to achieve predictable esthetics every time, and to accomplish this, we have chosen a methodical approach to solving esthetic problems: identifying the problem, visualizing the solution and then choosing the appropriate technique. The 'appropriate technique' is that which is most conservative in achieving our vision, and thus, minimally invasive porcelain veneers are a perfect solution to many esthetic problems.[1]

The porcelain veneer technique was first developed in 1980 by Adrian Jurim, a young porcelain technician working with Harold Horn at NYU, John Gwinett at Stony Brook and then John Calamia also working at NYU.[2–4] The Stony Brook team, with John Gwinett, set out to determine if the bond strength to etched dental porcelain was sufficiently strong enough for it to be a viable restorative material. The results were extremely encouraging, as the team found that the bond strength to etched porcelain exceeded the bond strength to etched enamel. The next step was to figure out clinical and laboratory requirements for restorations of this nature, including what the minimum thickness of porcelain veneers should be. The fabrication of the veneer by adapting the platinum foil technique proved to be accurate, predictable and efficient. The porcelain veneer was an incredible breakthrough that would change dentistry profoundly.[2]

Composite bonding, a very noble and revolutionary concept in the late 1970s and early 1980s, initiated the first steps in the evolution of esthetic (and adhesive) dentistry. However, at the clinical level, a high percentage of dentists did not enjoy or feel secure with the responsibility of incrementally reconstructing teeth – a responsibility that had until now belonged solely to the laboratory technician. Discomfort with this new challenge was one reason composite bonding was not completely embraced as the ideal solution for anterior esthetics. Additionally, although composites were and still are ideal for small anterior repairs, their relatively high wear potential and possibility for discolouration made them less than perfect for extensive anterior alterations.

Porcelain veneers provided a more durable, more esthetic solution than composite bonding, and thus their introduction catalysed a revolution in esthetic dentistry. The technique was overwhelmingly welcomed and absorbed into the profession, becoming the ideal standard of esthetic treatment. The porcelain veneer has proven to be one of the most conservative and successful options available to our patients, and it continues to evolve as we obtain new knowledge, materials and techniques.

ARMAMENTARIUM FOR VENEER PREPARATION

1. Reduction guides. The use of reduction guides when preparing teeth for veneers allows the clinician to be as minimally invasive as possible, and oftentimes reveals a tooth to need very little preparation. Reduction guides can be made from a number of materials, including the classic method of a clear vacuum stent (Fig. 8.1A,B), but the authors favour the use of polyvinyl siloxane putty. Typically, two putty indexes are taken of the diagnostic wax-up; one is trimmed to reveal proposed incisal length and edge position (Fig. 8.2A–C) and the other is trimmed to show facial clearance (Fig. 8.3A–C). The guide should extend onto several teeth distal to those being prepared, and the incisal guide should also extend to the palate for more stability.[5]

By working backwards from this index of the diagnostic wax-up, the guide enables the reshaping of the teeth prior to the final preparation if needed. This need for pre-preparation enameloplasty is common in reductive scenarios (i.e. overlapped or rotated teeth) and cases where the midline is to be shifted or the mesiodistal dimensions of teeth have to be changed.[5]

CLINICAL TIP

Reduction guides allow visualization of the final incisal edge position and an understanding of the final tooth form. In prepping cases with any reductive aspects, i.e. correcting a rotation, before any space can be made for porcelain, the reduction guide must sit passively on the teeth.

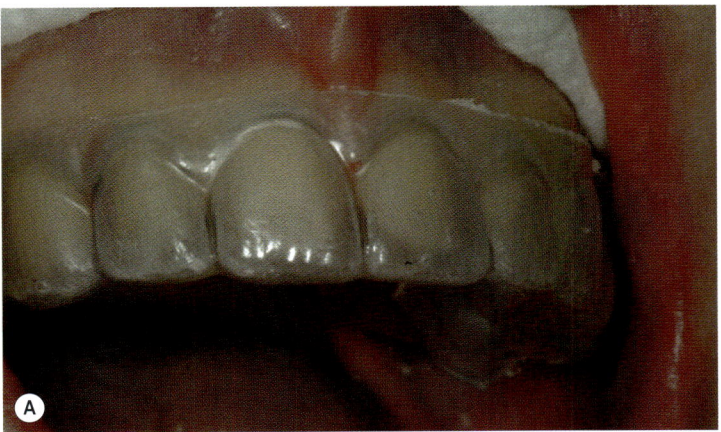 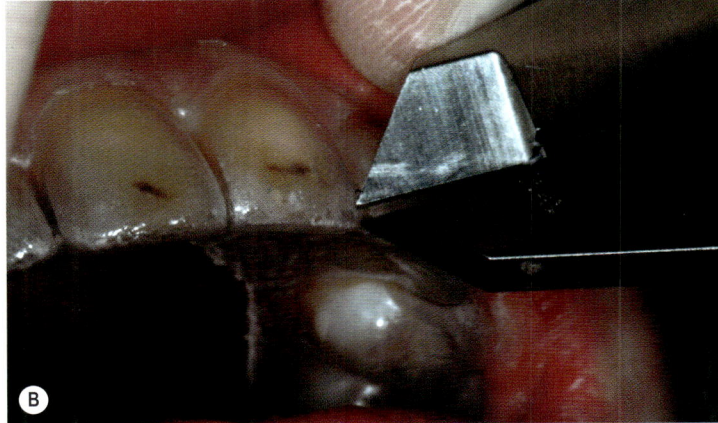

Fig. 8.1A,B A classic vacuum-style stent (made on a cast of the wax-up and not the wax-up itself). A digital caliper is used to measure clearance or a periodontal probe can be placed through holes in the plastic stent.

ARMAMENTARIUM FOR VENEER PREPARATION

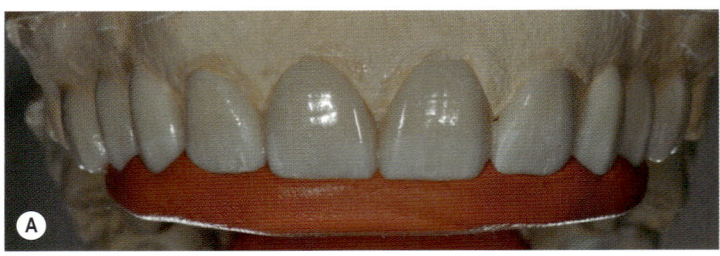
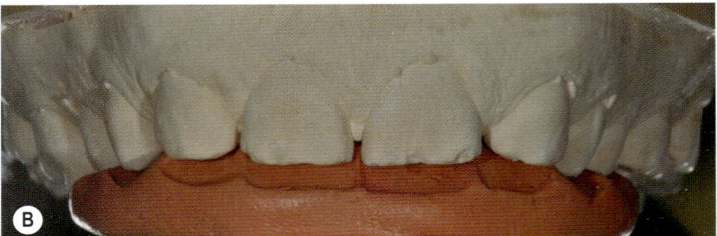
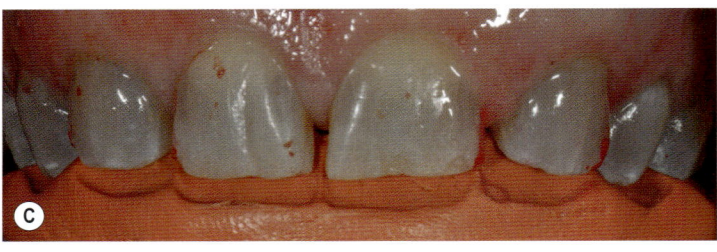

Fig. 8.2A–C   A PVS reduction guide, based on the wax-up and trimmed to show incisal clearance and proposed incisal edge position. Note the areas marked with red pencil, which lie outside the proposed tooth forms and must be trimmed prior to veneer preparation.

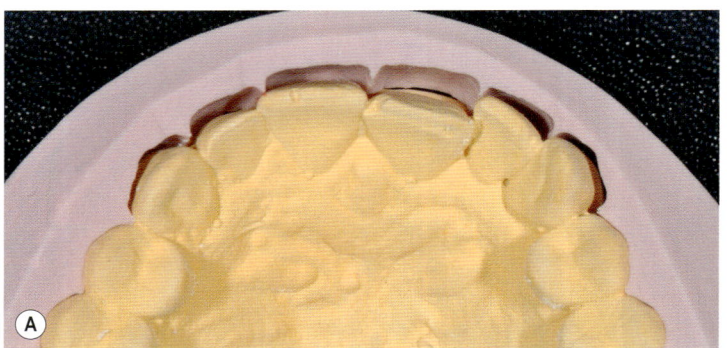
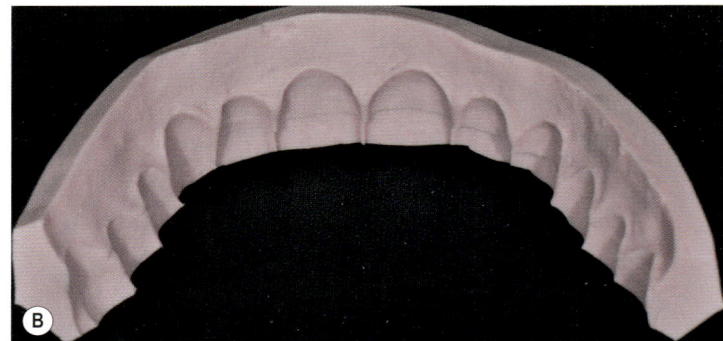
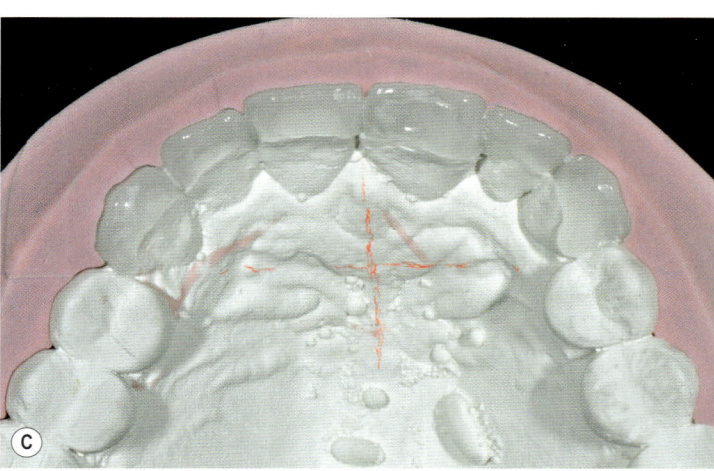

Fig. 8.3A–C   A PVS reduction guide trimmed to show facial clearance. In this case, the distal aspect of #8 tooth can be seen lying outside the proposed tooth form and must be reduced before veneer preparation begins.

Chapter 8
Anterior Bonded Restorations

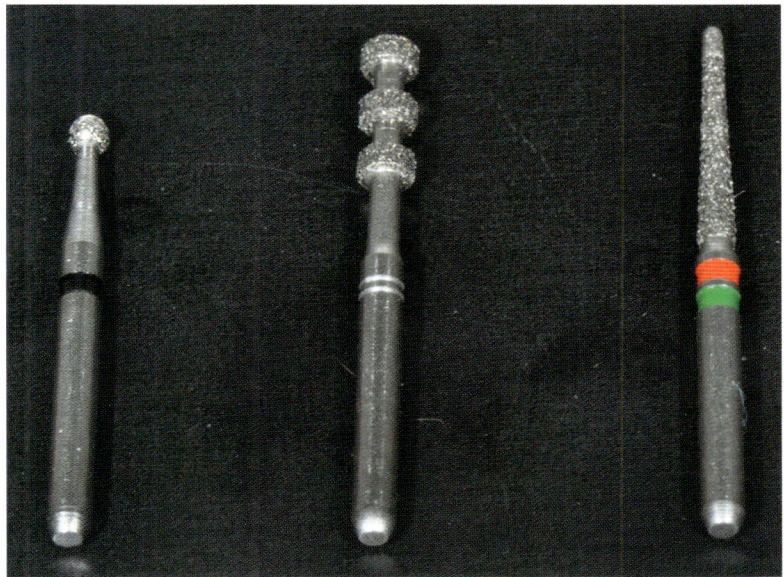

Fig. 8.4 For optimal efficiency, each of these burs should be picked up only once and used on each tooth before moving onto the next bur.

2. The 1 mm round diamond bur (Brasseler 5801.31.016) (Fig. 8.4) acts as a compass, tracing the gingival and proximal finishing lines. The bur should be placed halfway into the enamel, resulting in a 0.5 mm demarcation. One benefit of using a round bur is that the handpiece can be orientated in any direction, and the bur's cutting edge remains centered. This bur is also used to make incisal reduction depth guides, which vary depending on the proposed length of the final restoration. Note that the diameter of this bur must always be measured with a digital caliper, as they are not always consistent.

3. A self-limiting depth reduction bur (Brasseler 834.31.016 and 834.31.021) (Fig. 8.4) with three doughnut-like circles will give proper labial reduction on three planes (ginvigal, body and incisal). The clinician holds the bur parallel to each plane to assure proper reduction in that plane, and the 'bald' areas of the bur ensure that the bur does not penetrate further than the desired depth. These burs are available in 0.3 or 0.5 mm versions, and several other variations have been recently introduced.

4. A two-grit gross reduction bur (Brasseler 6844.31.016) (Fig. 8.4) is used to connect all of the depth reduction grooves and smooth out all the transitional angles. Additionally, the gingival and interproximal finish lines are refined with the fine-grit portion of this bur, as the clinician confirms gingival margin placement and makes sure the interproximal margin ('elbow') is sufficiently out of view. A third use for the gross

reduction bur, as described above, is at the very beginning of any reductive case, when enameloplasty must be performed to seat the teeth within the preparation guide passively.

5. Rubber wheels, 3M discs and thin metal proximal strips to further round all transitional areas and edges.

GUIDELINES FOR VENEER PREPARATION

To begin the discussion of the 'ideal' veneer preparation (Fig. 8.5) some crucial guidelines must be established first:

- The thickness of the porcelain laminate veneer should not be less than 0.5 mm ideally for feldspathic porcelain, and 0.3 mm for lithium disilicate (IPS e.max Ivoclar Vivadent).

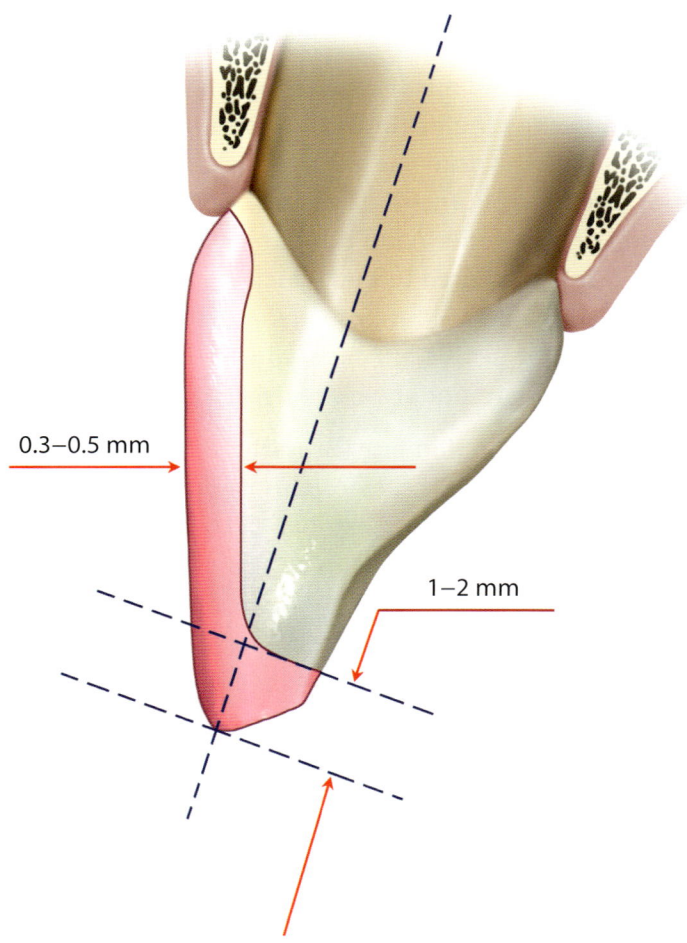

Fig. 8.5 **The ideal veneer preparation for a maxillary incisor.**

- The porcelain should be 1.0–1.5 mm thick in high stress bearing areas (i.e. incisally). Adequate incisal reduction also permits a positive seat during insertion and cementation and hides incisal margins.

- Sharp line angles anywhere in the preparation will create stress points and can eventually fracture the porcelain laminate veneer.

- Proper reduction at the gingival third of the tooth is essential to prevent overcontouring of the porcelain. Sufficient reduction in this area will give the laminate a natural emergence profile, which is crucial to both esthetics and periodontal health.

- Proximal preparation permits concealment of the interproximal finishing line and additional wrap-around for greater bond strengths (i.e. more enamel to be in contact with the porcelain). Furthermore, the increased thickness of the porcelain edges makes the restoration less likely to chip during insertion.

STEP-BY-STEP VENEER PREPARATION

PRE-PREPARATION ENAMELOPLASTY

After anaesthesia has been administered, seat the reduction guide(s) intra-orally and check that the existing dentition sits passively within the outline of the preparation guide. If not, reshape the teeth just enough to accomplish this. The areas in question can be marked in red while the guide is seated, and then adjusted accordingly with the guide out of the mouth. Once this has been achieved, the 1 mm round diamond bur is used to scribe the intended gingival and interproximal margins, and to make incisal depth cuts (Fig. 8.6).

PLACEMENT OF GINGIVAL MARGINS

The determining factors for gingival margin placement of the restoration are the height of the lip line, the colour of the prepared tooth you are covering and the periodontal biotype (thin or thick).

In a high smile line patient, absolute symmetry of the gingival margins of the central incisors is critical for esthetic success. Moving away from the midline, the importance of symmetry decreases. The margin placement for the central incisors needs to be exactly even, and this is done by getting in front of the patient and using a coloured pencil to line up the zenith points of the preparation margins (as is known, the zeniths should also both be placed slightly distal to each central's midline.)

STEP-BY-STEP VENEER PREPARATION

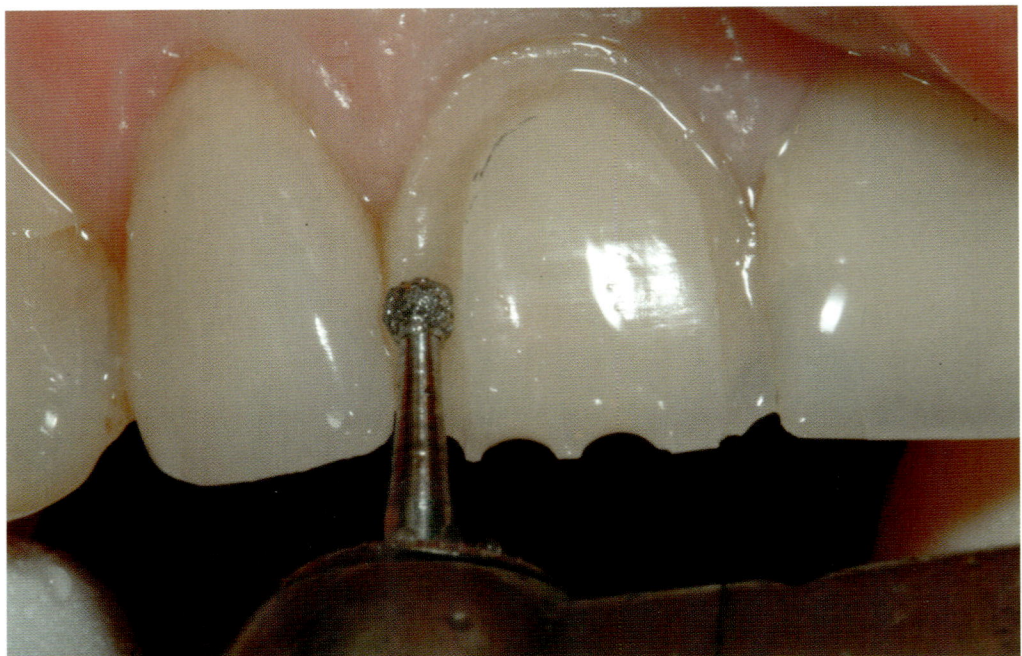

Fig. 8.6 Making incisal depth cuts.

CLINICAL TIP

Although the soft tissue height on one central might be more apical than the other, by levelling the finish lines the eye will go to that levelled preparation (Fig. 8.7).

If the goal is for the final restoration to be the same shade as the prepared tooth, then the gingival finishing line can always be kept supragingival. In a situation where the colour difference between the prepared tooth and the restoration is not that drastic, an equigingival placement of the finishing line is acceptable. Finally, in a situation where the difference in shade between the stump shade and the finished restoration is great, a subgingival or even intracrevicular finishing line is critical for preventing a dark halo from surrounding the restoration. Intracrevicular preparation is defined as the clinician probing the sulcus and not exceeding greater than 50% apical margin placement within the healthy sulcus. Once the sulcus is probed, the margin placement can be done carefully without injuring the soft tissue and it is still possible to achieve predictable soft tissue esthetics.

CLINICAL TIP

A good rule of thumb for a subgingival preparation is: the greater the contrast between the starting and desired shades, the further the finish line is placed within the sulcus for a maxillary porcelain laminate veneer (Fig. 8.8).

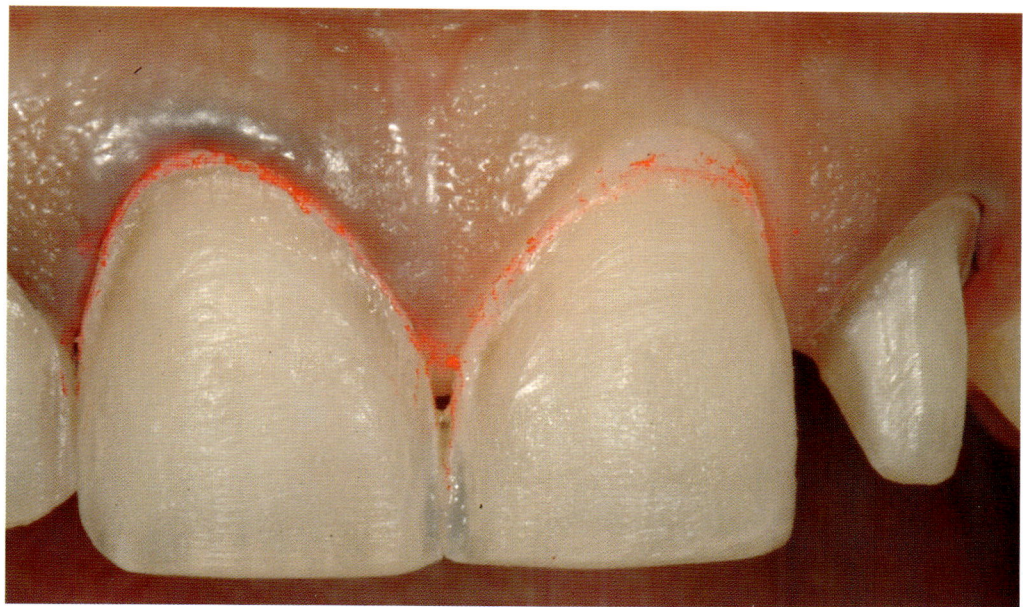

Fig. 8.7 In a high smile line patient, absolute symmetry of the gingival margins of the central incisors is critical for esthetic success.

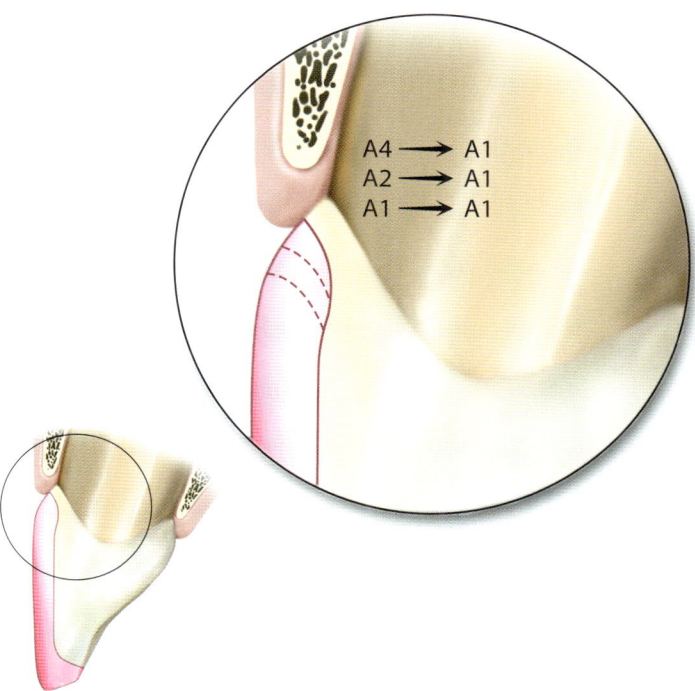

Fig. 8.8 Three different shade shift scenarios and the appropriate gingival margin placement.

The third important consideration in gingival margin placement is the patient's periodontal biotype, or whether the gingival tissue is thick or thin. This is determined by placing a periodontal probe into the sulcus; if you can see the colour of the probe through the tissue, this is a thin periodontal biotype and is more prone to recession. With a thin biotype patient, be as atraumatic as possible, especially if the intracrevicular preparation is indicated. In the thick periodontal biotype, insulting the tissue will usually result in an inflammation of the tissue and the tissue growing coronally, not apically.

CLINICAL TIP

With all the above points considered, the 'perfect storm' of an esthetic challenge is the combination of high smile line, discoloured and/or dark root, thin periodontal biotype and an asymmetry at the gingival margin of the central incisors.

PLACEMENT OF INTERPROXIMAL MARGINS

Like the gingival finish line, the position of interproximal finishing lines for veneers varies depending on the final esthetic goal.

When contact points between teeth can be maintained (as they should be unless tooth positions are being shifted), the teeth are prepared with at least a 0.5 mm deep chamfer interproximally, with an 'elbow' region tucking in just apical to the contact point. Ideally, the finishing line should be brought as far lingual as possible without breaking contacts (Fig. 8.9). Problems arise when this margin is not placed lingually enough and the junction between the porcelain restoration and tooth is noticeable. This is esthetically unacceptable, especially in cases with a drastic shade change.

When contact points are missing due to the presence of a diastema, the interproximal finishing line concept changes considerably. In these situations, a straight finishing line or 'slice prep' at the interproximal next to the diastema is preferred over a chamfer. Figure 8.10 demonstrates how the interproximal finishing line for a porcelain laminate veneer varies depending on the presence of contact points. The illustration shows a straight finishing line on the mesial of teeth numbers 8 and 9 due to the presence of a diastema, while the contact points on the distal of those teeth were left intact with a conventional deep chamfer interproximal finishing line.

Figure 8.11 highlights the proper interproximal straight wall finishing line preparation when a diastema is present (tooth #8) in comparison to the incorrect chamfer preparation (tooth #9). The straight finishing line on the mesial of tooth #8 allows the technician to build up the porcelain so that there is a smooth transition from the porcelain laminate veneer to the lingual contour of

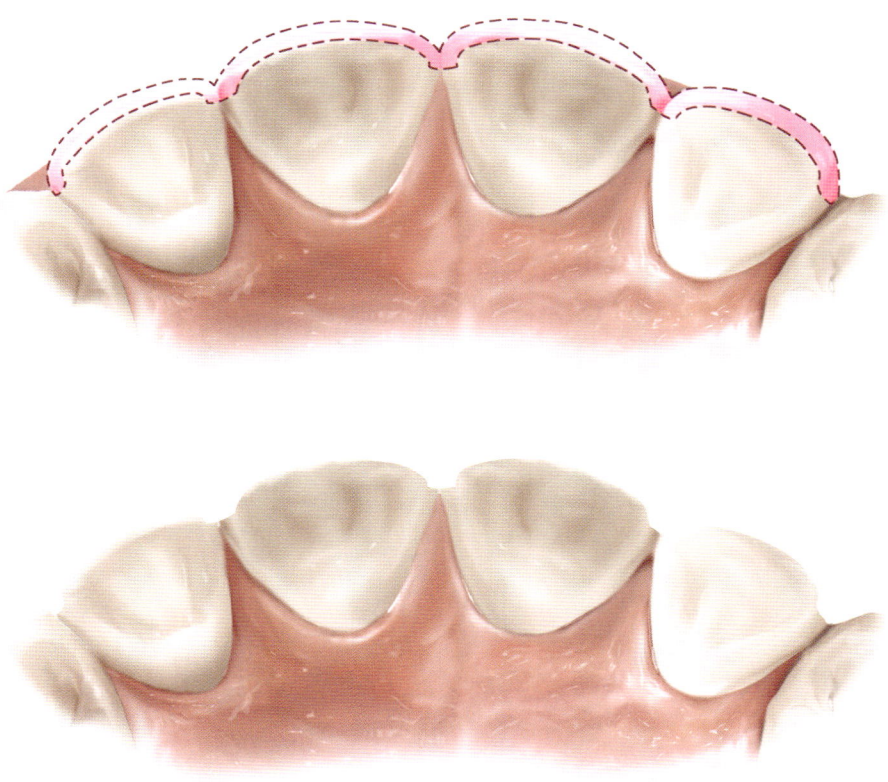

Fig. 8.9 The finish line is brought as far as possible in the lingual direction without breaking contact.

the tooth. However, the sharp line angle created by the chamfer preparation on the mesial of tooth #9 prevents the technician from being able to bring the porcelain into continuation with the tooth's lingual contour while trying to close the diastema. The resulting ledge of porcelain becomes both an irritant to the tongue and a plaque trap, stressing the importance of adapting a straight interproximal finishing line in cases where a diastema is present.

In other cases where tooth proportions (i.e. mesial and distal widths) are to be altered to achieve an esthetic smile balance (tooth-to-tooth proportion), contact points must be broken during tooth preparation so that placement of the mesial and distal extents of the teeth can be modified. In such cases, the interproximal finishing lines are once again a straight wall 'slice prep' so that the final porcelain veneers smoothly meet the lingual contour of the teeth.

Particular attention must also be paid to the reduction at the gingival–interproximal junction. When this area is reduced less than the required 0.5 mm, the finished case will look overcontoured and impingement of the papilla is very possible.

STEP-BY-STEP VENEER PREPARATION

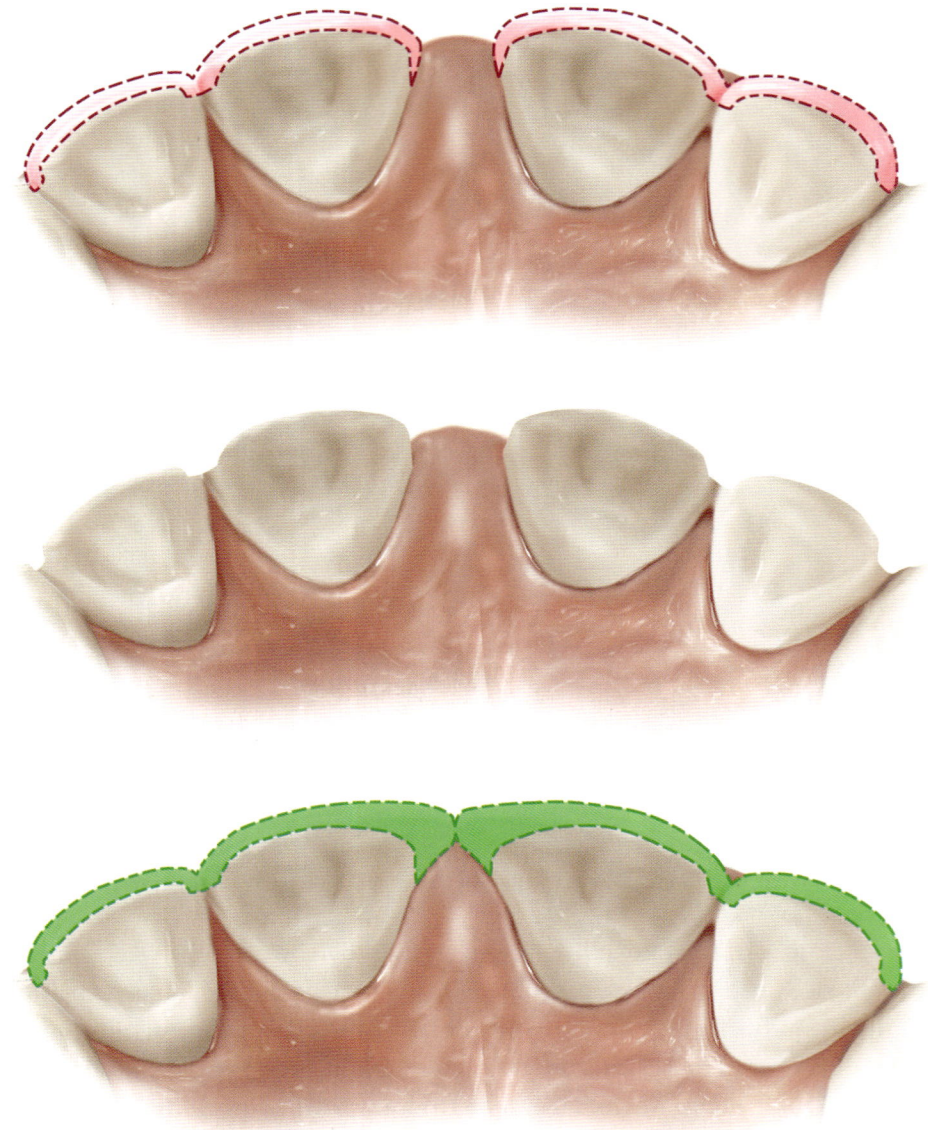

Fig. 8.10 When closing a diastema the 'slice' preparation is used.

INCISAL REDUCTION

Still using the 1 mm round diamond bur, create depth grooves for incisal edge reduction (Fig. 8.12) with the following considerations in mind:

- Conventional incisal preparation calls for a 1.0–1.5 mm thickness of porcelain to be present at the incisal edge, such that when a force is applied

ANTERIOR BONDED RESTORATIONS

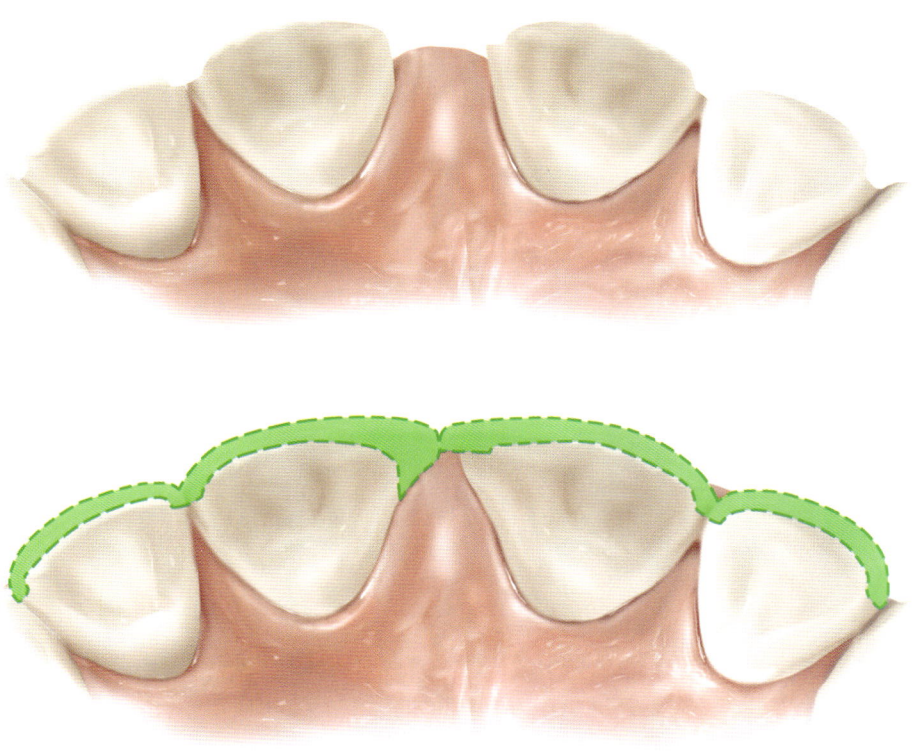

Fig. 8.11 A correct versus incorrect preparation for diastema closure.

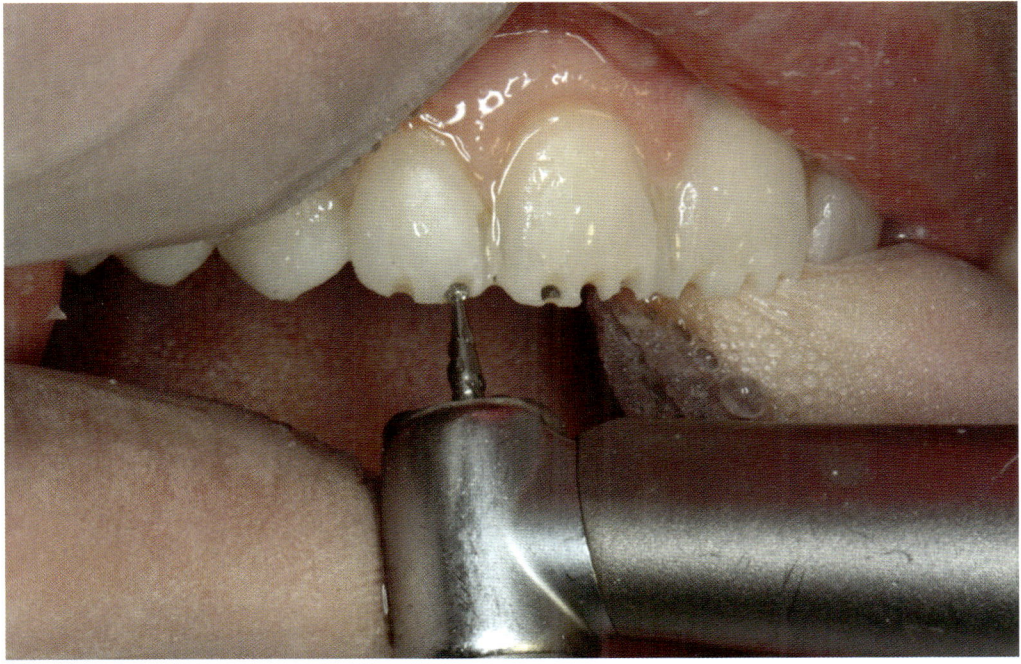

Fig. 8.12 Depth grooves for incisal edge reduction.

227

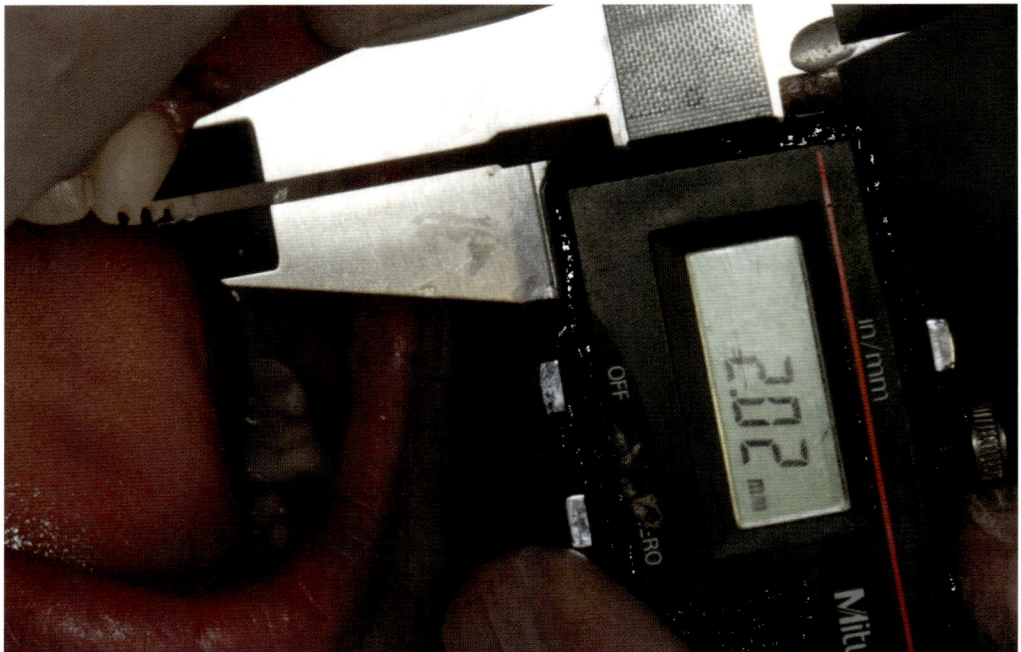

Fig. 8.13   A digital caliper being used to verify proper incisal reduction.

incisally it is compressive in nature and not a peeling force. If naturalness (i.e. incisal translucency or incisal edge contour) is desired, the incisal reduction should be closer to 2 mm.

- If the incisal position of the existing tooth is being changed, then it must be prepared as defined by the diagnostic wax-up to allow the technician to place it in the desired final position. The use of digital calipers, to measure precisely where you want to go, together with the incisal edge reduction guide help to achieve the precise reduction. The authors use the digital caliper for esthetic diagnostics and all through treatment, and 'will not leave home without it' (Fig. 8.13).

- The occlusion should be considered as the incisal reduction is performed. Ideally, the centric stops of the teeth being prepared should be marked before preparation and not violated. However, if a tooth must be reduced into the area of an occlusal contact, ensure that the resulting contact will be completely on porcelain. This might require slightly more reduction than the reduction guide dictates. In other words, contact on enamel is preferred, followed by contact on porcelain, but the contact should never be at the porcelain–enamel junction.

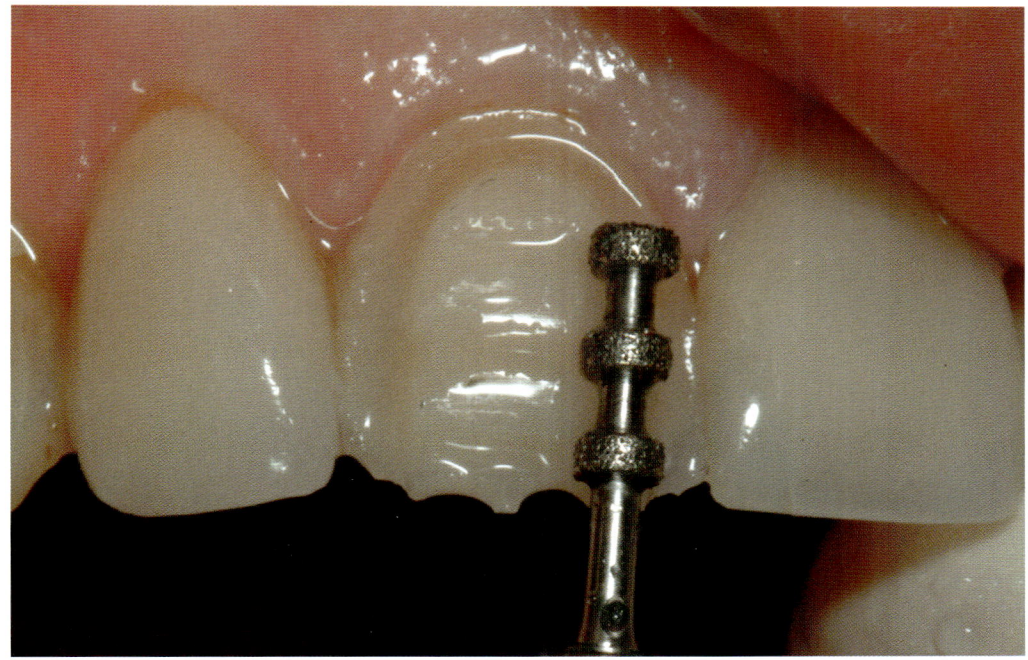

Fig. 8.14 Facial depth cuts.

FACIAL PREPARATION

After the gingival, proximal and incisal limits of the preparation have been defined, facial depth cuts are performed with the 0.3 or 0.5 mm reduction bur (depending on degree of shade shift and material selection), holding the bur parallel to the tooth's gingival third, middle third and then the incisal third (Fig. 8.14). The three planes are depicted in Figure 8.15. At this stage, the labial reduction guide should be seated to verify where facial reduction is needed and where it is not actually necessary.[5]

CONNECTING THE DEPTH CUTS AND FINISHING

The facial and incisal depth cuts are then connected and smoothed with the medium-grit body of the two-grit gross reduction bur (Fig. 8.16), while the fine-grit end of the bur refines the finish line. Care should be taken to ensure there are no undercuts or sharp angles as the preparation transitions from the finishing line to the facial and incisal surfaces of the tooth.[5]

The incisal depth cuts should be joined and blended at an angle perpendicular to the long axis of the tooth. If the incisal reduction is done on an apically sloping angle on the lingual (Fig. 8.17) instead of being perpendicular to the tooth's long axis, the resulting acute line angle acts as a chisel and can fracture

STEP-BY-STEP VENEER PREPARATION

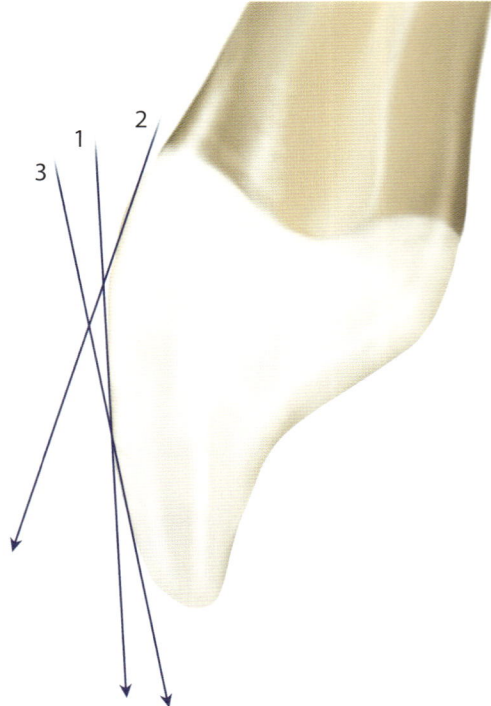

Fig. 8.15 The three planes of facial reduction.

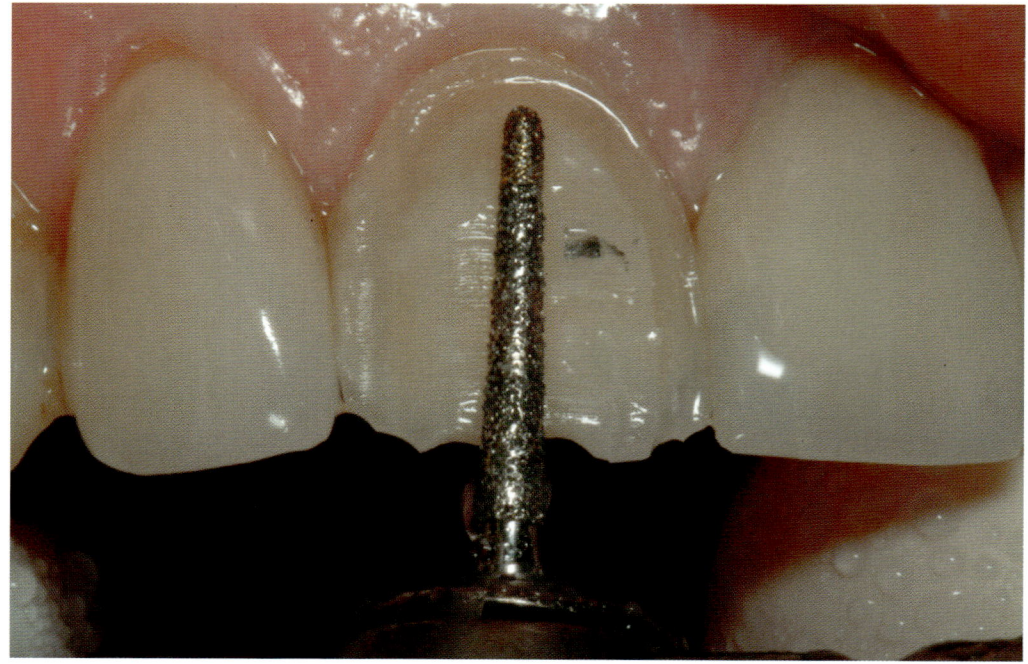

Fig. 8.16 The two-grit bur connects the depth cuts and refines the finish line.

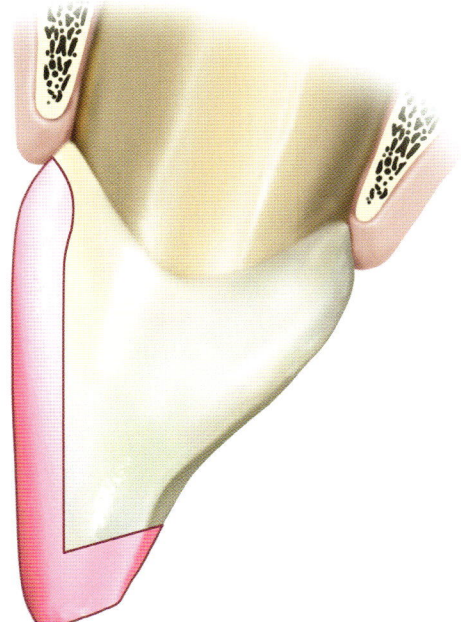 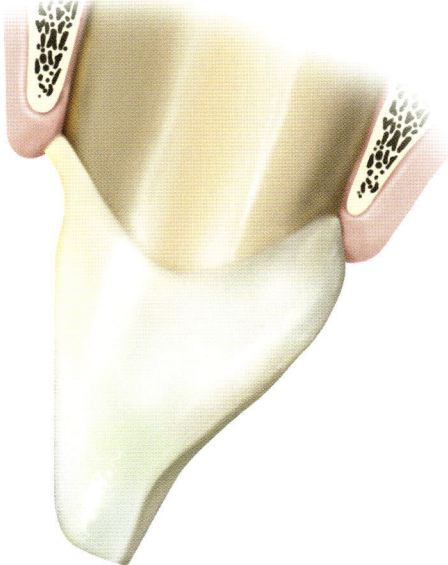

Fig. 8.17 Acutely angled, apically sloping incisal reduction can lead to porcelain fracture over time.

Fig. 8.18 The appropriate angle of incisal reduction, with a rounded labial–incisal angle and a lingual–incisal butt joint.

the porcelain over time. Figure 8.18 shows the appropriate angle of incisal reduction.

It is also critical that the preparation's labial–incisal angle is rounded, while the lingual–incisal finishing line remains a sharp butt joint (Fig. 8.18). When the labial–incisal angle is not rounded off, the sharp internal angle invites porcelain fracture.

A second consequence of an unrounded labial–incisal angle is an acute demarcation of colour between the restoration's incisal and body shades. This is demonstrated in Figure 8.19A, where light reflects off an improperly prepared tooth but travels through the restorative porcelain at the incisal edge. Figure 8.19B reveals how the rounded labial–incisal line angle in a properly prepared tooth reflects light in all directions, yielding an ideal transition of the restoration's shade from body to incisal colour.

It is very difficult to definitively seat porcelain laminate veneers on teeth lacking any incisal preparation, and so, even in cases where the teeth are being lengthened and already have adequate porcelain space (i.e. no incisal depth cuts needed), it is prudent to at least flatten the incisal edge and round off the labial–incisal angle.

Once the preparation is further refined and smoothed with 3M discs, rubber wheels and interproximal strips, the stump shade is recorded (Fig. 8.20) and the impression is ready to be taken.

CONSIDERATIONS FOR SHADE SELECTION

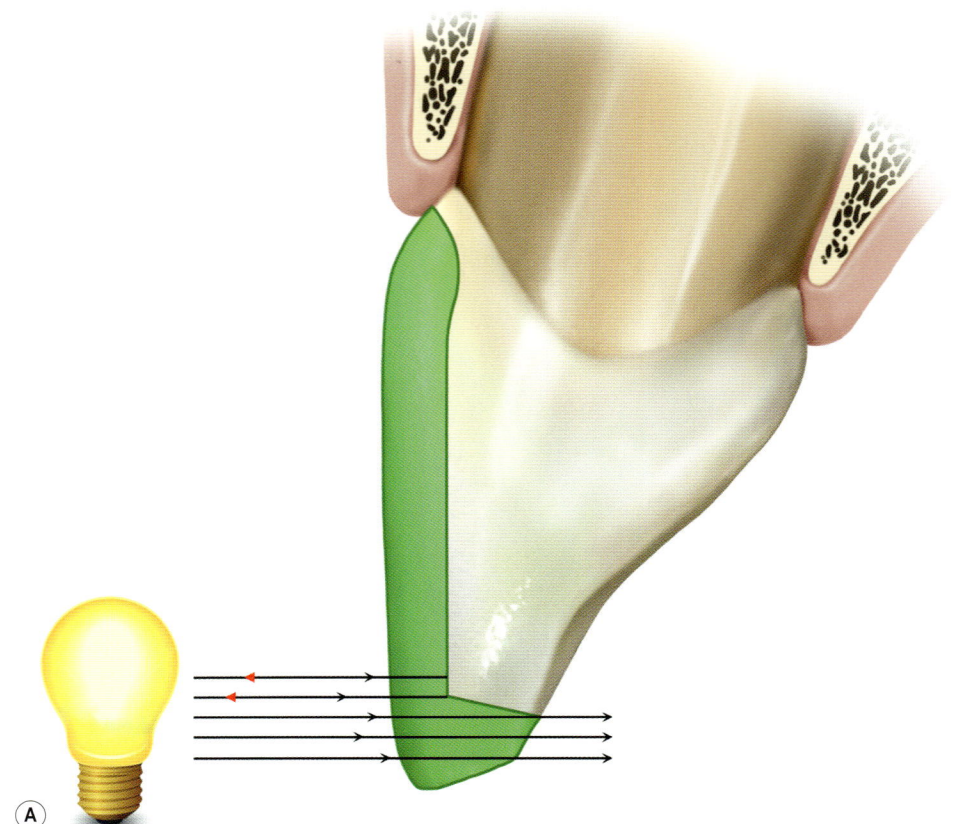

Fig. 8.19A,B Demarcation of UR (unrounded) labial–incisal angle between the restoration's incisal and body shades.

CONSIDERATIONS FOR SHADE SELECTION

As discussed in the diagnosis chapter (see Chapter 1), patients' preferences are the most important factor to consider when choosing the shade of restorations. However, it is the responsibility of the clinician to educate and guide patients towards an appropriate shade.

The starting shades of both arches are noted on the esthetic evaluation form at the first visit. This information, along with the answer to the 'straight, white and perfect' versus 'clean, healthy and natural' question, helps with selection of a shade for the next step in the esthetic process, the bis-acryl mock-up. The mock-up enables testing of different incisal edge positions, tooth shapes, positions and colours. There are admittedly fewer shades available in bis-acryl than for actual porcelain, but the choices available are certainly enough to begin to understand the patient's concept of colour early on. The patient is asked to

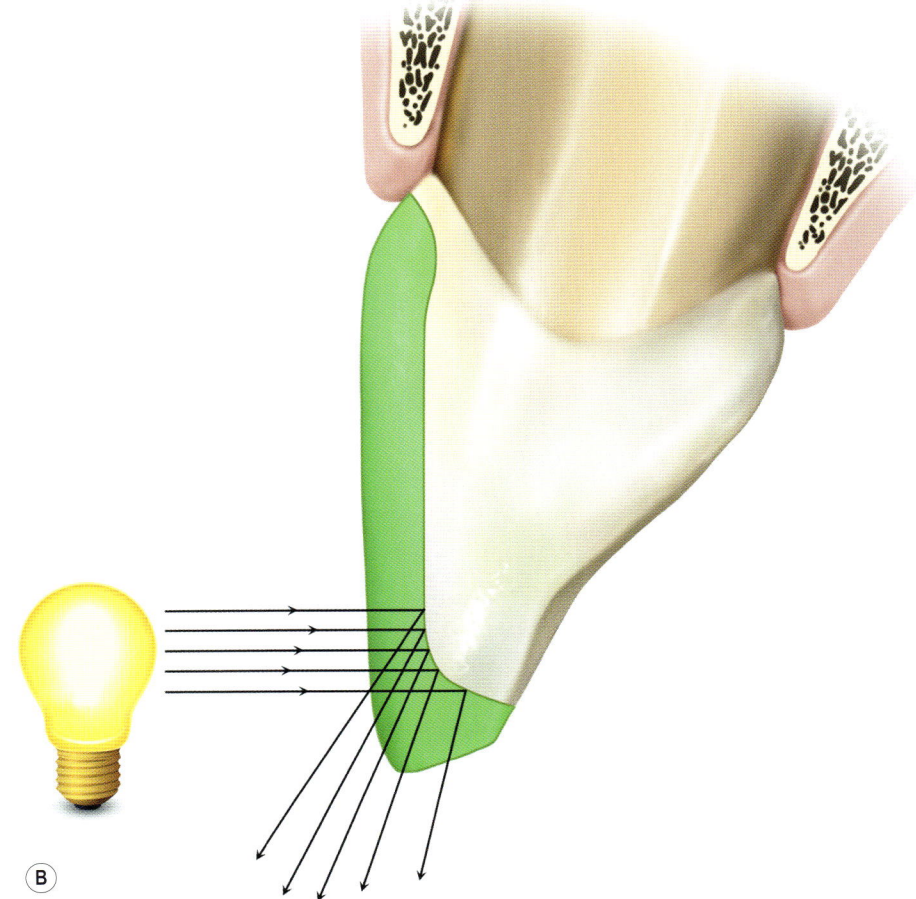

Fig. 8.19A,B *Continued*

consider the proposed shade's relation to the other teeth in the arch, as well as how this colour relates to the opposing arch and the overall esthetics. This is often the perfect time to mention whitening of the teeth not being veneered, which is best performed prior to veneer preparation. Indeed, even whitening a tooth to be veneered is beneficial, as the less drastic the shade change attempted, the less invasive the preparations will be.

Several guidelines to bear in mind during this conversation are as follows:

- Generally, the teeth should never be made whiter than the whites of the eyes. This discrepancy is very noticeable to the observer and will diminish the believability of the restorations.

- No tooth in the esthetic zone should ever be higher in value than the maxillary central incisors.

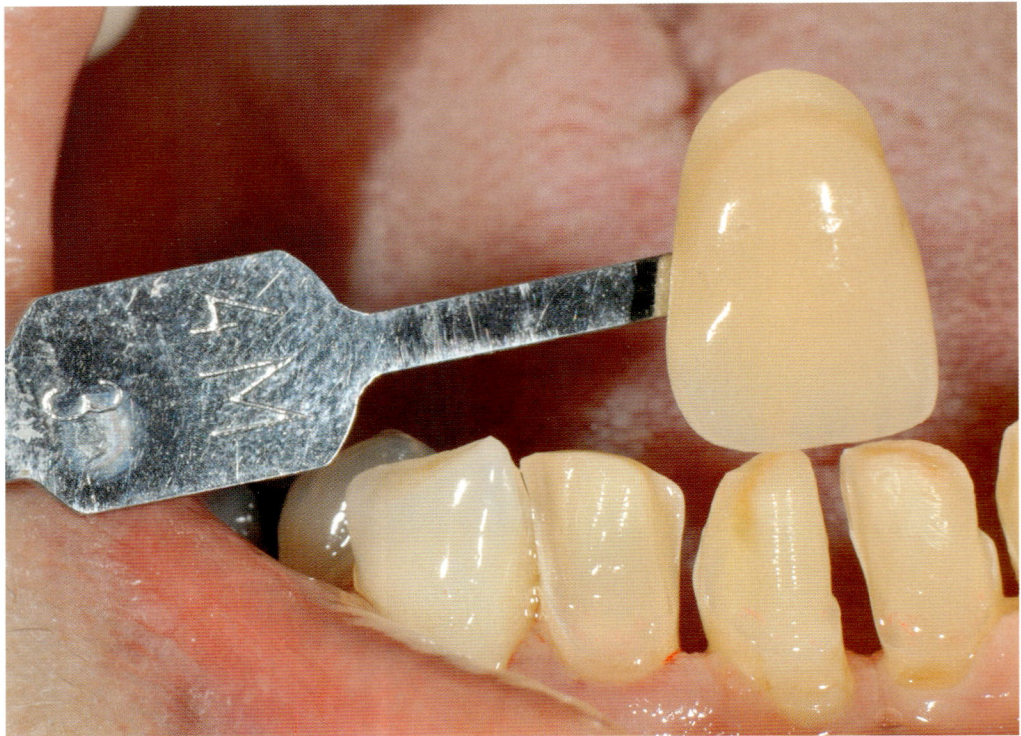

Fig. 8.20 **The critically important stump shade photograph.**

- Those patients with darker skin tones should be advised to select naturally occurring tooth shades, as opposed to bleach shades, as the increased contrast between skin and teeth will make even a natural shade appear very white. It follows that those with fairer skin tones can 'get away' with very light bleach shades.

- If a patient does opt for extremely white restorations, the inclusion of incisal translucency and increased surface characteristics will help minimize an artificial look.

On the day of tooth preparation, the shade of the teeth to be matched should be taken at the beginning of the appointment, before desiccation occurs and value falsely increases. Two shade tabs, one of the desired shade and one directly above or below in value, are held directly beneath the teeth to be matched and photographed. This provides the laboratory technician with a reference against which the computer can be calibrated. Additionally, the stump shade photograph (Fig. 8.20) is critically important for any all-ceramic restoration, especially a thin veneer. This communicates the underlying shade of the tooth, which will be considered as the technician aims for the final desired shade. A very dark or chromatic stump shade will often indicate that colour blocking is necessary.[6]

The period during which the patient is wearing their provisionals is the ultimate opportunity to assess the esthetics and for a real 'dress rehearsal' prior to porcelain fabrication. Once the patient has worn the provisionals for a few days and the lip posture and soft tissue has adapted to any new changes, the overall esthetics are analysed by the dental team. Questions are asked and answered with the patient at this critical assessment appointment to see what works well and what needs tweaking to meet patient desires. Depending on the patient's vision of perfection versus naturalness, the elements of esthetics are reviewed again for this dress rehearsal appointment.

Texture, incisal edge contour and position, embrasures, special effects at the incisal edge and line angles, base shade and transitional shade are discussed with the patient and digital photography and over communication will drive esthetic predictability. Using Skype with your ceramist, sharing videos or having the ceramist in your office all increase the chances of esthetic success.

THE APT PREPARATION TECHNIQUE

In the quest for minimal reduction, Dr Galip Gurel introduced the Aesthetic Pre-Evaluative Temporary ('APT') technique in 2003. This is a preparation method wherein the teeth are prepared directly through the bis-acryl mock-up, ensuring minimal removal of tooth structure. The APT technique is indicated in esthetic cases where the arch is being expanded or length and volume are being added to the teeth, although it can be used in a reductive scenario as long as pre-preparation enameloplasty is first performed (i.e. first making all teeth fit within the putty matrix).[5]

Once the mock-up (Fig. 8.21) is applied intra-orally at the preparation visit, phonetics, esthetics and function are again assessed. Once all are deemed satisfactory, anaesthesia is administered and tooth preparation can commence.

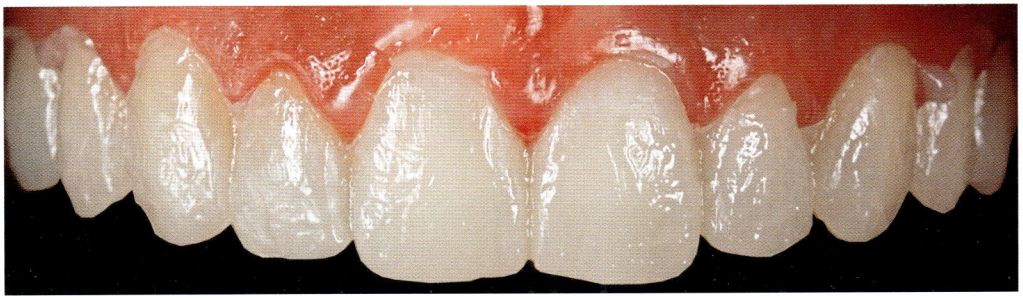

Fig. 8.21   The bis-acryl mock-up, applied for the Aesthetic Pre-Evaluation Temporary technique.

RETRACTION AND IMPRESSIONING

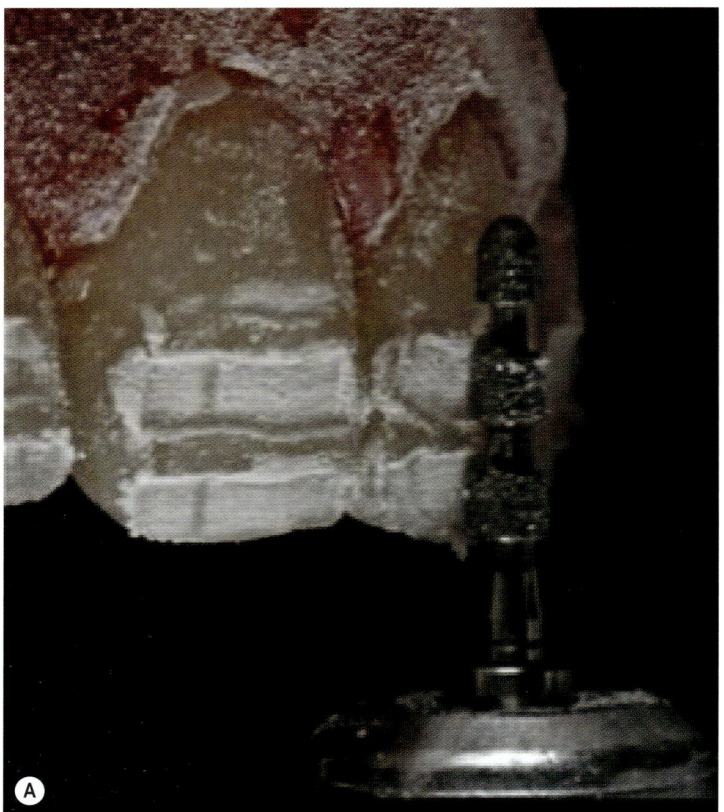
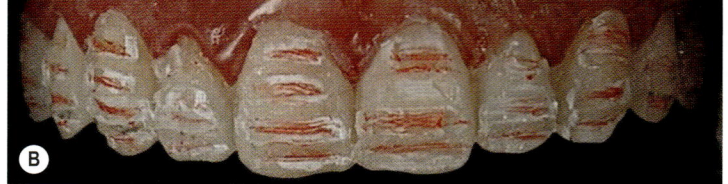

Fig. 8.22A,B Depth grooves of 0.3 and 0.5 mm.

Depending on the restorative material and degree of shade shift, either 0.3 or 0.5 mm depth grooves are decided upon and made in a horizontal fashion along the cervical, middle and incisal aspects of the teeth (Fig. 8.22A,B). Pencil marks are made to indicate the extent of the facial depth grooves, so that the mock-up can be removed and the depth cuts blended until all pencil marks disappear (Fig. 8.23A–C). Incisal depth cuts should be made prior to mock-up removal as well. Removing the mock-up will reveal that certain surfaces of the tooth remain completely untouched (i.e. any structure that is approximately 0.6 mm away from the facial extent of the APT), and therein lies the beauty of this method. Once the mock-up is removed, the interproximal and gingival margins can be defined and the preparations are complete (Fig. 8.24).

RETRACTION AND IMPRESSIONING

The same fundamental rules apply to impressioning for veneers as for full coverage preparations. The margin placement determines the need for retraction and

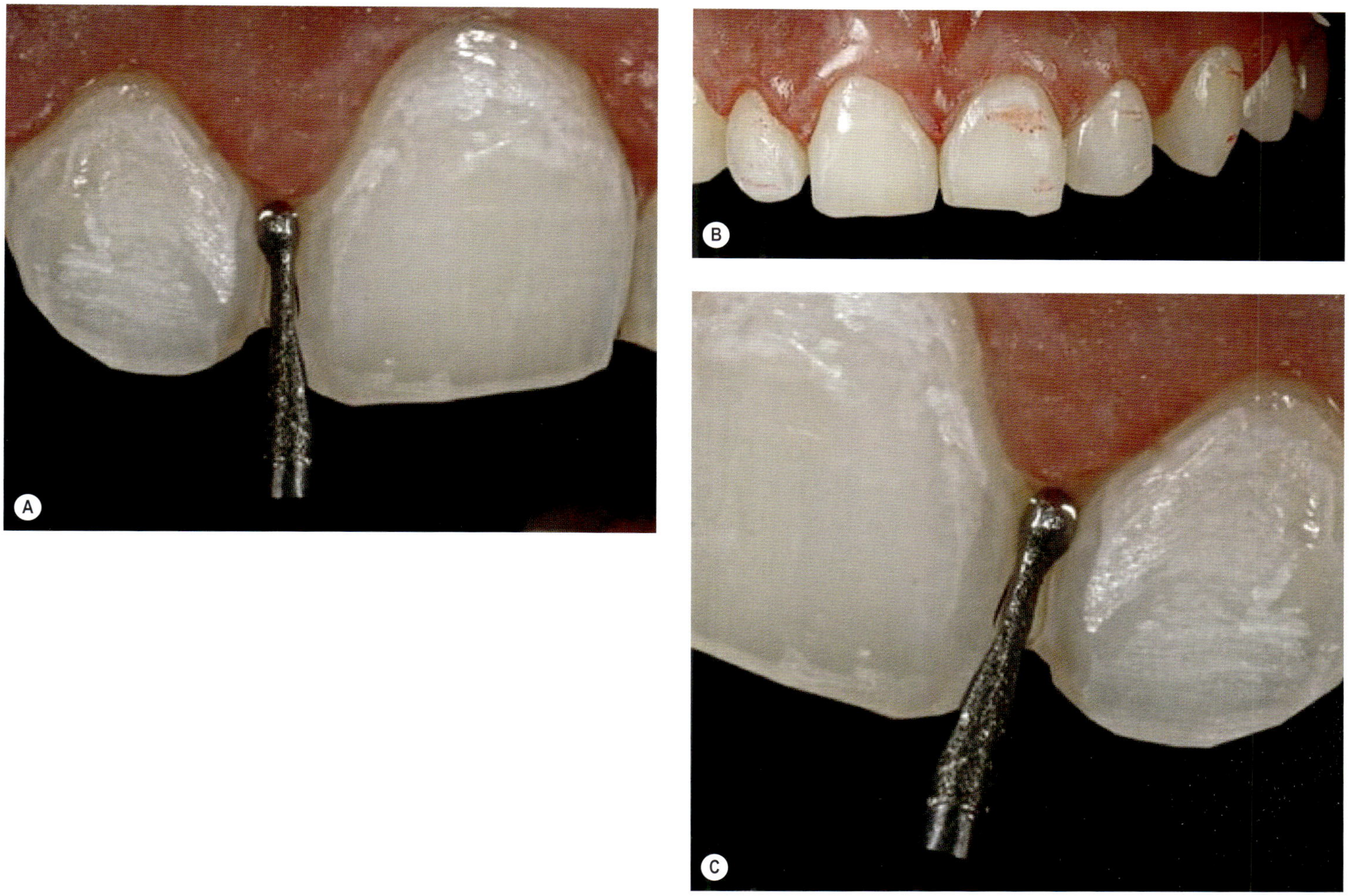

Fig. 8.23A–C Once facial and incisal depth cuts are blended (after removal of the mock-up), the gingival and interproximal margins are defined.

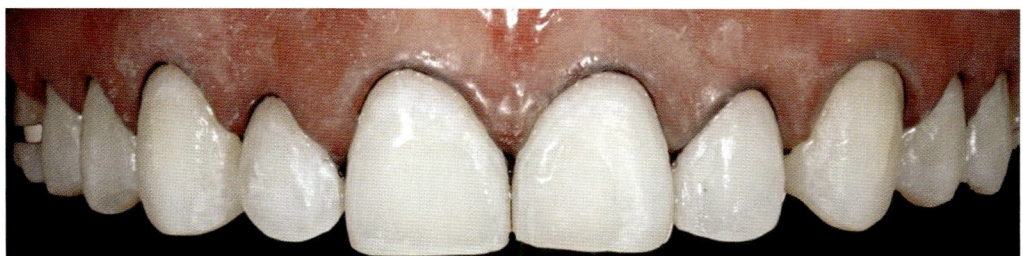

Fig. 8.24 The completed preparations (shown with retraction cord placed) are minimal and entirely in enamel.

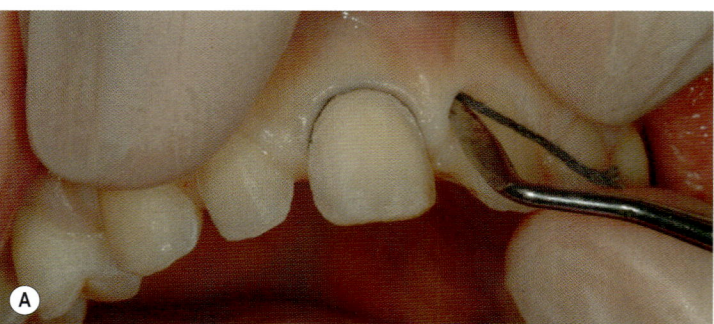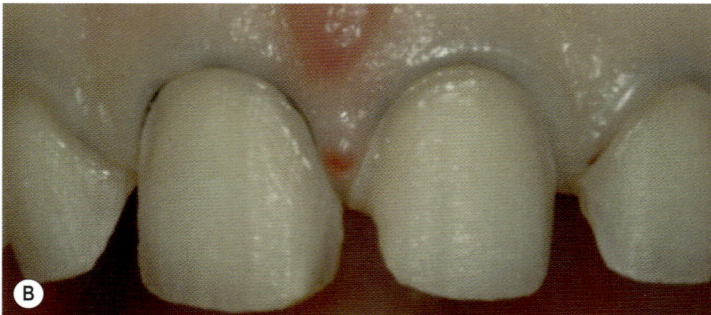

Fig. 8.25A,B Cord is placed gently to expose the margin.

the rule of thumb is: 'what you see is what you get'. If you can see the margin, you do not need retraction cord; if you cannot see the margin, you need to create space. Supragingival and equigingival scenarios, as long as a custom tray is used, do not require cord retraction. The subgingival or intracrevicular margin will need retraction and the goal is atraumatic cord placement; therefore, start with 000 or 00 cord to see the margin once the cord is placed. The retraction technique is to apply gentle pressure to roll the tip of the packing instrument, allowing the cord to be placed under the sulcus without bleeding (Fig. 8.25A,B).[7] The direction of force needs to be 'from where the cord issues', in other words, back on itself. This allows for visualization of the furthest extent of the preparation, plus retraction in an atraumatic way.

CLINICAL TIP

A custom tray is always fabricated to allow for a more detailed impression in all situations, as it supports the impression material and creates a hydraulic effect as it is seated (Fig. 8.26).

PROVISIONALIZATION

Provisional veneers serve as a time-tested functional and esthetic 'dress rehearsal' for the final restorations. With the exception of complex colour mapping and texturing, the provisional veneer mimics the final restoration almost exactly, most importantly establishing the new incisal edge position and contour. Encouraging patients to live in and approve their new smiles before committing to the final restorations creates a high energy, collaborative conversation that sets up for success.

In veneer provisionalization, the provisionals should be retained but not so strongly that they must be aggressively cut off at the delivery appointment. Doing so could alter the underlying surface of the preparation and cause an imprecise fit of the porcelain. The technique is to 'spot etch' and 'spot bond' just

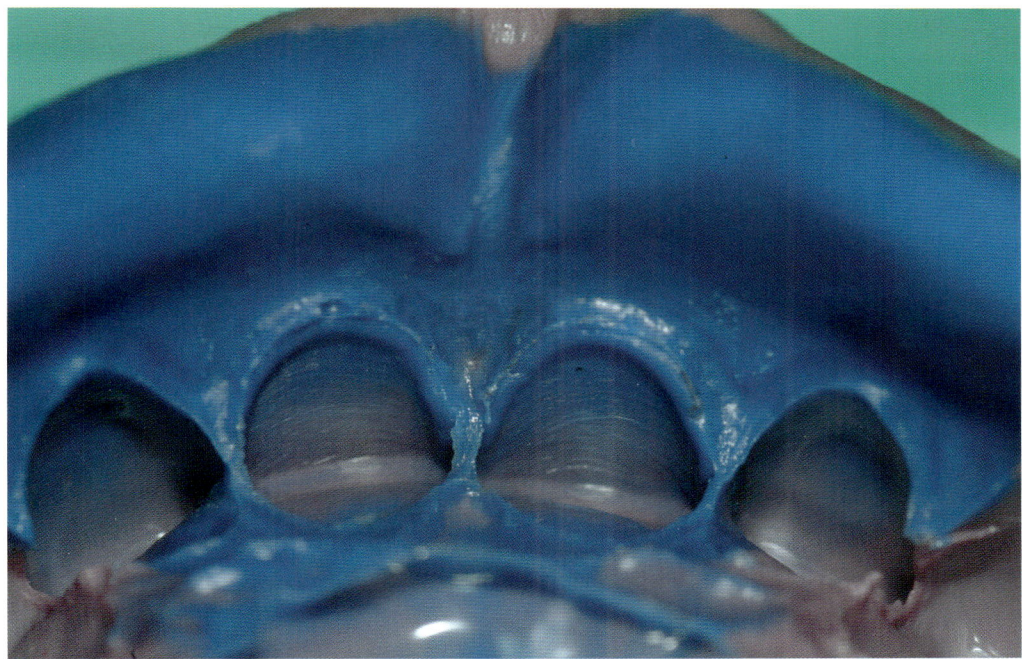

Fig. 8.26 A final impression obtained in a custom tray. The custom tray must always be used to support the impression material and create a hydraulic effect.

a small area of each prep, and to achieve significant mechanical retention in the embrasure spaces (while still creating open areas for cleansability and a proper emergence profile for soft tissue health).

Once the impression has been obtained, the preparations are cleaned with Tubulicid or any bactericidal agent, and spot etched with phosphoric acid just in the midfacial and along the incisal edge. The etchant is then rinsed off and bonding agent is applied to the spot-etched regions and cured. Next, a putty matrix of the wax-up, either clear or solid silicone (Figs 8.27 and 8.28), is filled with a bis-acryl material of the appropriate shade (e.g. Protemp by 3M and Integrity by Dentsply) and seated on the preparations. The matrix should be held firmly against the teeth while the material sets, so that the resulting 'flash' is minimal once the matrix is removed.

Any excess can be easily trimmed away with a #12 sickle-shaped scalpel and, if needed, fine composite-trimming carbides such as an ET4 by Brasseler. Additionally, flowable composite with filled resin can be added and contoured if there are areas that are deficient.

Alternatively to the 'direct' provisionalization technique described above, the preparations could be coated in a light layer of lubricant (i.e. Vaseline) prior to

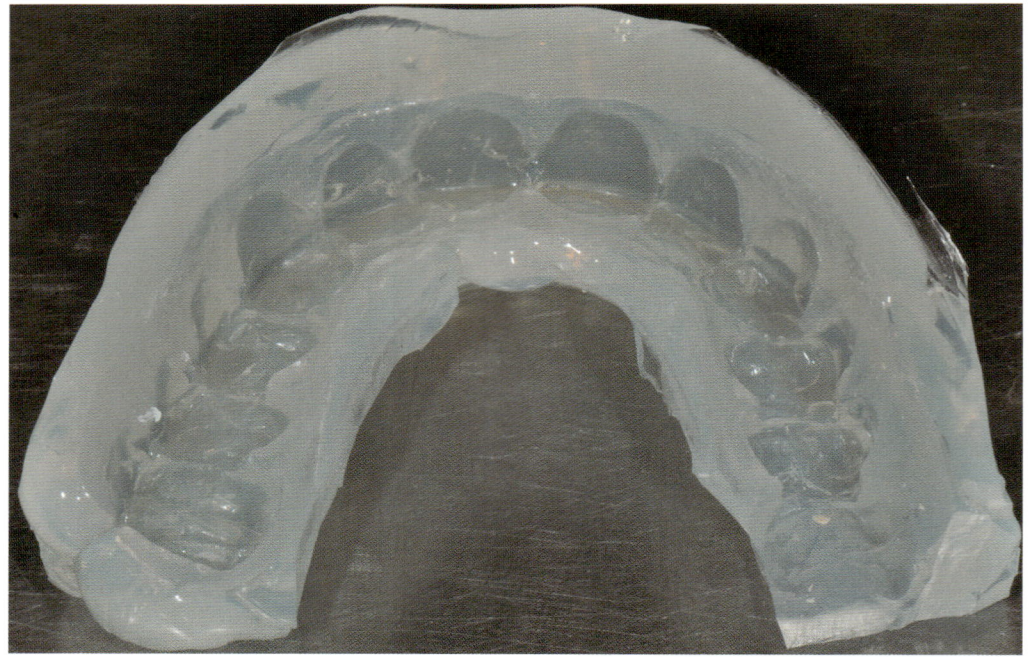

Fig. 8.27 A clear silicone provisional matrix, which can be used with light-cured provisional material.

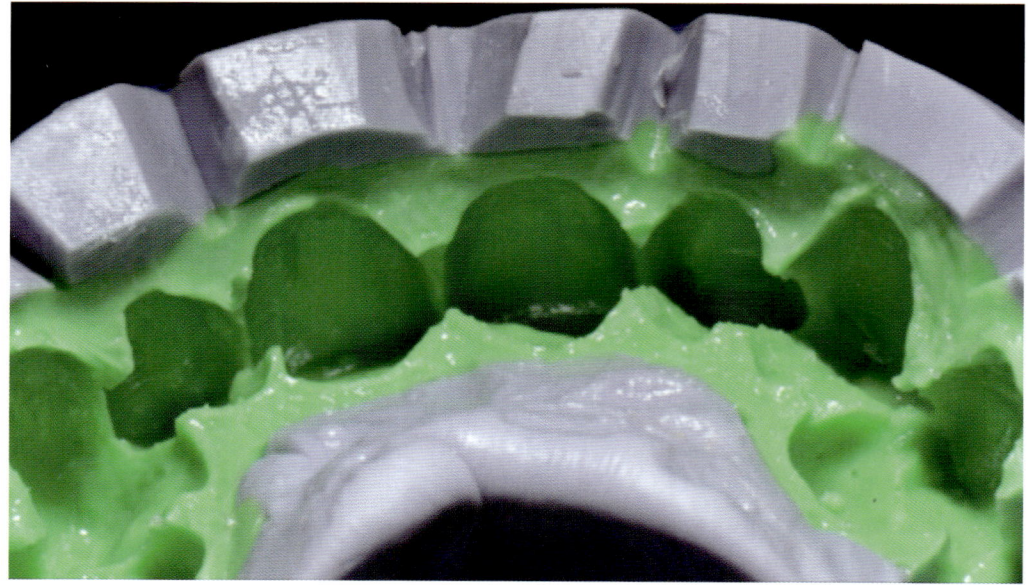

Fig. 8.28 A putty matrix for provisional veneers, with an inner layer of light body impression material for maximum detail. V-shaped notches at each papilla allow for the escape of excess material and the matrix extends onto the palate for accurate seating.

matrix seating, allowing the provisionals to be removed once the bis-acryl sets and then trimmed and finished outside the mouth. In this indirect scenario, the lubricant is then cleaned off the preparations, spot etching is performed and the finished provisionals are adhered with light-cured flowable composite. In the authors' opinion, the indirect and direct provisionalization techniques work equally well, although the direct method is usually faster.

Once the provisionals have been adhered to the preparations and finished (Fig. 8.29A–C), it is time to once again step back and engage the patient in the conversation. Esthetics are assessed (although there should be little surprise at this point, considering that the provisionals are an exact replica of the mock-up and wax-up), as are phonetics and function. Centric contacts are balanced, and all excursive movements are adjusted to achieve ideal mandibular movement and the least amount of force on the incisal edges. Any further alterations are made until both patient and clinician are completely satisfied, at which point an alginate impression is taken. After the alginate is obtained, the provisionals can be glazed for added effect.[7]

The poured alginate of the provisionals will serve as the new template for the laboratory technician to follow and must be included with the case materials (along with photographs of the provisionals, the final impression and the bite registration). The technician will use this model to fabricate an incisal index, which should enable duplication of the 3-dimensional position of the incisal edges exactly (Fig. 8.30A–D). Before sending this model to the laboratory, a duplicate is made to create a vacuum-formed temporary nightguard, which will help the provisionals resist any dislodging forces at night.[1]

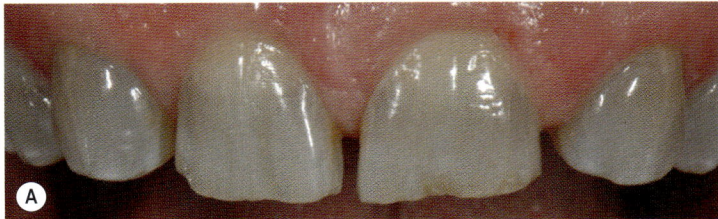
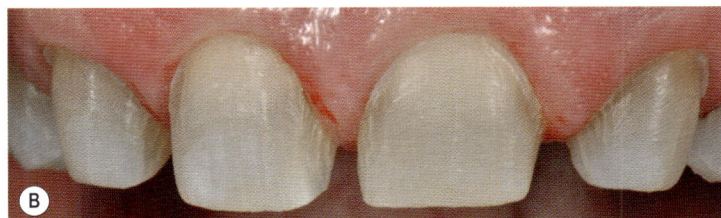
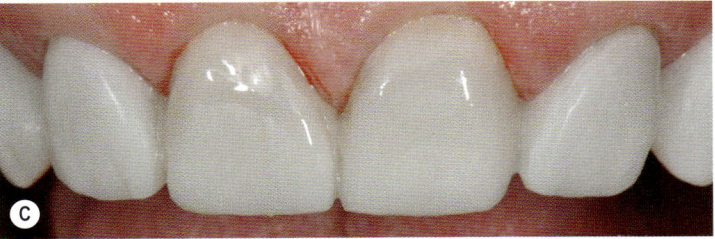

Fig. 8.29A–C Finished and glazed provisional veneers (shown with pre-operation dentition and preparations). Because the light body/putty matrix was so well adapted, there was very little 'flash' to remove.

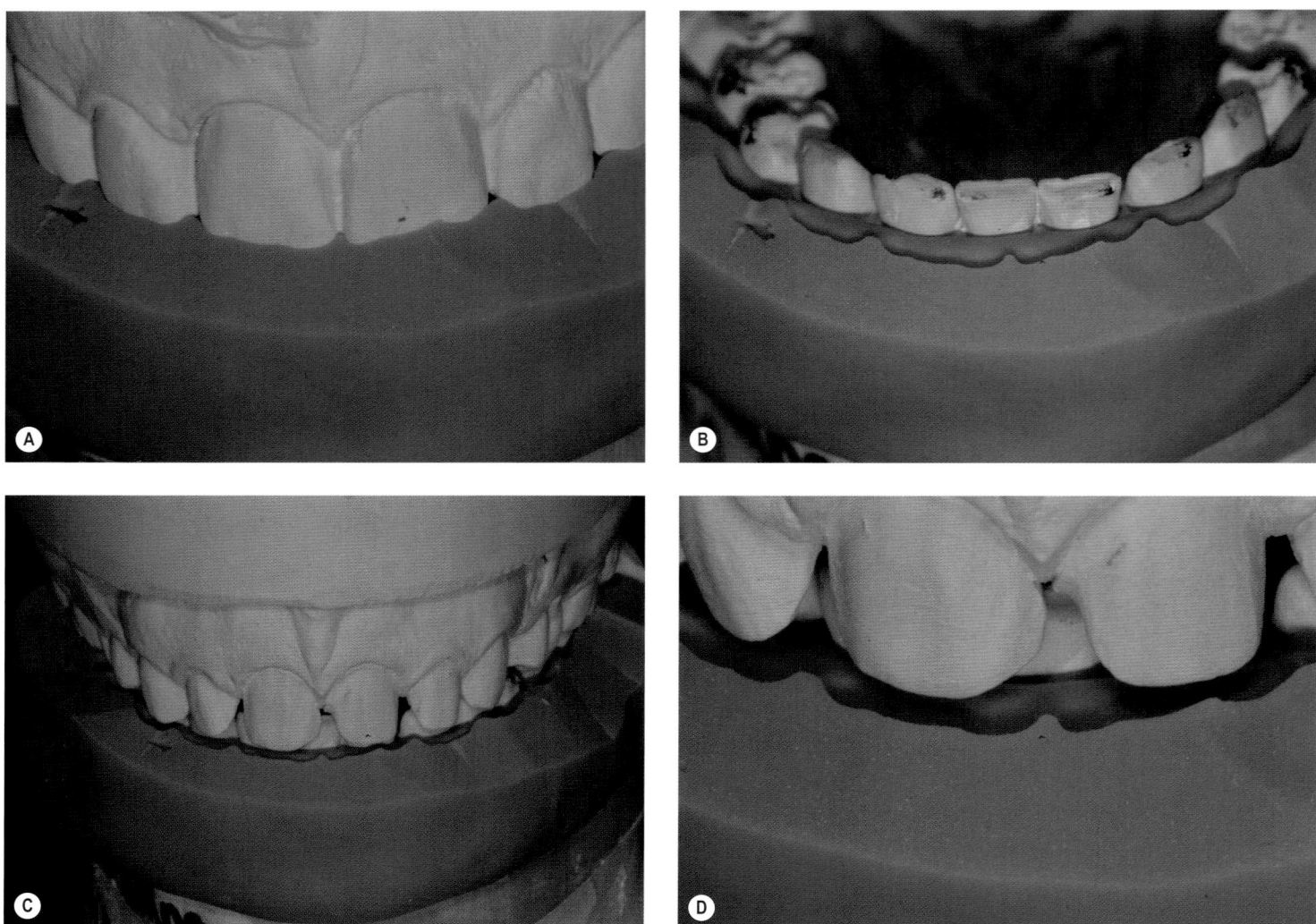

Fig. 8.30A–D An incisal edge index, fabricated when the model of the provisionals is mounted against the counter model. The technician then seats the master model into this index and can replicate the labial, incisal and palatal surfaces of the teeth exactly as desired. This index contains all the information necessary for predictable esthetics, phonetics and occlusion.

The final evaluation of the provisionals is done a week later, once the patient has lived in their new smile for a week; at this point, the patient should be able to give valuable feedback on colour and contour. Additionally, as the patient is no longer anaesthetized, the clinician can observe phonetics and smile dynamics more accurately than at the preparation appointment. As the aim is to harmonize the dental esthetics with the lips and the face, waiting a week also allows the orofacial muscles and lips to adapt to the new incisal edge position – or not.

If need be, any esthetic or functional modifications can be made to the provisionals (additively with flowable composite or reductively with 3M discs). At this point, of course, a new alginate would be taken and sent to the technician.

If the week-later evaluation of the provisionals is skipped and committing to porcelain occurs too soon, a valuable opportunity to test the visualized solution is lost. Allowing the provisionals to be 'time tested' is one more way to ensure predictability and success.

CONSIDERATIONS FOR ANTERIOR MANDIBULAR VENEERS

The same principles that apply to maxillary anterior porcelain laminate veneer preparation hold true for the mandibular anterior porcelain laminate veneer preparation but with some variations. The facial reduction is 0.3–0.5 mm and is completed in multiple planes, and the incisal reduction must be 1.5 mm such that the final porcelain restoration is of adequate thickness to withstand the forces of occlusion (Fig. 8.31).

A major difference between mandibular veneer preparation and maxillary preparations is that the gingival region is usually not visible in mandibular teeth due to labial coverage; as such, the gingival finish line can be kept supragingival to maintain optimal periodontal health.

CONSIDERATIONS FOR POSTERIOR VENEERS

Many esthetic cases involve restoring 10 or even 12 teeth per arch, extending deep into the posterior area. Since the maxillary buccal cusp is a nonfunctional cusp, the porcelain laminate veneer preparation of maxillary posterior teeth is very similar to what has been discussed regarding the ideal preparation thus far (Fig. 8.32). The 0.5 mm buccal surface reduction is carried onto the occlusal surface where it ends in a 0.5 mm deep chamfer placed halfway between the buccal cusp tip and the central fossa. The preparation is completed with a 1.0 mm reduction of the cusp tip and then the rounding off of the two planes of reduction.

The preparation of mandibular posterior teeth for porcelain laminate veneers is more demanding than that of their maxillary counterparts, since mandibular buccal cusps are functional in nature and their occlusal tables are visible. Usually, the buccal margin can finish on the inner incline of the buccal cusp (similar to the maxillary scenario). In extreme colour change situations, the

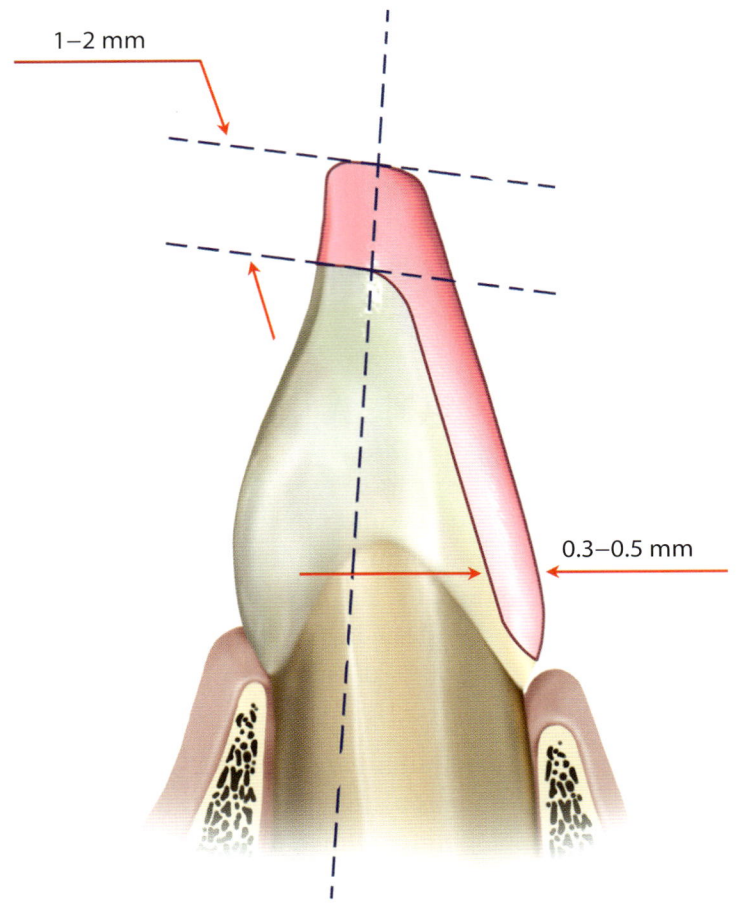

Fig. 8.31 An ideal mandibular anterior veneer preparation.

margin should be placed into the central fossa with 1.5 mm thickness of porcelain to support the occlusal load. As such, the occlusal chamfer should extend up to and including the central fossa depending on the previous restoration that is being replaced. That is, if there is an old conservative occlusal filling, the new veneer combines into a veneer plus inlay and a solid 1.5 mm of porcelain must cover the mandibular buccal cusp to support its activity (Fig. 8.33).

Placement of the gingival finishing line for posterior porcelain laminate veneer preparations follows the same principles as those discussed for their anterior counterparts, with less importance on soft tissue esthetics and smile line. The location of the gingival finishing line for maxillary posterior porcelain laminate veneers depends on the contrast between the stump and the desired finished shades. On the other hand, the gingival finishing line for mandibular posterior porcelain laminate veneers is concealed and thus should be kept supragingival,

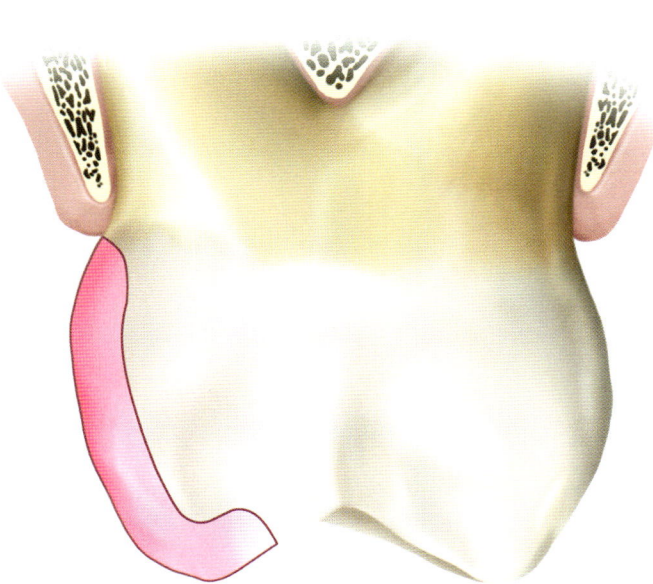

Fig. 8.32   An ideal maxillary posterior veneer preparation.

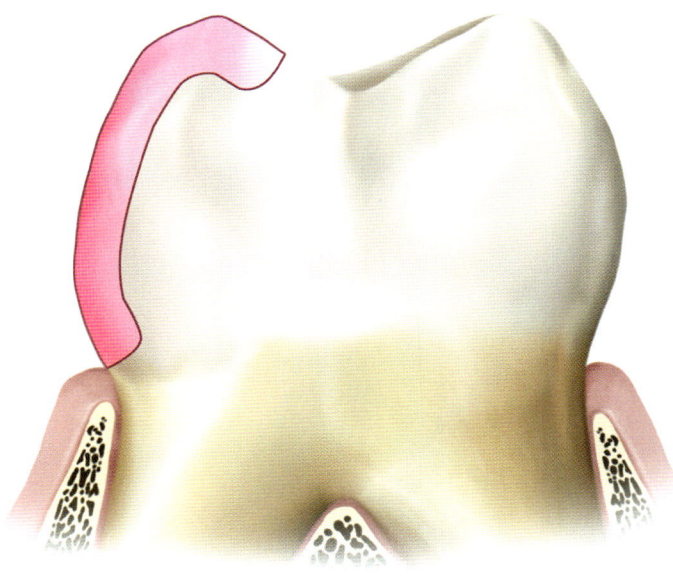

Fig. 8.33   An ideal mandibular posterior veneer preparation.

following the contour of the soft tissue so as to once again maintain maximal gingival health.

RESTORATION OF FRACTURED AND CARIOUS TEETH WITH PORCELAIN LAMINATE VENEERS

The porcelain laminate veneer is also a valuable tool for restoring fractured teeth to optimal esthetics. Many clinicians advocate first rebuilding the fractured area in composite and then conventionally preparing the tooth to receive a bonded porcelain laminate veneer to complete the restoration. The danger with this restorative method is that the flexure module (modulus of elasticity) of composite and porcelain are substantially different. Consequently, when a force is applied in the incisal area, the underlying composite gives a little and the inflexible porcelain without a rigid support will fracture. Instead, we recommend that the sharp edges of the fracture line should first be eliminated and then the tooth be prepared as outlined earlier to receive a porcelain laminate veneer. The porcelain laminate veneer fabricated for this type of restoration varies in thickness from 0.5 mm on the labial to upwards of 6.0 mm of solid porcelain in the fracture area. The skill of the ceramic technician is highly tested in fabricating such a restoration, but the resulting esthetic benefits are well worth it. In addition, because porcelain is strongest under

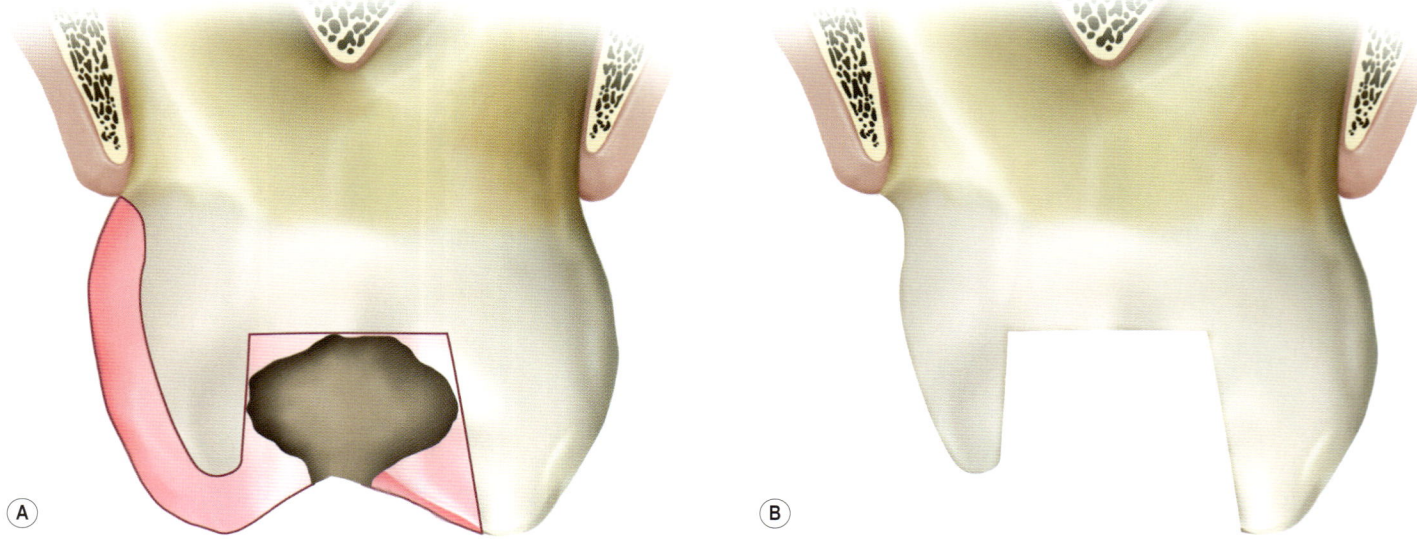

Fig. 8.34A,B Preparation for a veneer-onlay laminate veneer.

compressive forces, the solid porcelain does not run the risk of fracturing when a force is applied incisally.

The conservative nature of the porcelain laminate veneer preparation can also lend itself to the esthetic restoration of teeth with Class I or II caries. In the past, the tendency was for a posterior tooth to be treatment planned for a full coverage crown when an esthetic restoration was desired and the tooth had an existing large occlusal amalgam or composite filling. Instead, a variation of the porcelain laminate veneer called a veneer-onlay laminate veneer is recommended in such cases. The preparation for such a restoration requires the excavation of the entire old amalgam or composite and any remaining carious tooth structure, with the proximal walls diverging towards the occlusal so there is a path of insertion and withdrawal (Fig. 8.34A). The buccal surface is then prepared for a veneer, and the two preparations are merged, making sure that the buccal cusp tip is reduced by at least 1.0–1.5 mm. The resulting veneer-onlay laminate veneer restoration is not only highly esthetic but is extremely conservative since the healthy lingual portion of the tooth is left untouched (Fig. 8.34B). The authors refer to this as a 'Venlay' restoration.

MATERIAL SELECTION

When it comes to selecting a restorative material for veneers (or any restoration), the material must be decided upon prior to tooth preparation. The materials conversation between laboratory technician and dentist must begin in the diagnostic phase, and the following must be considered:

- What is the shade of the underlying tooth?
- Is a drastic shade change being planned?
- Are natural teeth or existing restorations to be matched?
- How much characterization is desired?
- Are there excessive forces anywhere in the mouth, i.e. bruxism or parafunctional habits?

At the time of this writing, when it comes to porcelain veneers, the two most common choices are either lithium disilicate (E. Max) or feldspathic porcelain. Bonded composite veneers are also indicated in certain scenarios; a detailed description of the natural layering freehand bonding technique will conclude this chapter.

Lithium disilicate (Fig. 8.35) offers several advantages over feldspathic porcelain: 360–400 mPa tensile strength (feldspathic has 90–100 mPa), a minimum required thickness of only 0.3 mm (versus 0.5 for feldspathic), and an increased ability to 'block out' a dark or yellow stump shade. Because of its increased resistance to fracture, lithium disilicate is more appropriate than feldspathic porcelain for veneer/Class III hybrid restorations, as well as veneer/onlay combinations.

Despite the numerous advantages of lithium disilicate, however, feldspathic porcelain is often the appropriate choice when a single veneer is being used to match heavily characterized natural teeth, or when matching an existing feldspathic restoration.

Bear in mind that when choosing the proper material, the clinician must also consider the strengths and limitations of the technician, as each material is different in different hands.

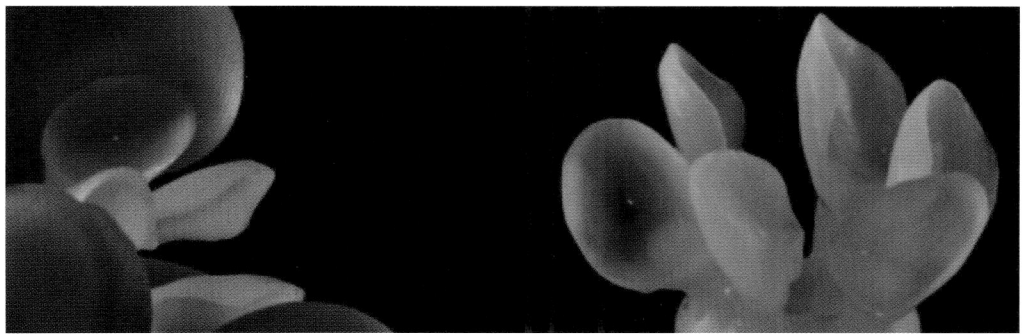

Fig. 8.35 Lithium disilicate veneers, a mere 0.3 mm thick.

INSERTION AND FINISHING

At the delivery appointment, anaesthesia is administered and the following steps are performed:

1. Remove the provisionals from the patient's teeth, either flicking them off with an instrument (Fig. 8.36A,B) or cutting grooves first with a thin bur (at the incisal edge or midfacial, but never interproximally). Be gentle with the gingiva to avoid bleeding.

2. Polish away any remaining spot bonding with a black polishing 3M disc (Fig. 8.37) or a fluted carbide bur. A finishing strip can be used to remove any interproximal remnants (Fig. 8.38).

3. Try in each veneer with water or Try-in paste (if wishing to adjust the value), individually and then all together (Fig. 8.39). Place a gauze throat pack while trying in the veneers. The patient is given a hand mirror and gives approval.

4. Isolate the teeth with cotton rolls or a rubber dam (i.e. Optragate by Ivoclar), pumice the teeth, and pack Hemodent-soaked #000 cord at each preparation (unless the finish line is supragingival and does not require cord) (Fig. 8.40A,B).

5. Prepare each veneer by:

    a. Etching internal surface with phosphoric acid for 30 seconds (assuming the laboratory has already etched the veneers with hydrofluoric acid), rinsing off and drying.

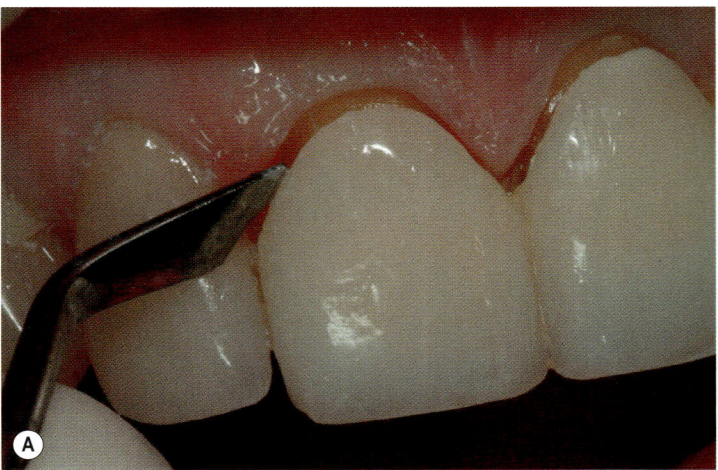 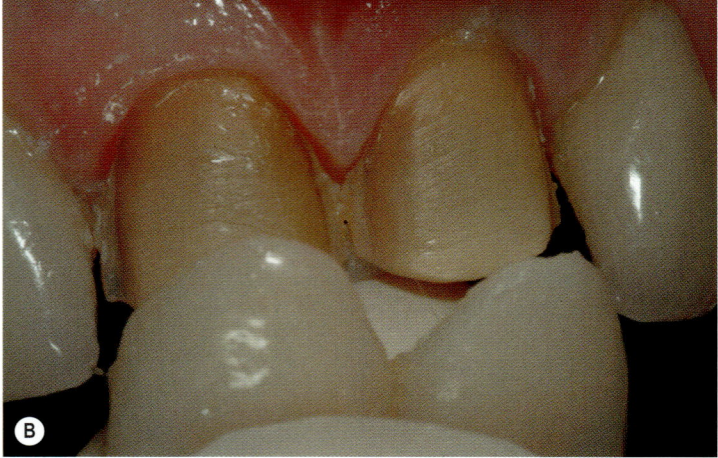

Fig. 8.36A,B Removal of the provisionals from the patient's teeth.

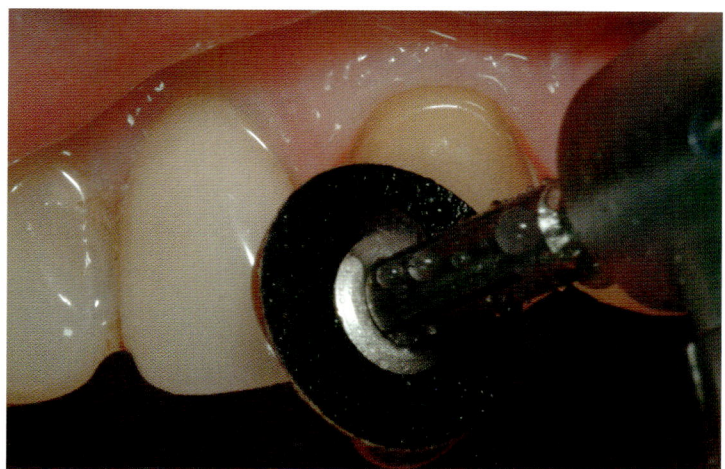

Fig. 8.37 Polish away any remaining spot bonding with a black polishing 3M disc.

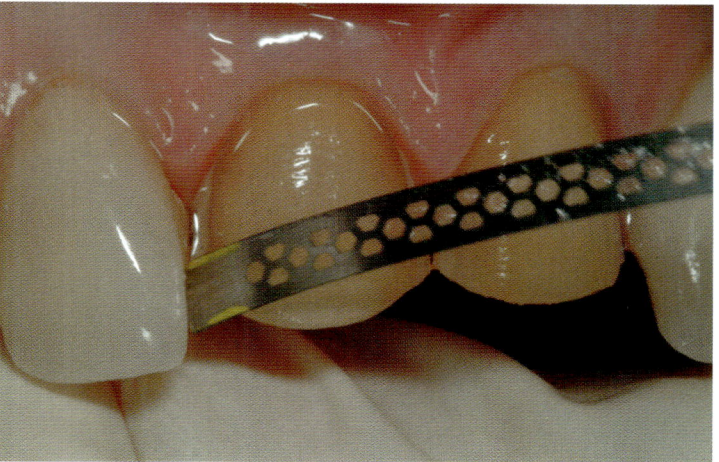

Fig. 8.38 A finishing strip can be used to remove any interproximal remnants.

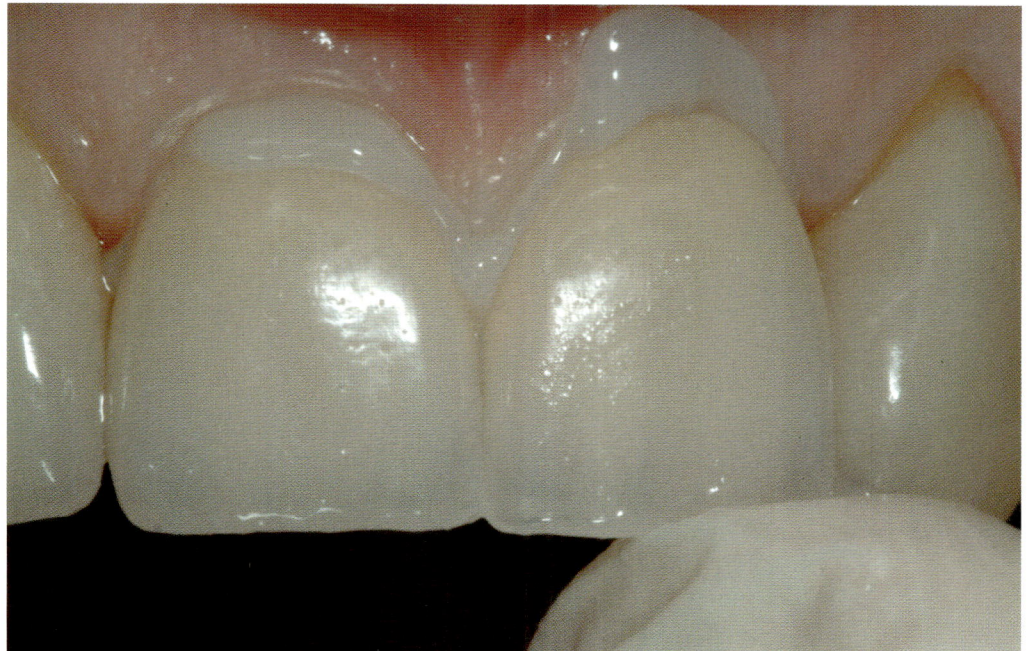

Fig. 8.39 Trying in the veneers.

b. Placing the veneers in a cup of alcohol and placing the cup in the ultrasonic bath for 1 minute (Fig. 8.41). This ensures removal of any Try-in paste residue, phosphoric acid or salivary proteins.

c. Adding a drop of silane to the intaglio of each veneer. Silanation is perhaps the most critical step when bonding porcelain to enamel. Add another layer of silane once the first layer evaporates.

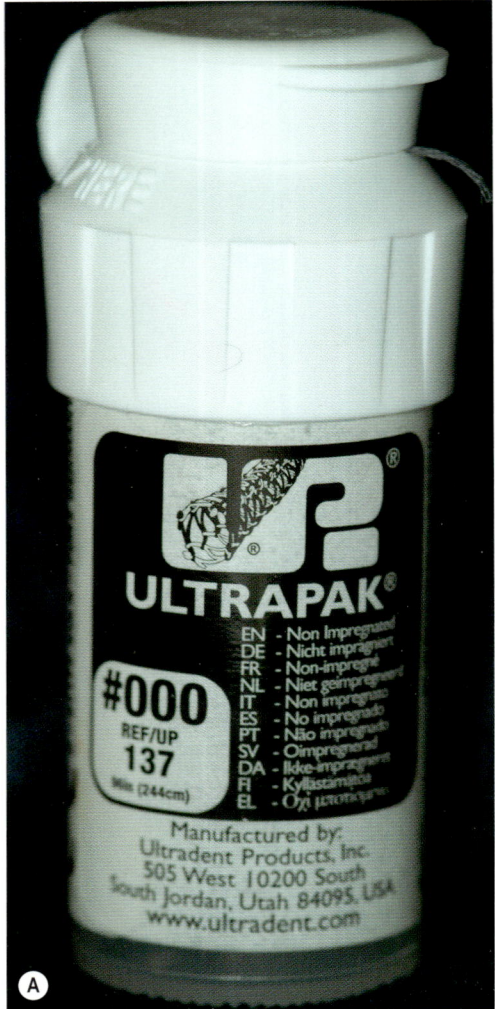
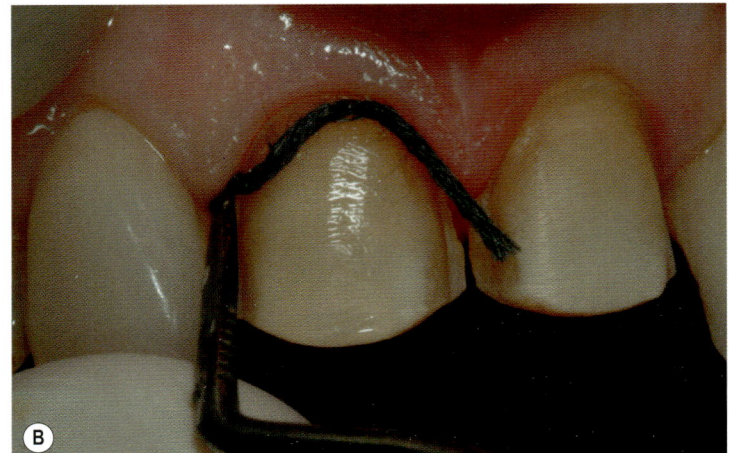

Fig. 8.40A,B (A) Rubber dam; (B) Hemodent-soaked cord.

6. Teflon plumber's tape can be placed for isolation on either side of whichever is first to be prepared (usually #8 and #9).

7. Apply Tubulicid (Fig. 8.42A) to the teeth with a cotton pellet to disinfect the enamel surface (Fig. 8.42B).[8]

8. Etch the teeth with 37% phosphoric acid (Fig. 8.43). Rinse and dry off (Fig. 8.44).

9. Apply bonding agent (i.e. Optibond by Kerr and Excite by Ivoclar) to the tooth, and to the intaglio of the veneer, but do not cure it (Fig. 8.45).

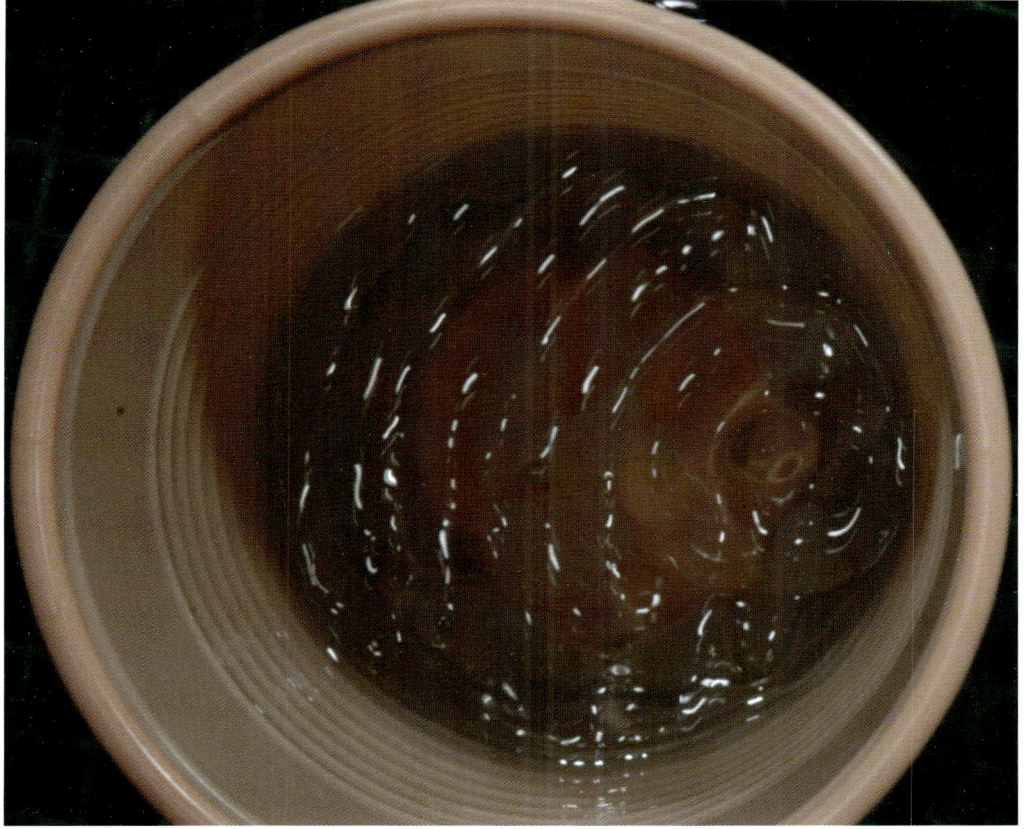

Fig. 8.41　The veneers are placed in an ultrasonic bath.

10. Inject veneer cement into the incisal area, margins and body of the veneer, with the tip in the whole time to avoid bubbles (Fig. 8.46). The authors favour using just the base component of Variolink veneer cement (Ivoclar) without the catalyst, as the base is solely light cured and will not set prematurely.

11. Seat the veneer and confirm its position (Fig. 8.47). Depending on each clinician's level of comfort and experience, the veneers can be cemented one by one, or all at once.

12. 'Tack' cure for 2 seconds only, while gently pressing veneer both incisally and facially. This brief curing locks the veneer into place, yet keeps the cement in a gel state. This makes cleaning up much easier than attempting to remove completely cured excess cement.

13. Remove excess cement with a rubber tip instrument (Fig. 8.48). You can also use a Mylar strip interproximally and pull it to the palate at this point.

INSERTION AND FINISHING

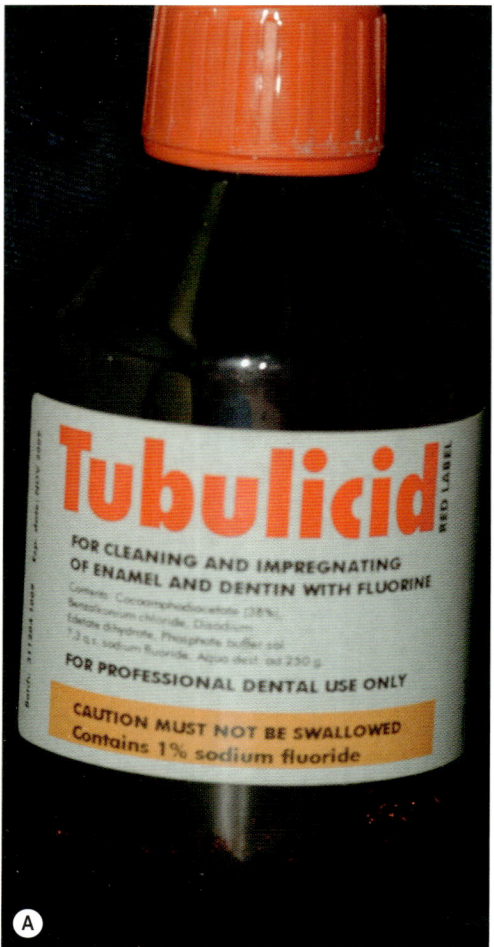
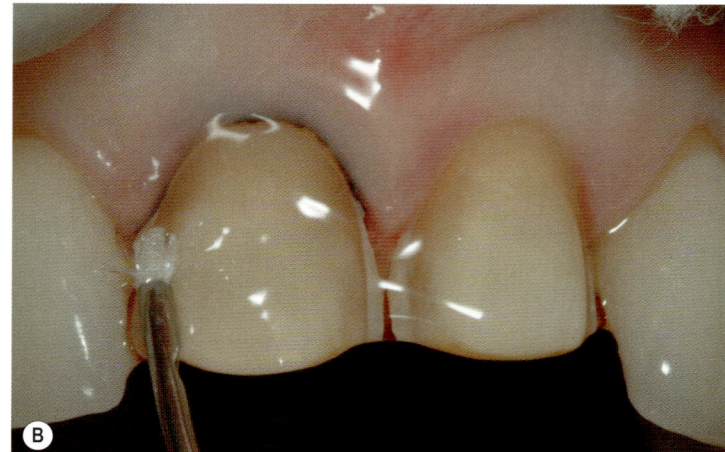

Fig. 8.42A,B (A) Tubulicid; (B) application to the teeth.

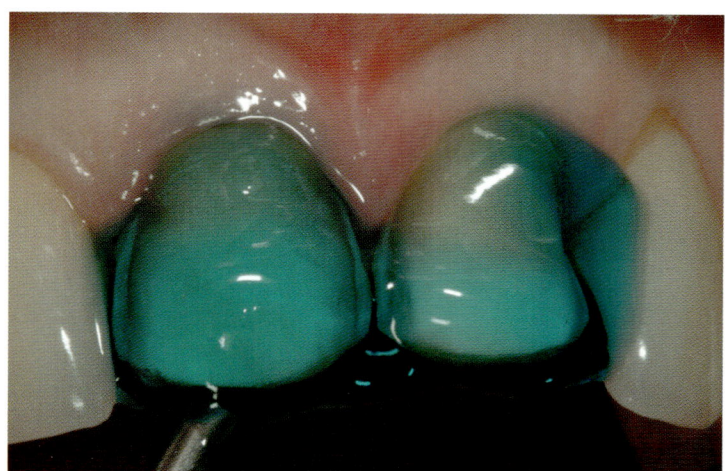

Fig. 8.43 Etching the teeth with phosphoric acid.

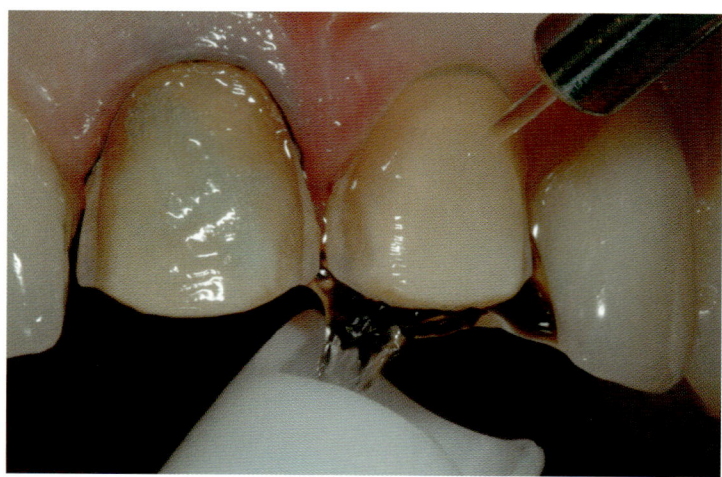

Fig. 8.44 Rinse and dry off.

ANTERIOR BONDED RESTORATIONS

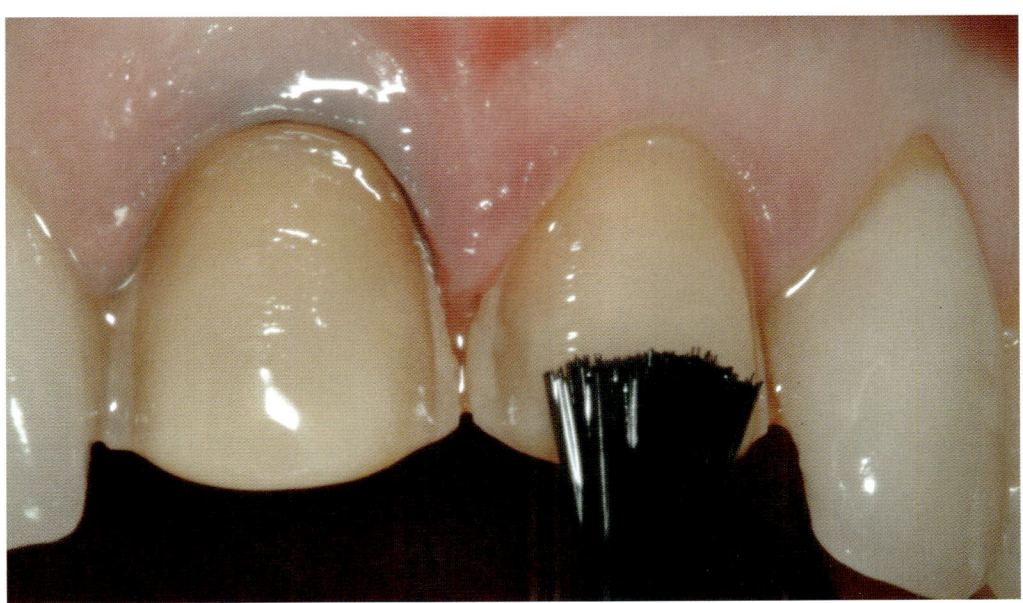

Fig. 8.45 Apply the bonding agent.

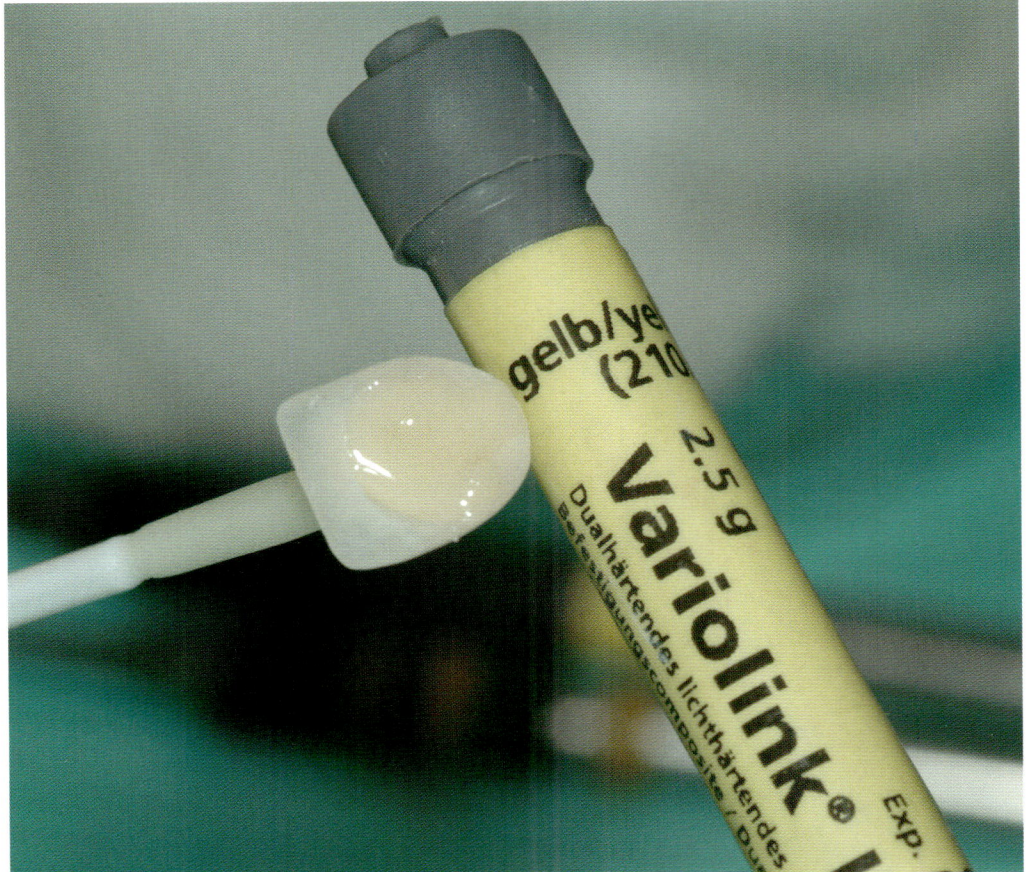

Fig. 8.46 Inject the veneer cement.

253

INSERTION AND FINISHING

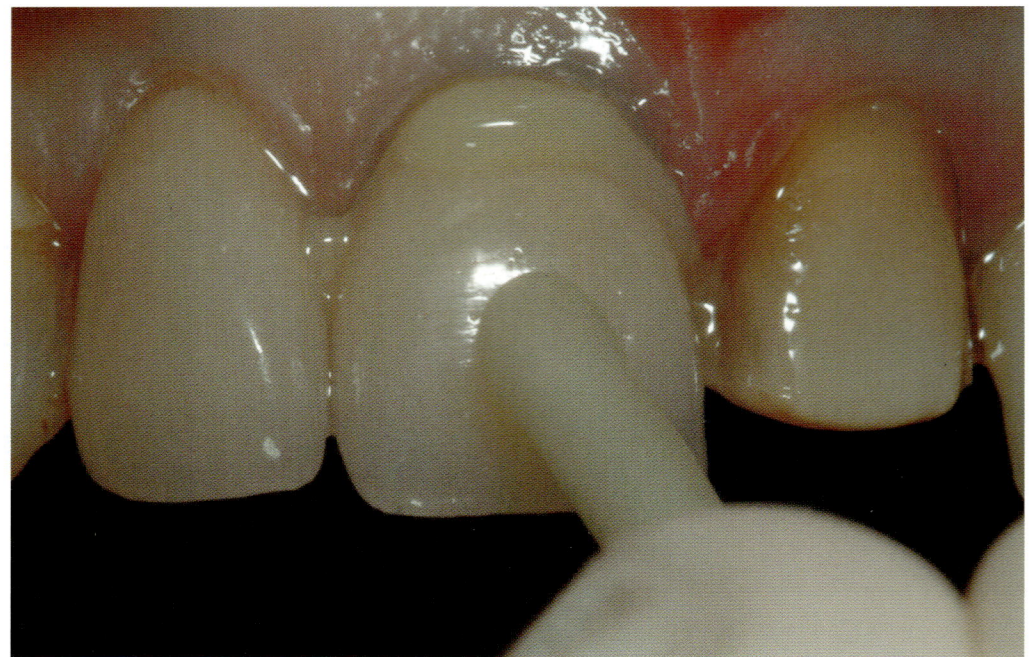

Fig. 8.47 Seat the veneer.

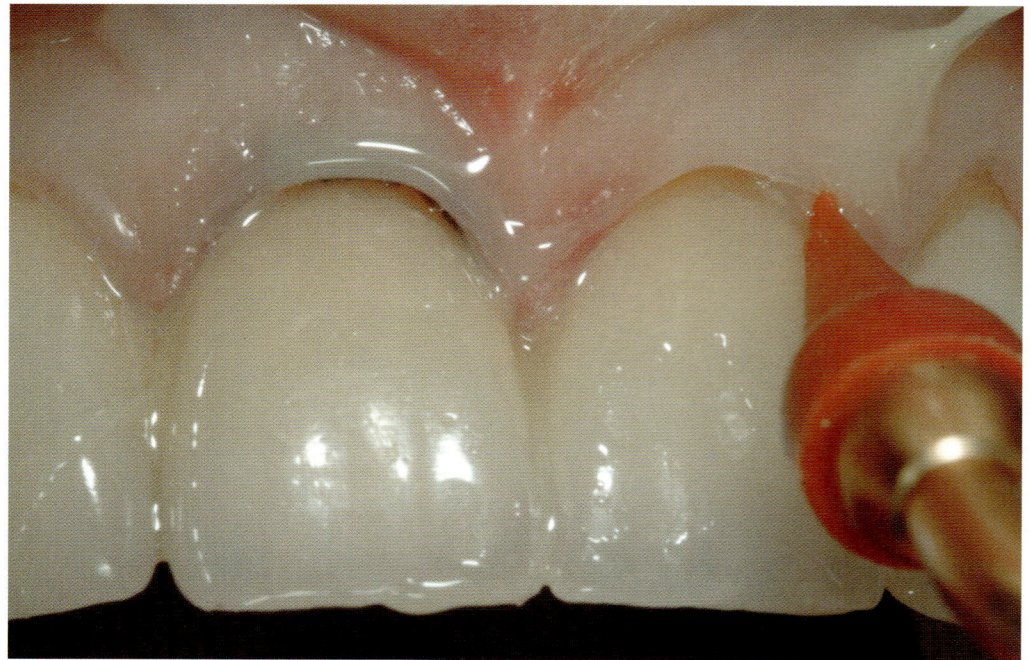

Fig. 8.48 A rubber tip instrument is used to clean up excess cement after tack curing.

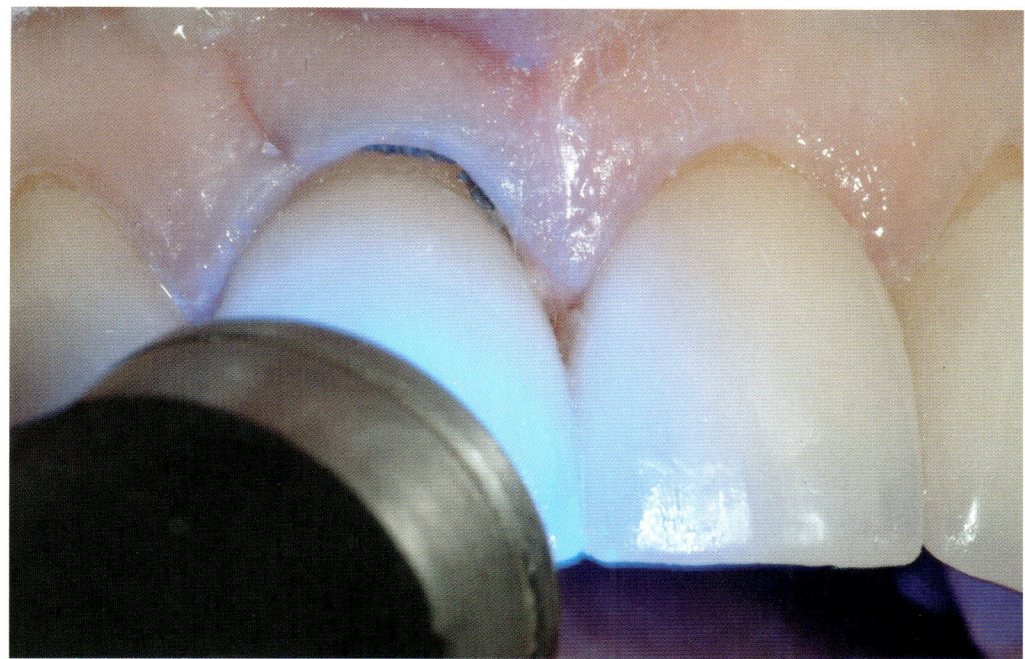

Fig. 8.49 Perform a full cure.

14. Perform a full cure for 20 seconds (Fig. 8.49) from the palatal first, then facial, being sure to keep the curing light moving. Keeping the light in one place for too long could cause porcelain fracture.

15. Remove the cord from the sulcus, which will remove any excess cement from the gingival margin region (Fig. 8.50).

16. Perform the final polishing and occlusal adjustments with finishing diamonds, discs (Fig. 8.51A) and yellow finishing strips (Fig. 8.51B). Recall that the centric stops must be either on porcelain or tooth but never at the junction of the two. Remove any interproximal cement with a QwikStrip Serrated Strip from Axis Dental (i.e. Cerisaw or serrated interproximal strip) and floss (Fig. 8.51C).

17. Take photographs (Fig. 8.52) and an alginate impression for a protective nightguard.

CONTINUOUS CARE

Both forces and plaque will break down natural teeth and the artificial tooth surface. By controlling both of these, patients can have restorations for decades.

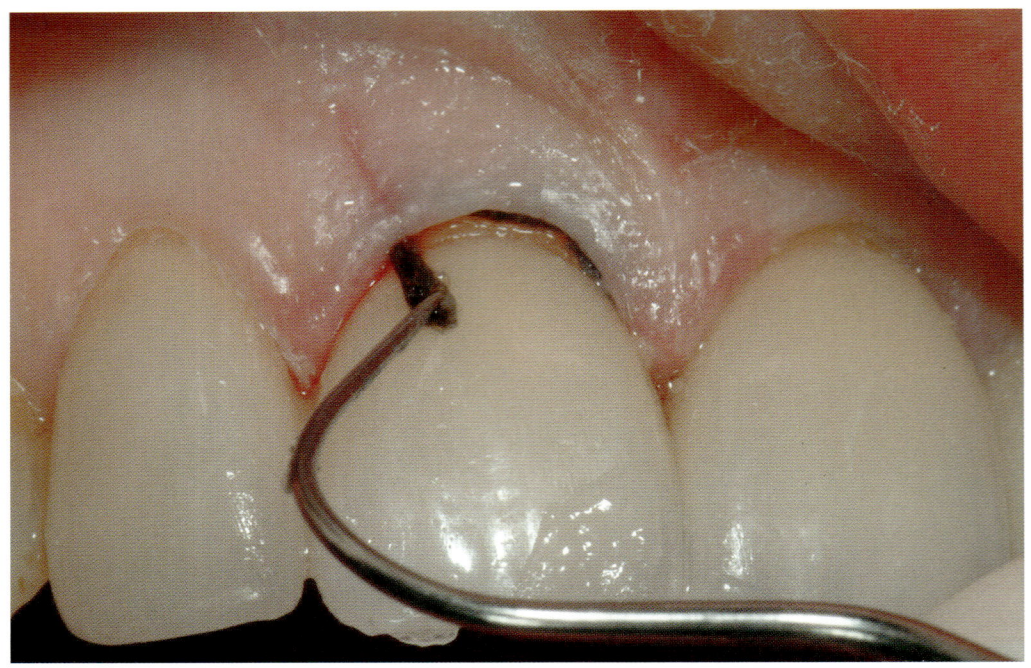

Fig. 8.50 Remove the cord.

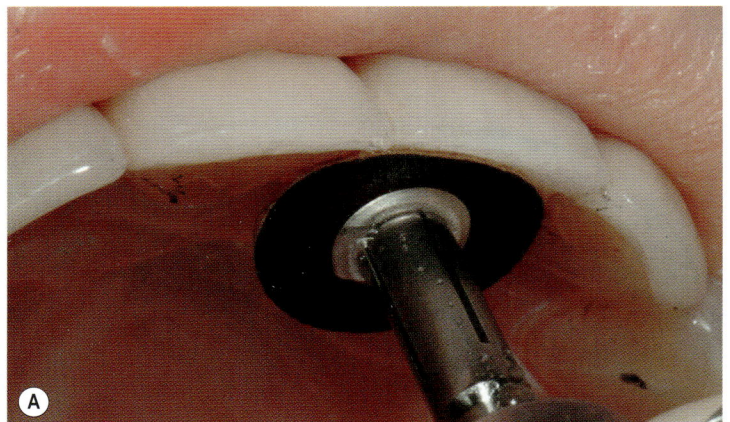

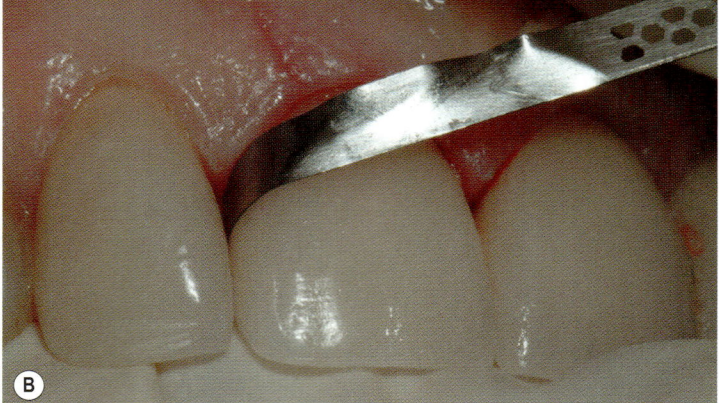

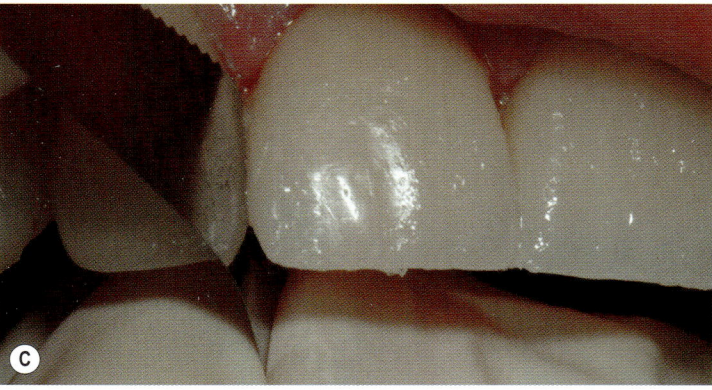

Fig. 8.51A–C Final polishing and occlusal adjustments.

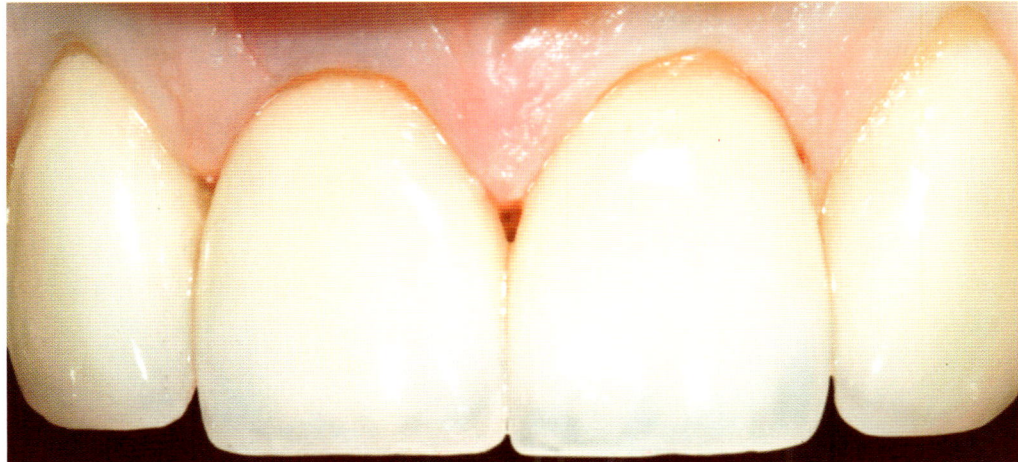

Fig. 8.52 Cemented veneers on insertion day. The patient will return for a final assessment and final photographs in 2 weeks, after the gingiva has healed completely.

ESSENTIALS

- Reduction guides allow visualization of the final incisal edge position and an understanding of the final tooth form. In prepping cases with any reductive aspects, i.e. correcting a rotation, before any space can be made for porcelain, the reduction guide must sit passively on the teeth. This allows the clinician to work backwards from the visualized 3-dimensional design of the wax-up.

- Veneer preparation requires reduction guides, a 1 mm round diamond bur, a self-limiting depth reduction bur, and a two-grit gross reduction bur. Rubber wheels, 3M discs and finishing strips are used to round off any remaining transitional areas and edges.

- Gingival margin placement must be carefully considered. It is best to keep the finish line equi- or supragingival, but if a large shade shift is desired, the finish line is placed within the sulcus. Interproximally, an 'elbow' is prepped just apical to the contact point, to hide the veneer's finish line when viewed laterally.

- When contact points are missing (i.e. diastema closure), the veneer preparation becomes a 'slice' prep, allowing the technician to build up the porcelain so that there is a smooth transition from the porcelain laminate veneer to the lingual contour of the tooth.

- Provisional veneers serve as a 'dress rehearsal', and are made from a matrix of the same wax-up that will guide the final porcelain. To ensure even more predictability, an alginate of the provisionals in the patient's mouth is taken and sent to the laboratory. This is especially critical if the shape of the provisionals has been altered in any way following patient feedback.

- Esthetic predictability is developed through a strategy to maximize the information flow from the patient to the esthetic dentist and the technology. This starts with the 3-step analysis and moves through treatment to a custom incisal edge index taken from the time-tested provisional, producing a predictable final result.

Having a substantial hygiene programme in the office for continuous care and so that any problems can be dealt with early is critical. The dentist and the hygiene team have the opportunity to evaluate the mouth from a standpoint of plaque control, forces and stresses patients can put on their teeth, and the health of the mouth. If the patient comes in routinely, a minimum of twice a year, the team can work with the patient on plaque control, proper oral hygiene technique of brushing and flossing and proper nutrition. If there are forces in the mouth that are above normal forces, a protective appliance, a nightguard (orthotic), is fabricated to protect the restorative dentistry.

PATIENTS' FAQS

Q. How much are you going to shave down my teeth?

A. The beauty of veneers is that they require minimal tooth reduction, or 'preparation' as we call it. If we did not make any space, the veneers would probably look bulky. The good news is that in most situations, the newest materials require minimal reduction – just half of what was required in the past.

Q. On preparation day, am I leaving here with anything on my teeth?

A. Yes! You will leave this appointment wearing your temporaries, i.e. provisionals, which are a plastic version almost identical to what the final veneers will look like. This is your 'dress rehearsal', and we actually want you to look very closely at your temporaries. Any changes you'd like to make (e.g. shade, length and shape of the teeth) can be discussed with our lab and addressed before they make the final porcelain.

Q. Are there any foods I should stay away from when I have my veneers?

A. Anything that will chip your teeth can also chip your veneers. We would advise against biting anything extremely hard, i.e. chicken bones or very hard bread crust. You shouldn't feel that you're 'walking on eggshells', but always remember that although the materials we have today are extremely strong, porcelain is inherently more brittle than a natural tooth.

Q. Should I whiten my teeth before receiving the veneers?

A. Yes! A porcelain veneer cannot be bleached, so before we select the colour for your veneers, we should make your other teeth (the ones that will not be receiving veneers) as white as possible, so we can match to that and have everything blend nicely. Additionally, if we whiten the teeth that are receiving the veneers, we can make the veneers as thin as possible (i.e. less tooth shaving) because we won't have to mask as dark a colour.

CLINICAL CASE 8.1

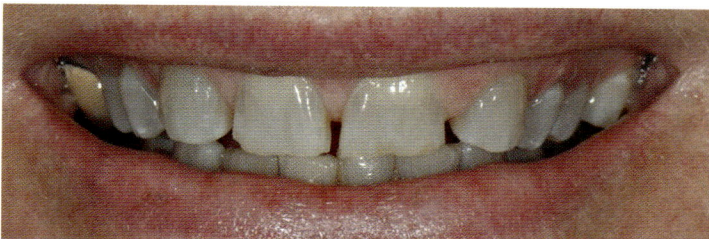

Fig. C8.1.1   Pre-operative dentition, dentofacial view.

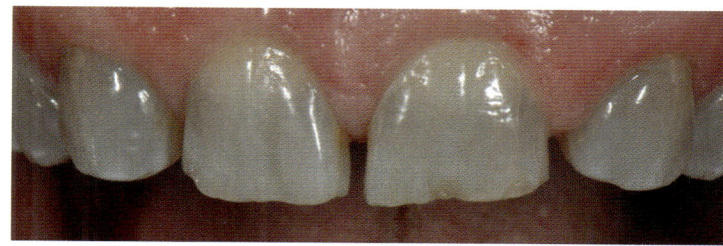

Fig. C8.1.2   Dental view of pre-operative dentition.

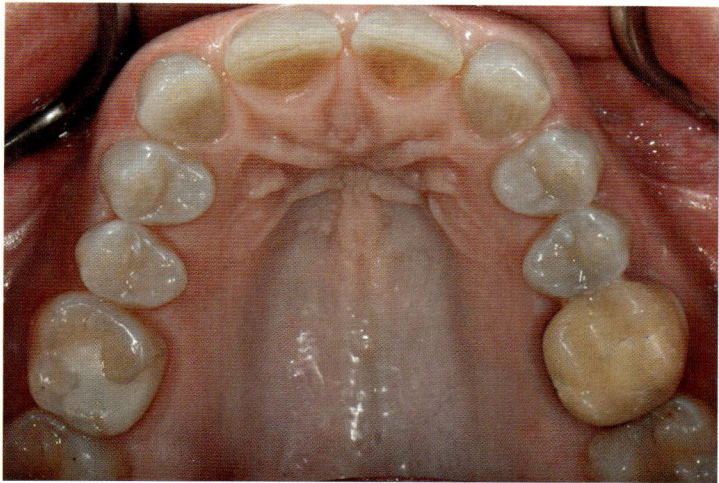

Fig. C8.1.3   Occlusal view of pre-operative dentition.

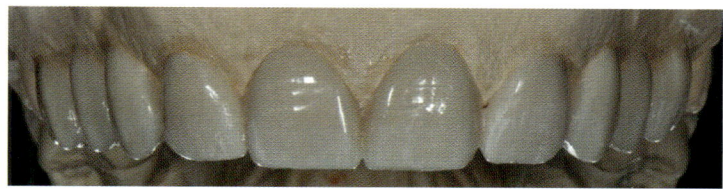

Fig. C8.1.4   The diagnostic wax-up.

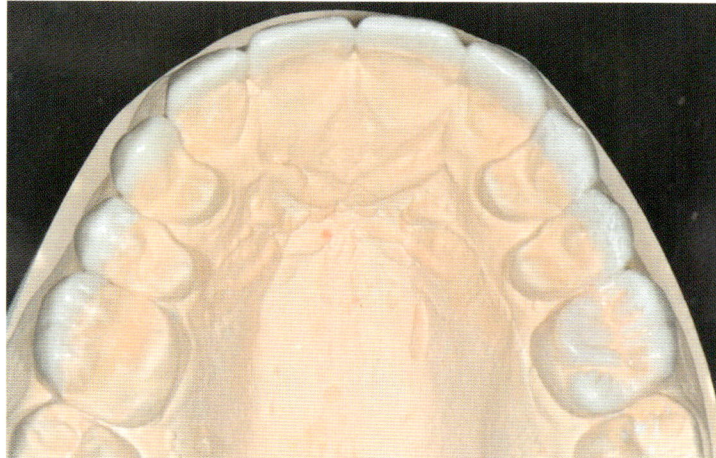

Fig. C8.1.5   Diagnostic wax-up, occlusal view.

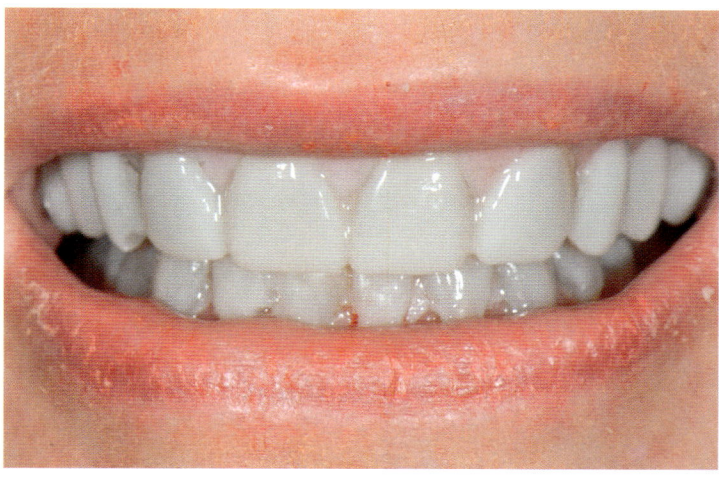

Fig. C8.1.6   The intra-oral mock-up (mandibular arch was treated as well).

CLINICAL CASE 8.1

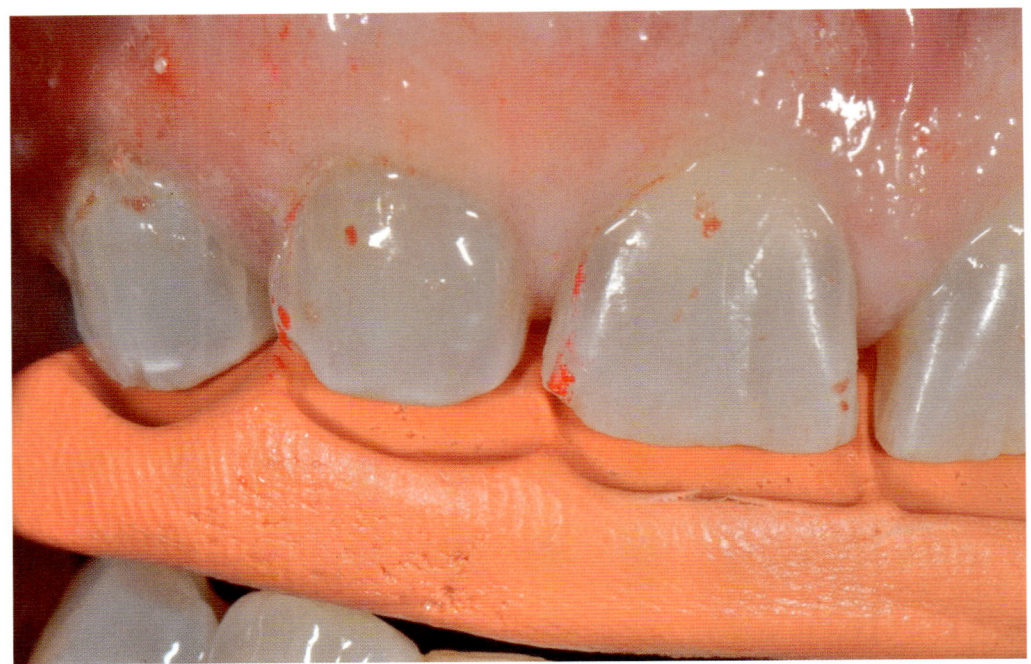

Fig. C8.1.7 PVS reduction guide showing the need for pre-preparation enameloplasty.

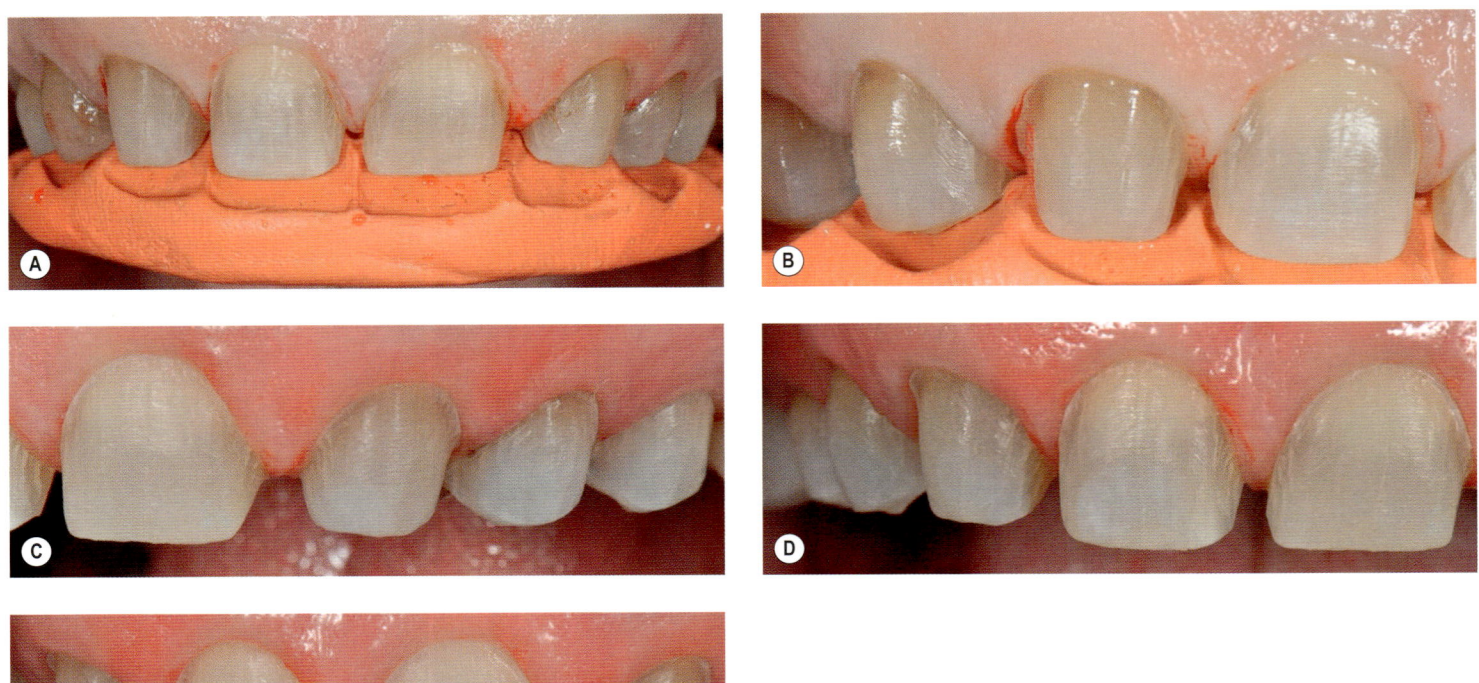

Fig. C8.1.8A–E Showing frontal and lateral views of completed preparations.

260

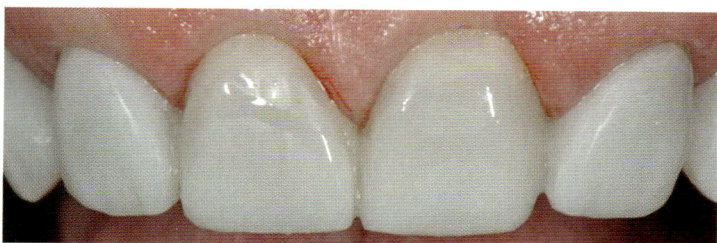

Fig. C8.1.9 Glazed provisional veneers.

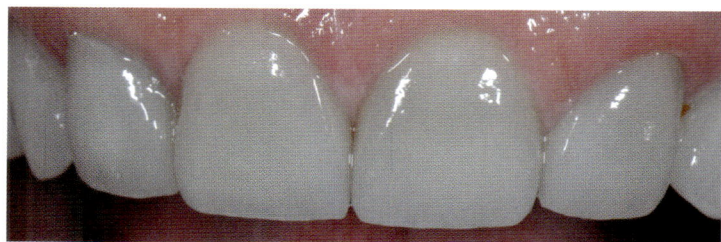

Fig. C8.1.10 Final veneers (photo taken 2 weeks after insertion), demonstrating healed gingival tissue. Note how closely the final restorations mimic the form of the provisionals.

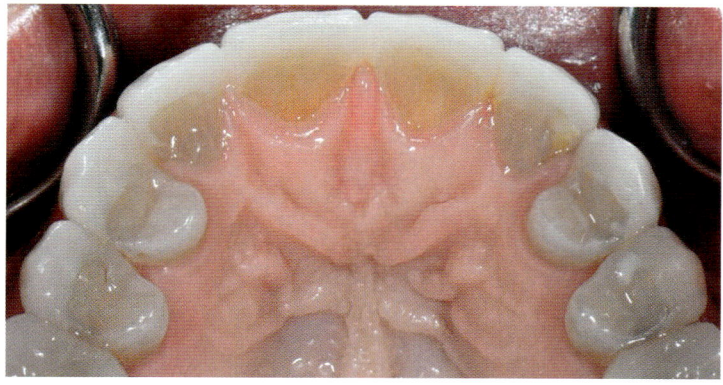

Fig. C8.1.11 Occlusal view of inserted veneers.

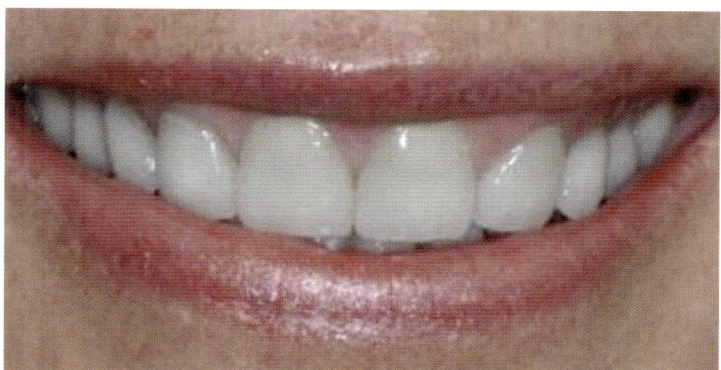

Fig. C8.1.12 Dentofacial view of inserted veneers.

CLINICAL CASE 8.2

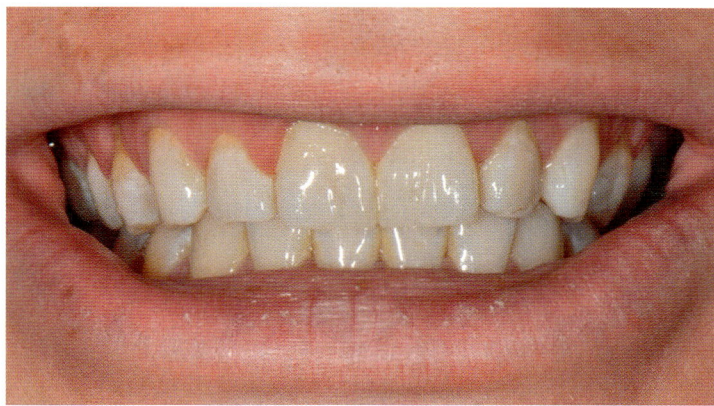

Fig. C8.2.1 A 20-year-old patient presents with discoloured teeth displaying severe anterior wear, which must be restored before posterior wear begins.

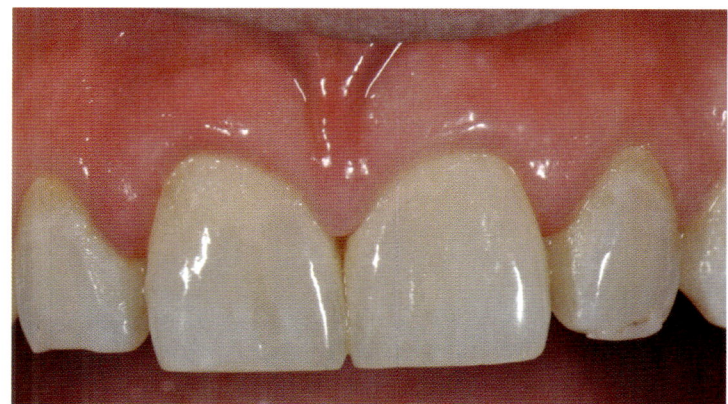

Fig. C8.2.2 A wear facet on #7, worn incisal edges on #8 and #9, and a failing composite restoration on the incisal edge of #10.

CLINICAL CASE 8.2

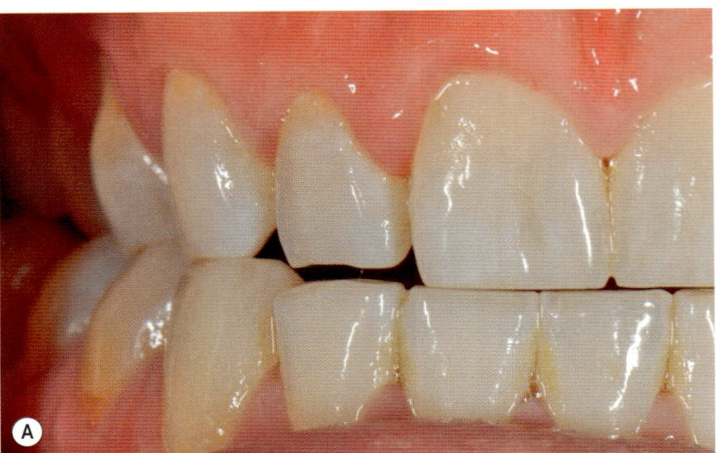 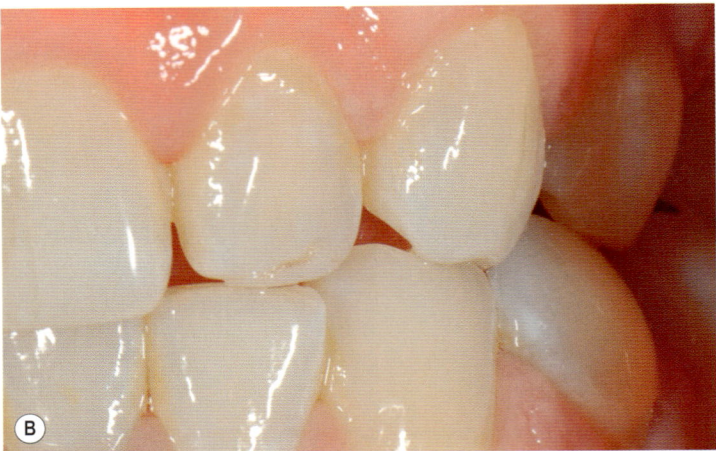

Fig. C8.2.3A,B Lack of canine guidance bilaterally, explaining the worn incisal edges of the anterior teeth. The canines should disclude the anterior teeth when the mandible moves into lateral excursions. Additionally, the posterior teeth are not separated when the patient is in the protrusive edge-to-edge position, which speeds up the wear of both the anterior and posterior teeth, and must be corrected.

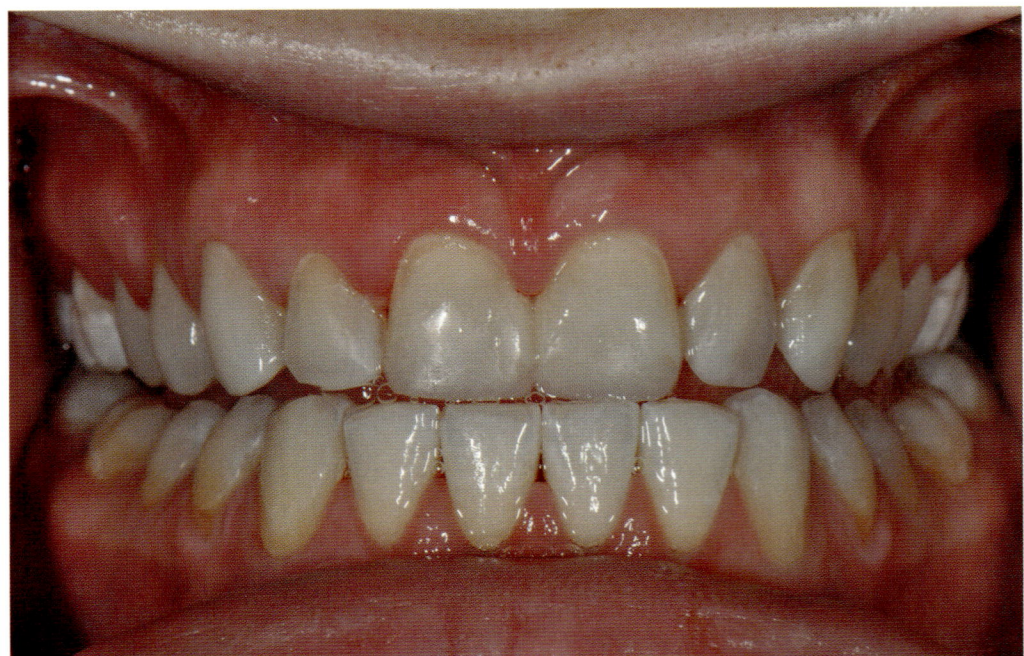

Fig. C8.2.4 The resin veneer provisionals (teeth #4–13) correct the occlusal issues, providing separation of posterior teeth when in edge-to-edge position (shown here) as well as bilateral canine guidance.

CHAPTER 8
ANTERIOR BONDED RESTORATIONS

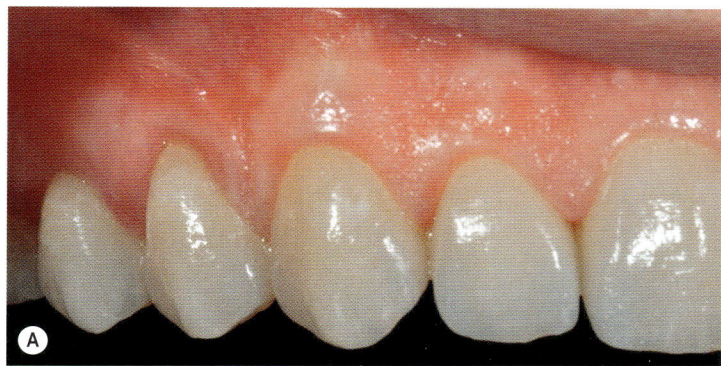
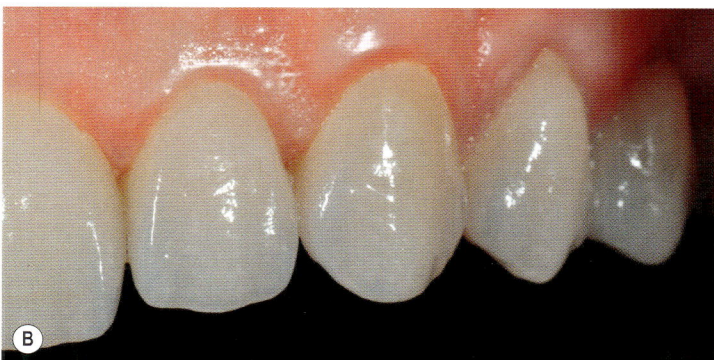
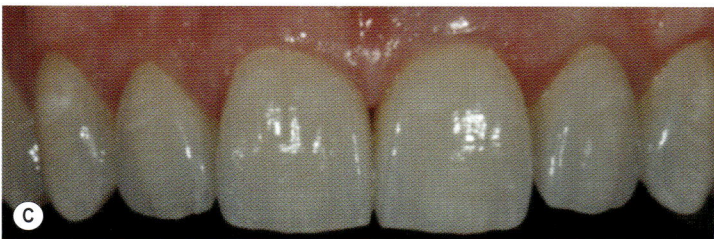

Fig. C8.2.5A–C   The final restorations, lithium disilicate veneers, display a high degree of naturalness and characterization as per the patient's desire. The perfected occlusal scheme that had been built into the original wax-up, and then the provisionals, has been transferred accurately and predictably into the final restorations.

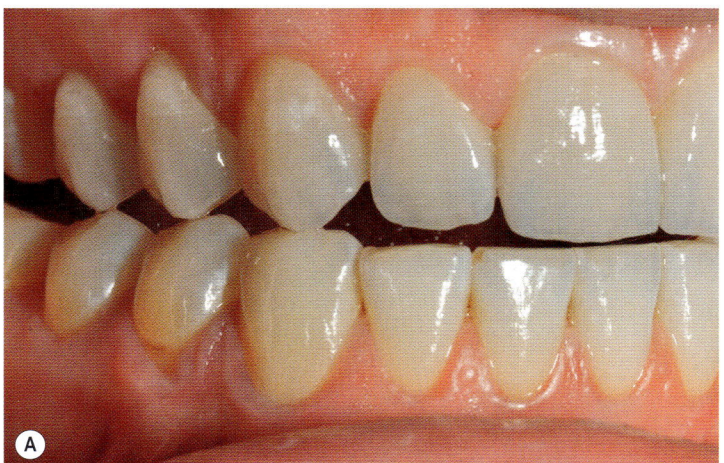
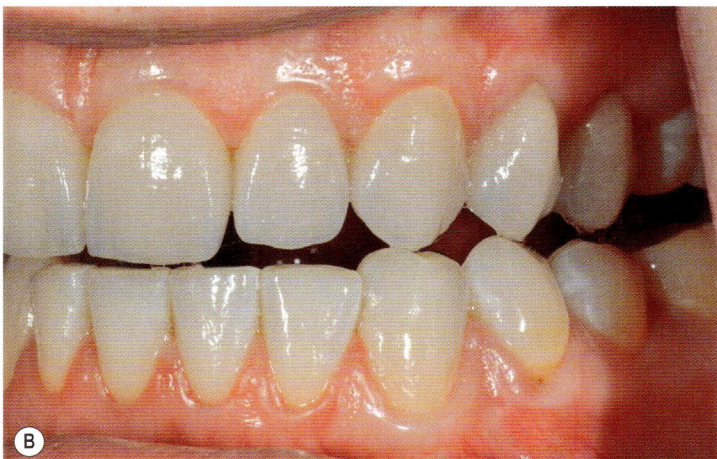

Fig. 8.2.6A,B   Left and right lateral guidance (carried on both the canines and premolars) will now protect the incisal edges of the anterior restorations.

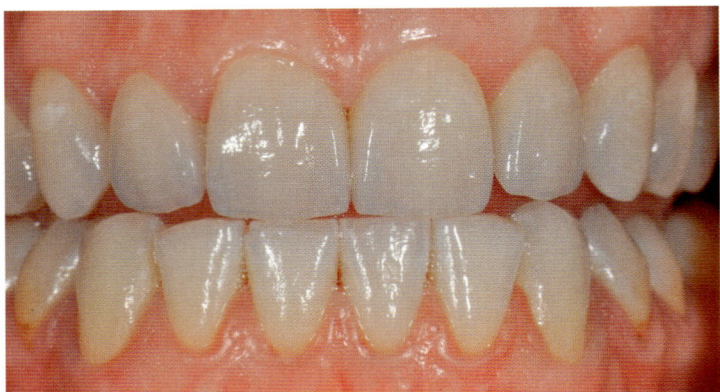

Fig. C8.2.7 Just as they had done in the provisionals, the maxillary central incisors separate the posterior teeth in the edge-to-edge position.

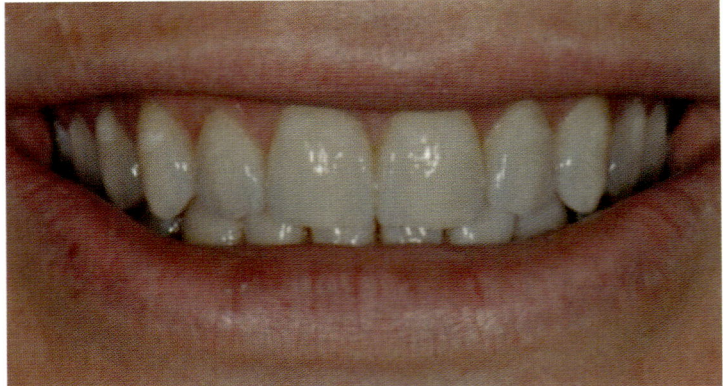

Fig. C8.2.8 The final outcome is a major esthetic improvement, yet completely natural looking and harmonious with the rest of the patient's dentition. The perfected occlusal scheme will ensure longevity of these restorations.

CLINICAL CASE 8.3

Freehand composite bonding (by Dr Newton Cardoso)

As excellent as feldspathic porcelain and lithium disilicate are, composite resin is sometimes the most appropriate material for esthetic improvement of the anterior teeth. One such case will be presented, utilizing the natural layering technique originally described by Dr Didier Dietschi.[9]

The Aesthetic Evaluation Form is filled out, paying attention to elements such as gingival display, lip support, negative space, length/width ratios, axial inclination and incisal embrasures.

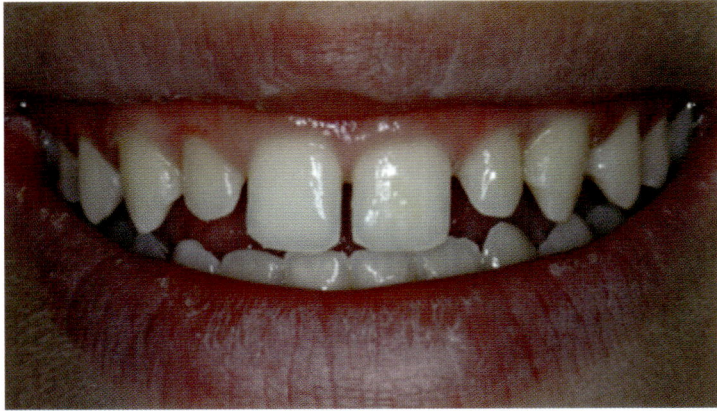

Fig. C8.3.1 A 17-year-old patient presents with the chief complaint of, 'I don't like my small, spaced-out teeth.' This patient had multiple diastemata despite previous orthodontics. She did not like her 'naïve' look and desired something more sensual and mature.

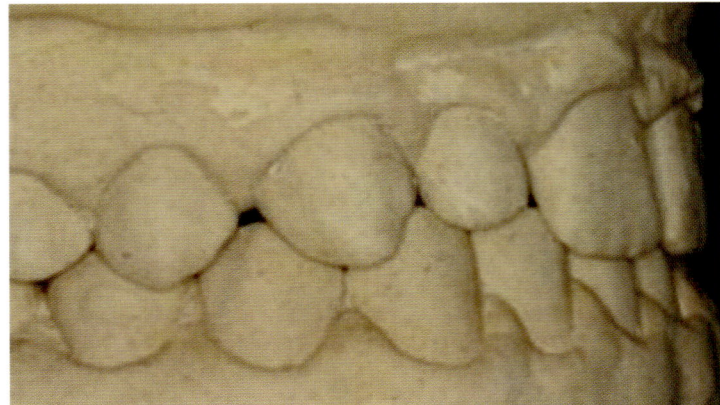

Fig. C8.3.2 The initial stone model shows the absence of lip support in the upper anterior area due to orthodontic compensation; there is a volume of tissue missing in the premaxilla, which will be compensated for by building out the cervical area of the teeth in the diagnostic wax-up.

The tri-dimensional position of the maxillary central incisor's incisal edge is assessed as well.

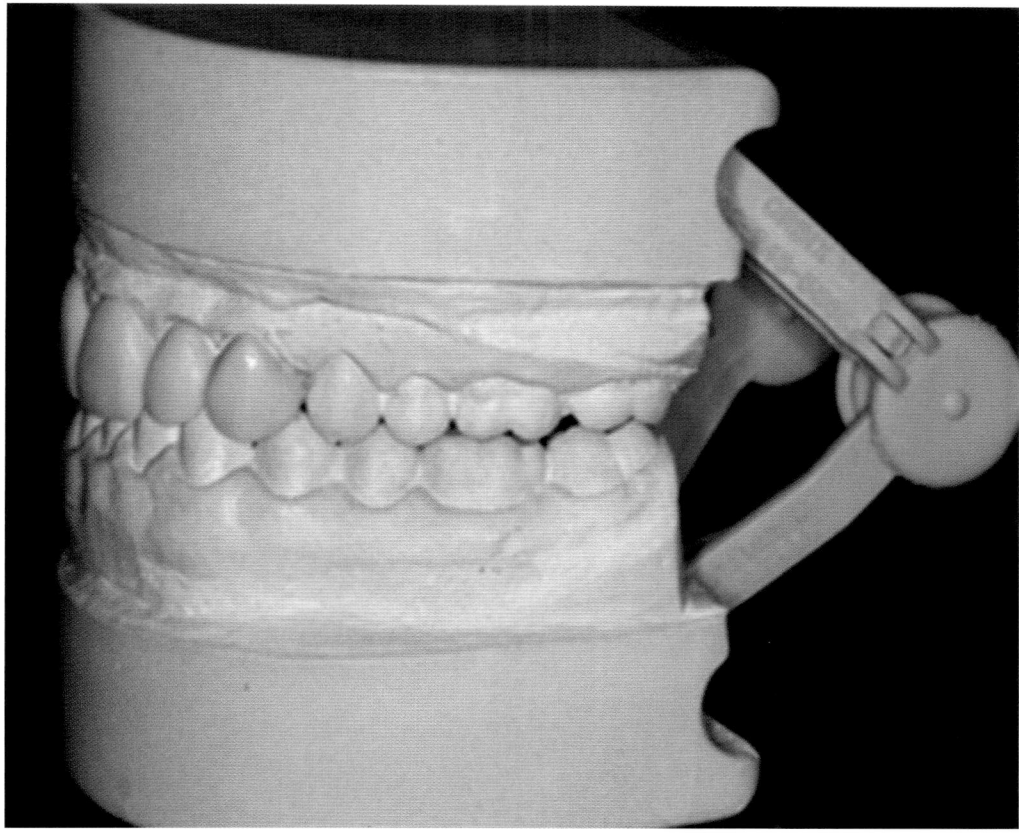

Fig. C8.3.3 Following the ideal zenith positions of the diagnostic wax-up, minor gingivoplasty is performed with an electrosurgery. The diagnostic wax-up here displays a thickness of material at the cervical edge of the teeth, to compensate for the deficient premaxilla bone support.

CLINICAL CASE 8.3

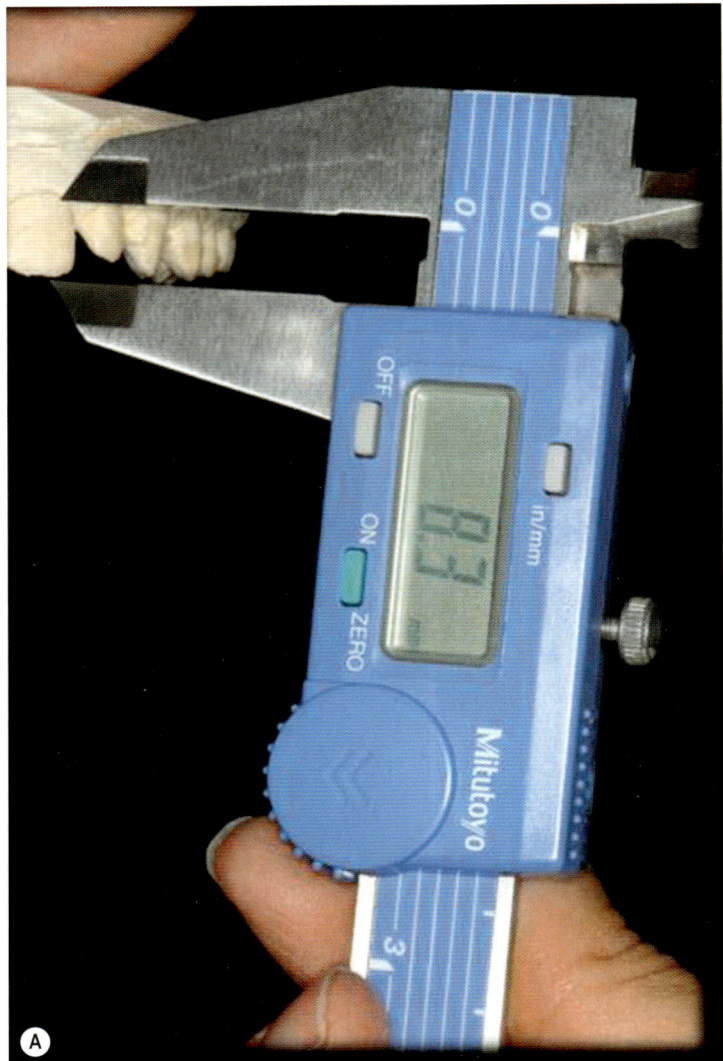

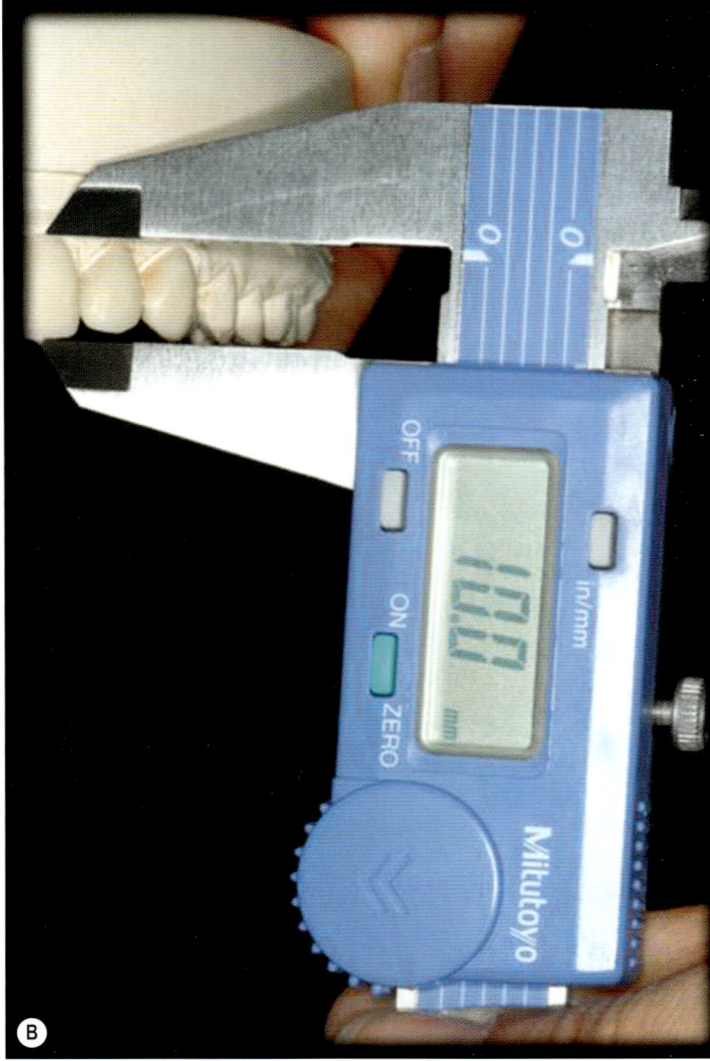

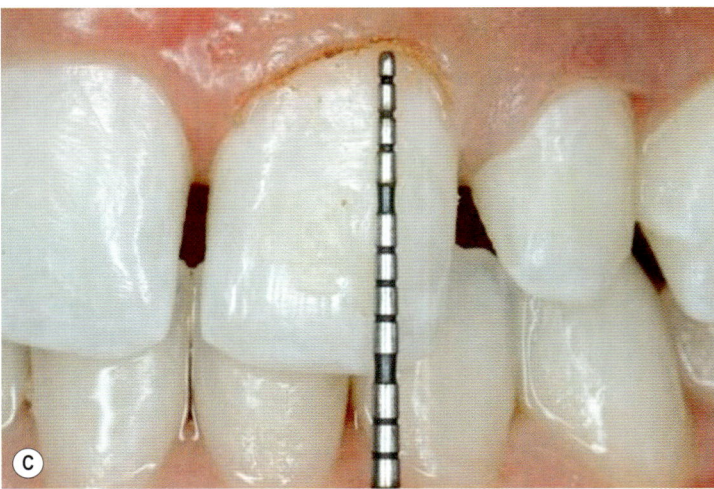

Fig. C8.3.4A–C The gingivoplasty is done without invading or compromising the biological width. The electrosurgery is also used to slightly thin out the interdental papillae where necessary. A digital caliper (A,B) is used to measure the study model and wax-up as well as the real tooth to be treated. Probing the gingival sulcus after gingivoplasty (C) confirms the presence of adequate biological width.

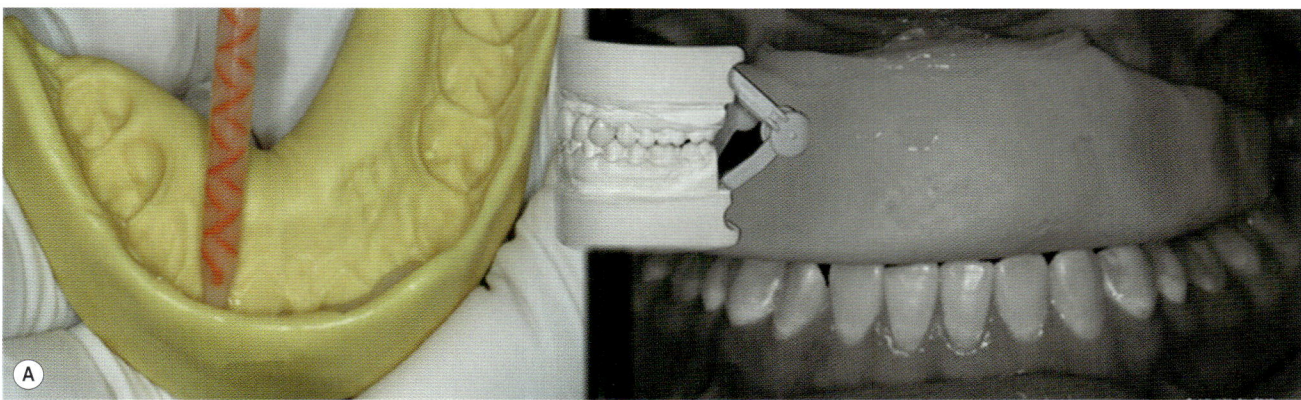

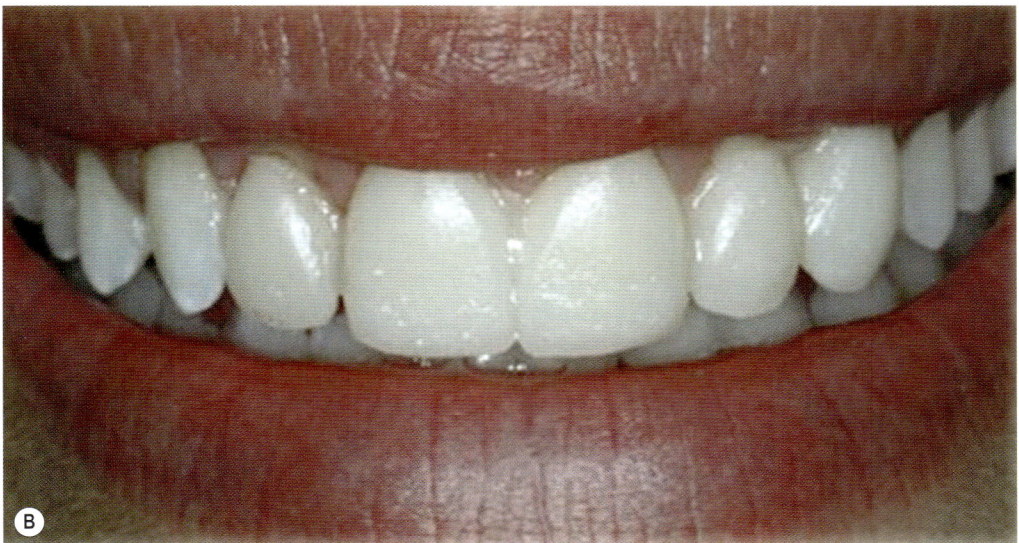

Fig. C8.3.5A,B Identical to the porcelain veneer process, the diagnostic wax-up is captured in a putty index and transferred to the teeth as a bis-acryl mock-up. This is the opportunity to 'visualize the solution', as information is gathered on esthetics, function, phonetics and whether the design is liked by the patient. Again, this is to ensure predictability and maximum communication among patient, clinician and technician.

CLINICAL CASE 8.3

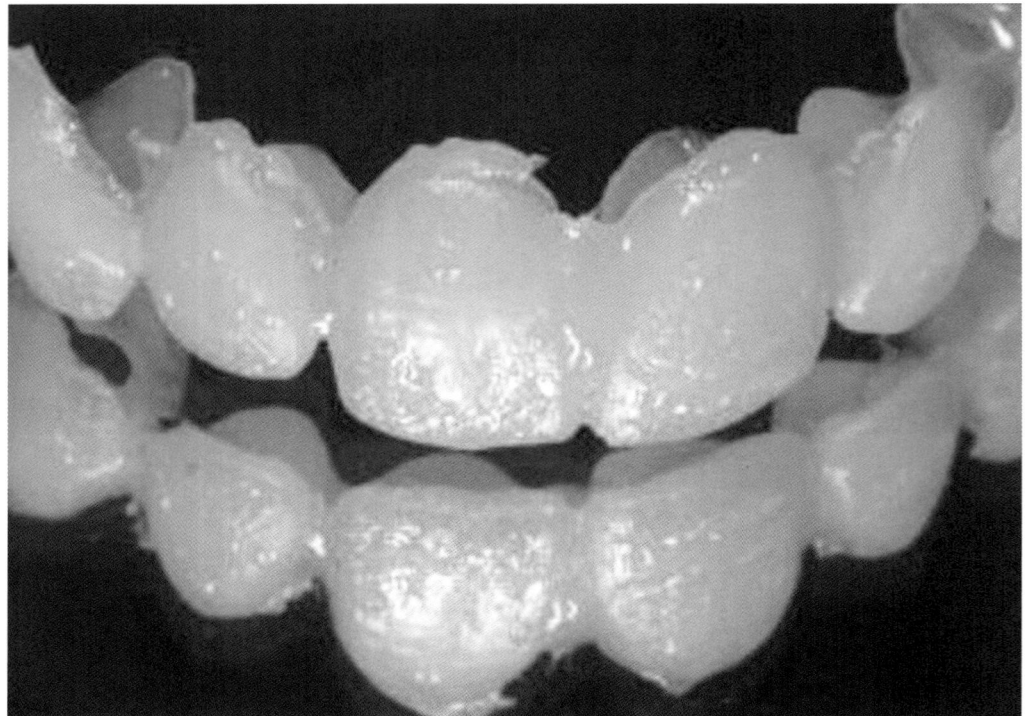

Fig. C8.3.6 Most of the time the intra-oral mock-up can be removed without being damaged. The thickness of the mock-up can be observed, giving valuable information as to exactly how additive the composite on each tooth will be. Knowing the composite thickness on each tooth is important, because that thickness must be split between a dental shade, an enamel shade and perhaps characterization and texture. Very often, clinicians are not cognizant enough of space limitations, adding in all sorts of effects, mamelons, tints, opaquers and translucency – only to remove it all when they reshape the restoration to the ideal final form. Respecting the space available is critical for these types of restorations. Do not forget that two bodies cannot occupy the same place in space.

With the mock-up perfected intra-orally and impressioned, a new model is created and a PVS index is fabricated.

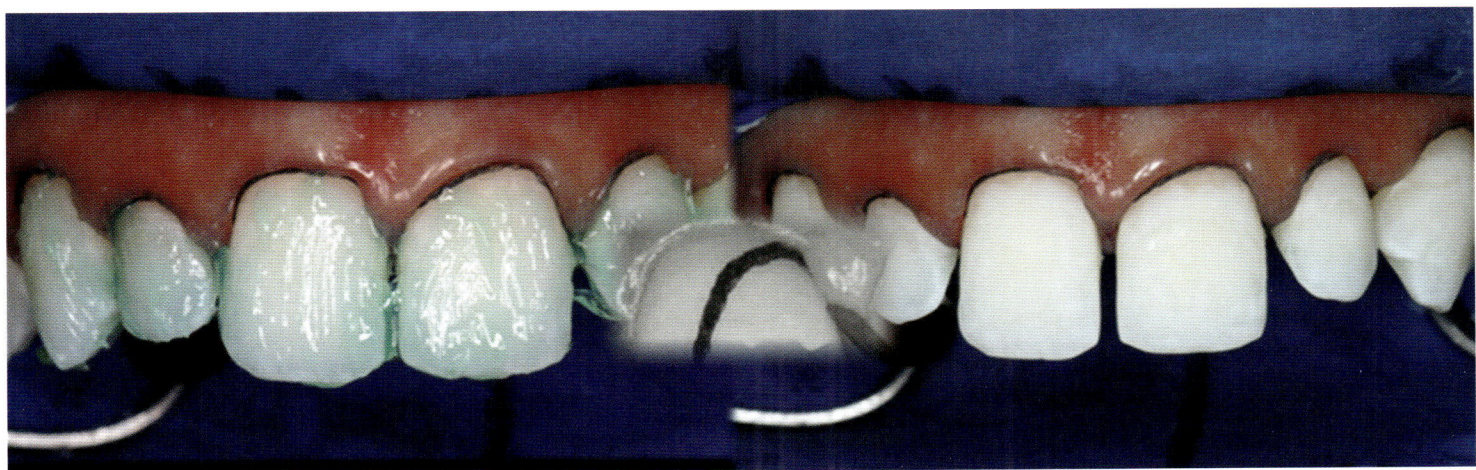

Fig. C8.3.7 Triple-zero cord is placed to prevent gingival exudate from contaminating the bond, a modified rubber dam is placed and the teeth are etched.

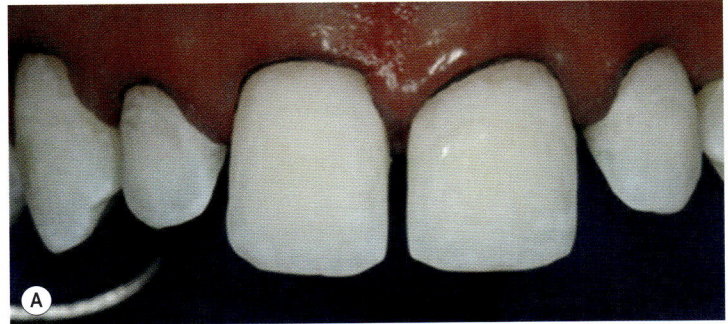 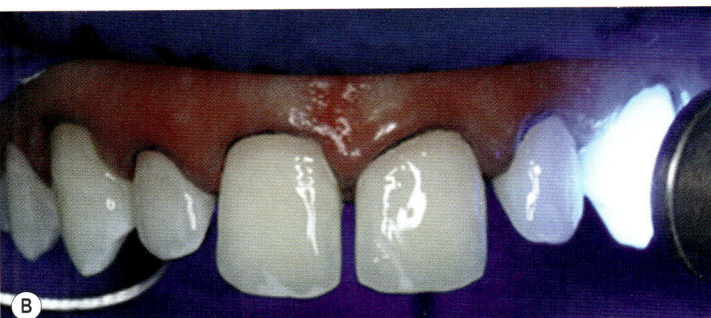

Fig. C8.3.8A,B Bonding agent is applied to all etched surfaces and cured.

CLINICAL CASE 8.3

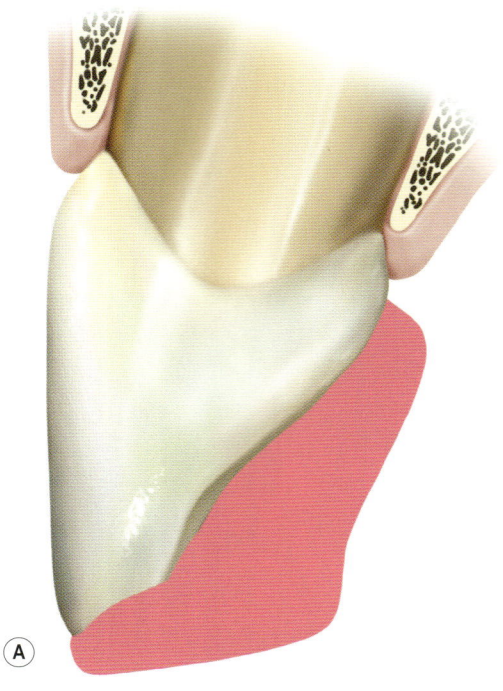

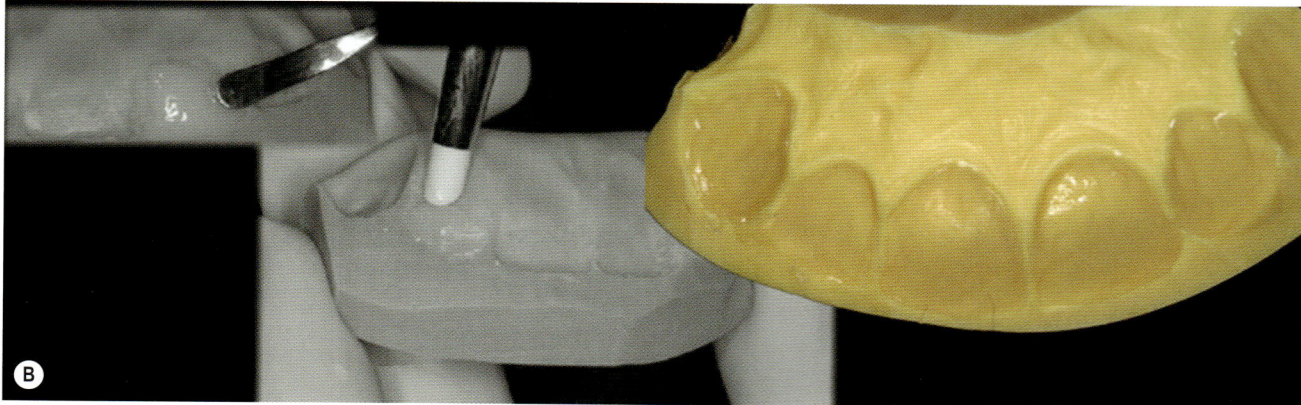

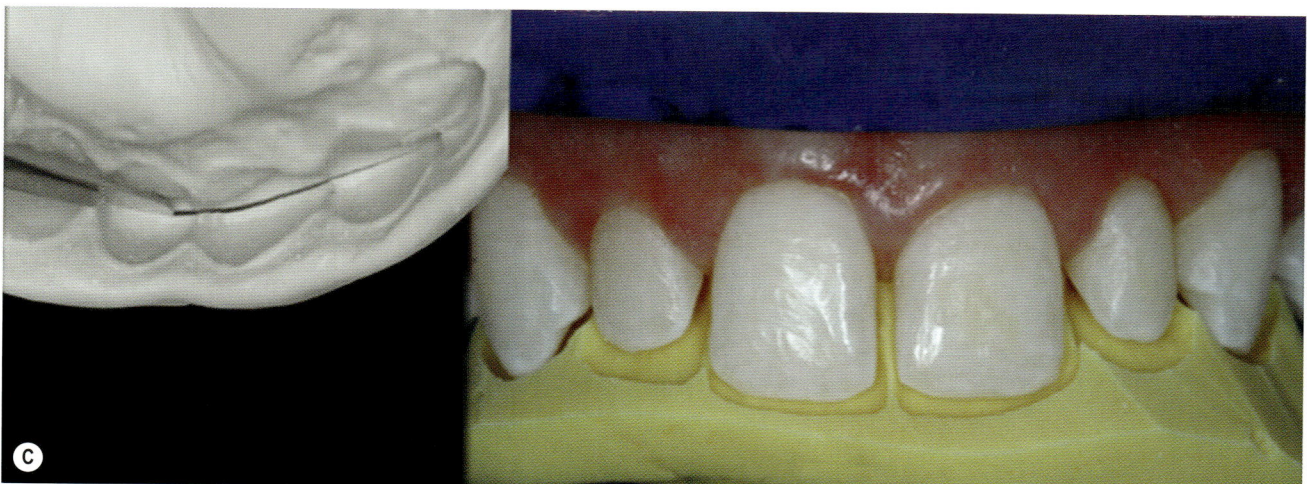

Fig. C8.3.9A–C The index is then placed and used to begin building up the lingual walls of the teeth.

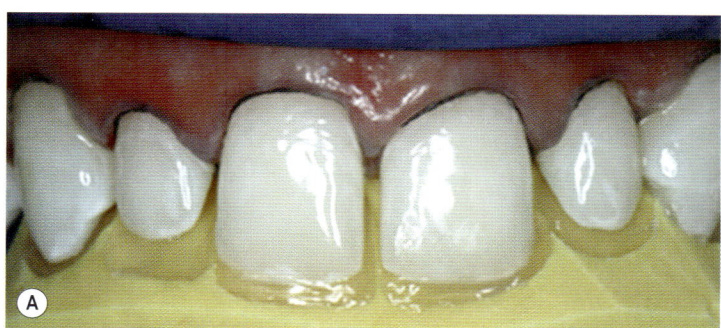
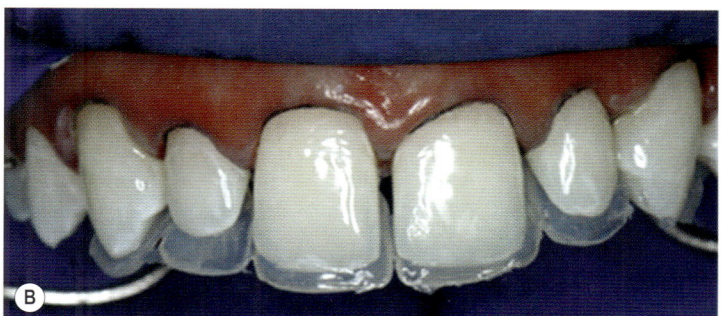

Fig. C8.3.10A,B A translucent enamel shade is used to build the lingual wall and incisal extent of the teeth, by flowing the material directly into the PVS guide.

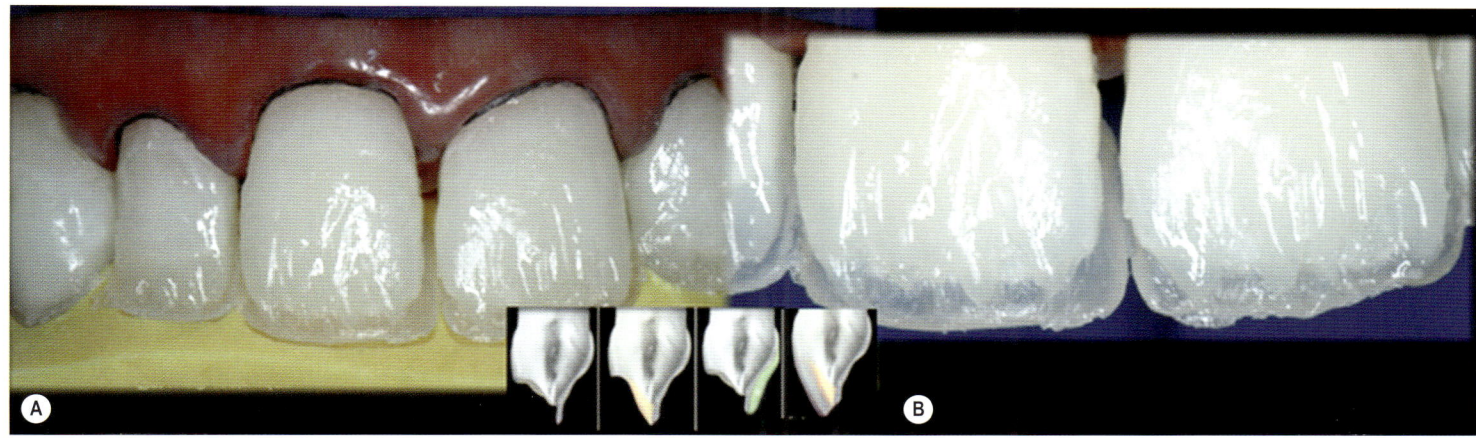

Fig. C8.3.11A,B After curing, the index is removed gently and the dentine layer can be built into the translucent enamel 'shell'. Mamelons can be built into this layer, with the space between them adding a translucency effect. The challenge here is modulating the amount of light to be transmitted or reflected, aiming to reproduce what is normally found in a natural tooth. Once the dentine layer has been created satisfactorily, another layer of translucent 'enamel' material is added to the facial surface, following the PVS index, and bringing the restorations to full contour.

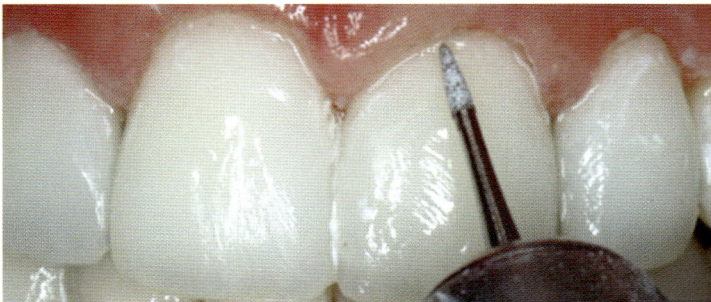

Fig. C8.3.12 Any texture can be added with a flame-tipped diamond bur and the line angles are defined with a red pencil and sandpaper discs. After the finest sandpaper disc is used, a final polish is applied with diamond polishing paste.

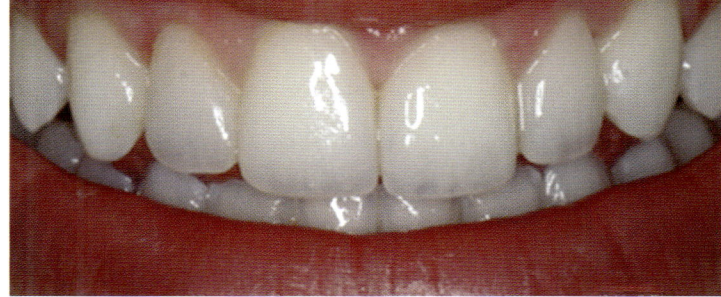

Fig. C8.3.13 The final outcome, created following a very conservative protocol, is functional, durable and highly esthetic compared to the pre-operative dentition (Fig. C8.3.1). Most importantly, the relative 'retrievability' of composite veneers, and their virtually noninvasive nature, makes this material an excellent choice for a younger patient requiring esthetic improvement.

Seminal literature

Chiche GJ, Pinault A. Esthetics of anterior fixed prosthodontics. Chicago: Quintessence; 1994.

Dawson P. Functional occlusion: from TMJ to smile design. St Louis, MO: Mosby Elsevier; 2007.

Feinman RA, Goldstein RE, Garber DA. Bleaching teeth. Chicago: Quintessence; 1987.

Gurel G. The science and art of porcelain laminate veneers. Chicago: Quintessence; 2003.

Muia PJ. The four dimensional tooth color system. Chicago: Quintessence; 1985.

Rufenacht CR. Fundamentals of esthetics. Chicago: Quintessence; 1990.

Scharer P, Rinn LA, Kopp FR. Esthetic guidelines for restorative dentistry. Chicago: Quintessence; 1982.

Tarnow DP, Chu SJ, Kim J. Aesthetic restorative dentistry, principles and practice. Mahwah, NJ: Montage Media Corporation; 2008.

REFERENCES

1. Dawson P. Functional occlusion: from TMJ to smile design. St Louis, MO: Mosby Elsevier; 2007. p. 150, 173.

2. Gwinnett AJ. Bonding basics: what every clinician should know. Esthetic Dent Update 1994;5:35–41.

3. Horn HR. A new lamination: porcelain bonded to enamel. NY State Dent J 1983; 49(6):401–3.

4. Calamia JR, Simonsen RJ. Effect of coupling agents on bond strength of etched porcelain. J Dent Res 1984;63:Abstract 79.

5. Gurel G. The science and art of porcelain laminate veneers. Chicago: Quintessence; 2003. p. 248, 249, 257, 260, 261, 485

6. Muia PJ. The four dimensional tooth color system. Chicago: Quintessence; 1985. p. 11–30.

7. Rufenacht CR. Fundamentals of esthetics. Chicago: Quintessence; 1990. p. 289–318, 348.

8. Brannstrom M. The cause of postrestorative sensitivity and its prevention. J Endod 1986; 12(10):475–81.

9. Dietschi D. Clinical application of the 'natural layering concept'. Dentsply; 2006.

CHAPTER 9

High-Performance Planning with Digital Design

NEWTON CARDOSO, PAULO BATTISTELLA

Digital smile design. 276
Laboratory technique 283
Clinical case 9.1 288
Clinical case 9.2 292
Conclusion 296
Acknowledgement 297

How do we maximize the effectiveness of the esthetic dental team for creating beautiful smiles? How can we use today's technology to connect the treatment room to the ceramist's bench, even when we are miles apart?

In previous chapters, we have spent a great deal of time discussing the flow of information from esthetic diagnosis to patient mock-up to provisionalization and then to the finished case. Using today's digital technology, we can improve the system. This chapter describes a digital protocol, first created by Christian Coachman, which improves communication and results in greater predictability for our esthetic cases.

DIGITAL SMILE DESIGN

We begin with the Aesthetic Evaluation Form and understanding our patient's needs and wants, followed by looking at the facial, dentofacial and dental views. A camera is used to document the facial view, analysing the general anatomical form and symmetry of the face (Fig. 9.1).

The next step is the dentofacial view (Fig. 9.2), where we analyse the positioning of the lips to the teeth, and then the dental view, which helps assess colour, tooth shape, translucency, value, zenith levels and the other micro-esthetic elements (Fig. 9.3).

After the complete series of photographs are obtained, we start our reverse digital planning, using the digital smile design methodology. The following

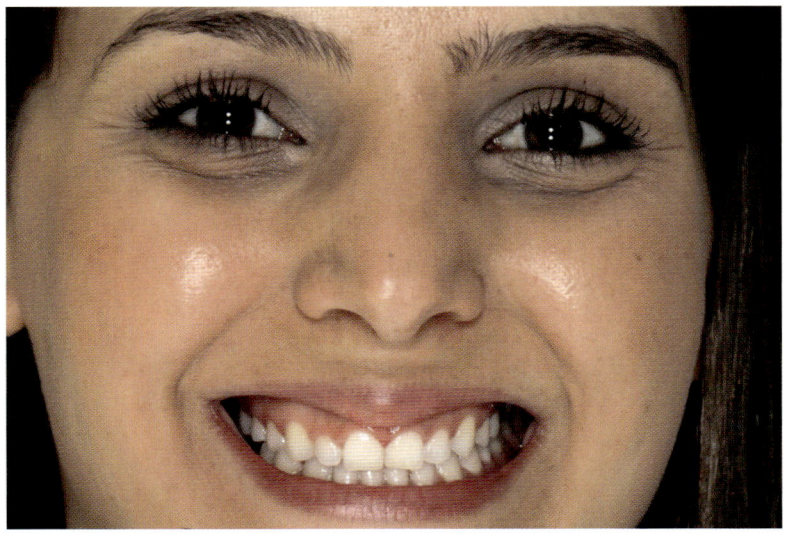

Fig. 9.1 Facial view.

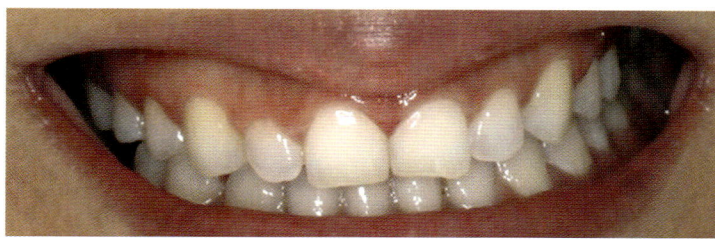

Fig. 9.2 The dentofacial view is used to assess the horizontal and vertical components of the smile, including buccal corridor, lip symmetry and the degree of gingival display while smiling.

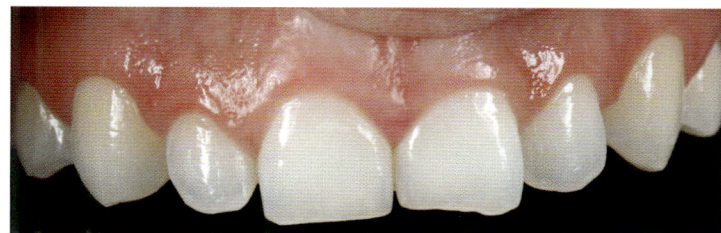

Fig. 9.3 The dental view (note the canted midline, orientated according to the facial view) helps analyse the micro-esthetic elements.

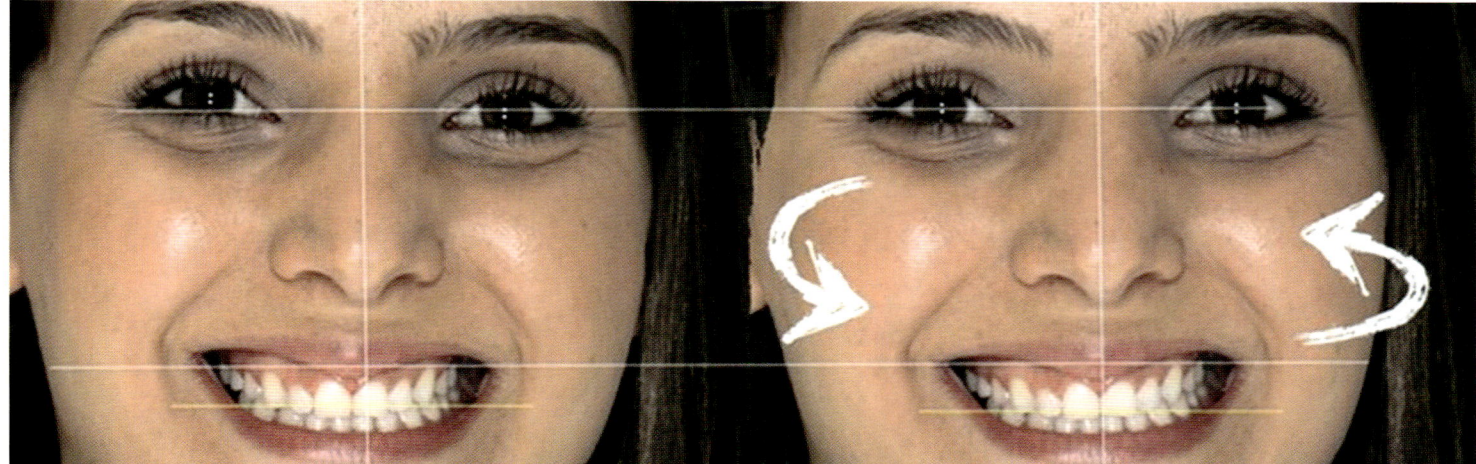

Fig. 9.4 The facial view with the head rotated so that the interpupillary line parallels the horizon. The midline, incisal line and zenith lines are drawn as well.

process utilizes Apple's Keynote software. For a photograph of the patient's full-face smiling, we first orient the head so that it is exactly straight up and down, that is, not leaning to the left or the right (Fig. 9.4). This will help orient the interpupillary line exactly parallel to the horizon. If this is not done correctly, the relationship of the incisal plane to the horizon will be incorrect, which might mask a canted maxilla.

Next, we zoom in and overlay the intra-oral photograph (Figs 9.5 and 9.6). We can now measure the size of the tooth on a physical model, and can calibrate an image of a ruler against the tooth in the photograph to correlate to the same height. For example, if the natural tooth is 10 mm high, we calibrate the ruler in the picture to be 10 mm in height. Next we carefully draw the outline

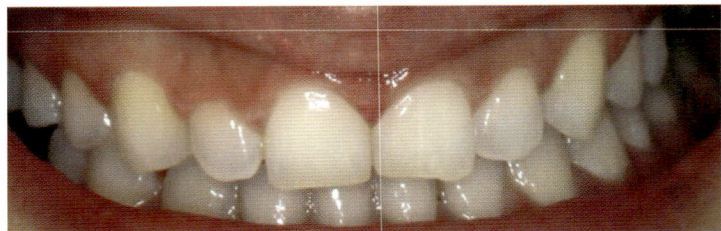

Fig. 9.5 The facial view is zoomed in upon, until we see just the dentofacial aspect.

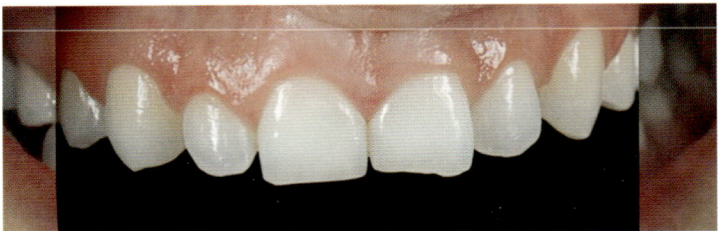

Fig. 9.6 The dental view is laid over the dentofacial view.

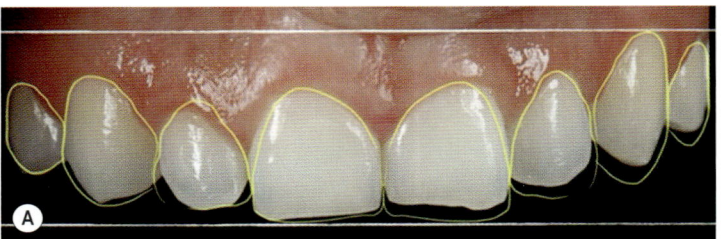

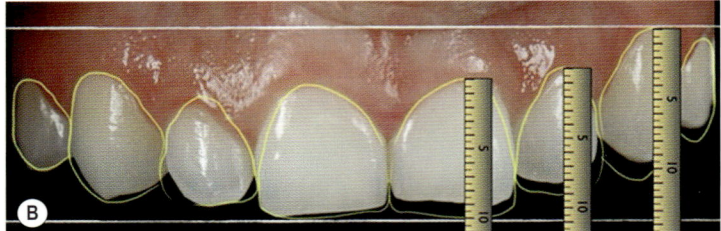

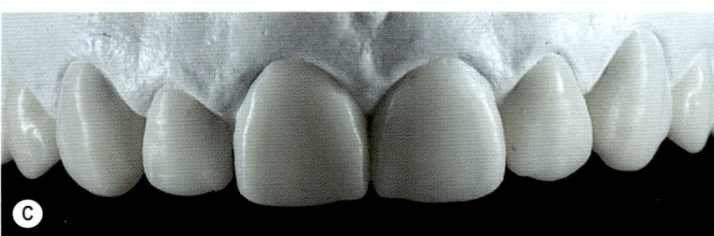

Fig. 9.7A–C The proposed changes to the tooth forms are measured with the calibrated digital ruler, and an exact replica is created in wax. Note that the wax-up does not reflect the changes to the gingival zeniths, which will be addressed only after the new incisal edge positions are tested via an initial mock-up.

of the new tooth forms, paying attention to the gingival zeniths, embrasures and incisal and proximal lines. The dimensions of these new tooth forms, the new extents of the 'white' and 'pink' zones, are measured via the digital ruler and the information is used to guide the wax-up (Fig. 9.7A–C). Figures 9.8A,B illustrate how the same digital ruler is used to measure changes in gingival height.

Prior to wax-up fabrication, the digital smile design can be tested virtually by simply cutting and pasting the new teeth into the patient's mouth (Fig. 9.9A–D). We observe the positioning of the lips, gingival zeniths, and shapes and sizes of the teeth. If both dentist and patient are satisfied, the wax-up can be fabricated and an intra-oral mock-up performed (Figs 9.9A,B, 9.10A,B and 9.11).

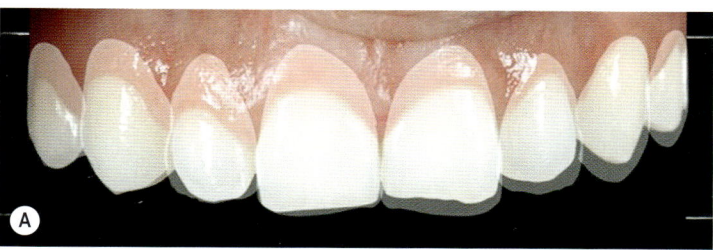
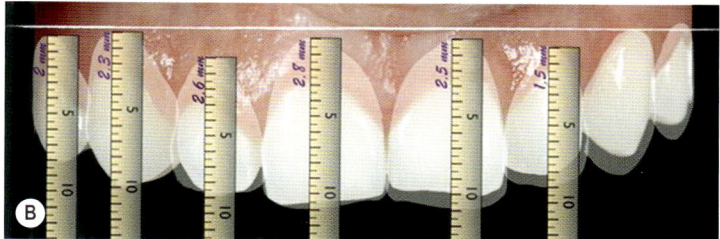

Fig. 9.8A,B The digital, calibrated ruler is used to measure the amount of length added to the incisal and gingival aspects of the teeth.

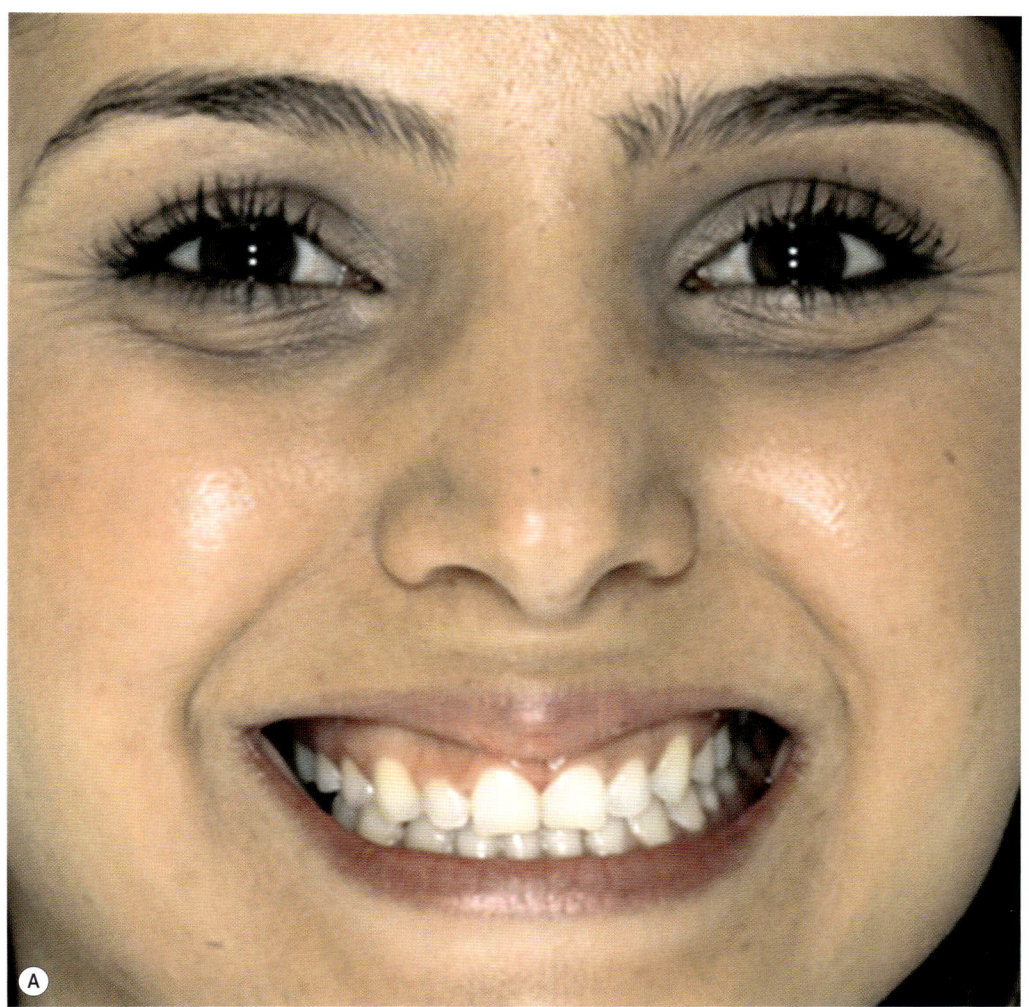

Fig. 9.9A–D Facial and dentofacial views of the digital mock-up.

Continued

DIGITAL SMILE DESIGN

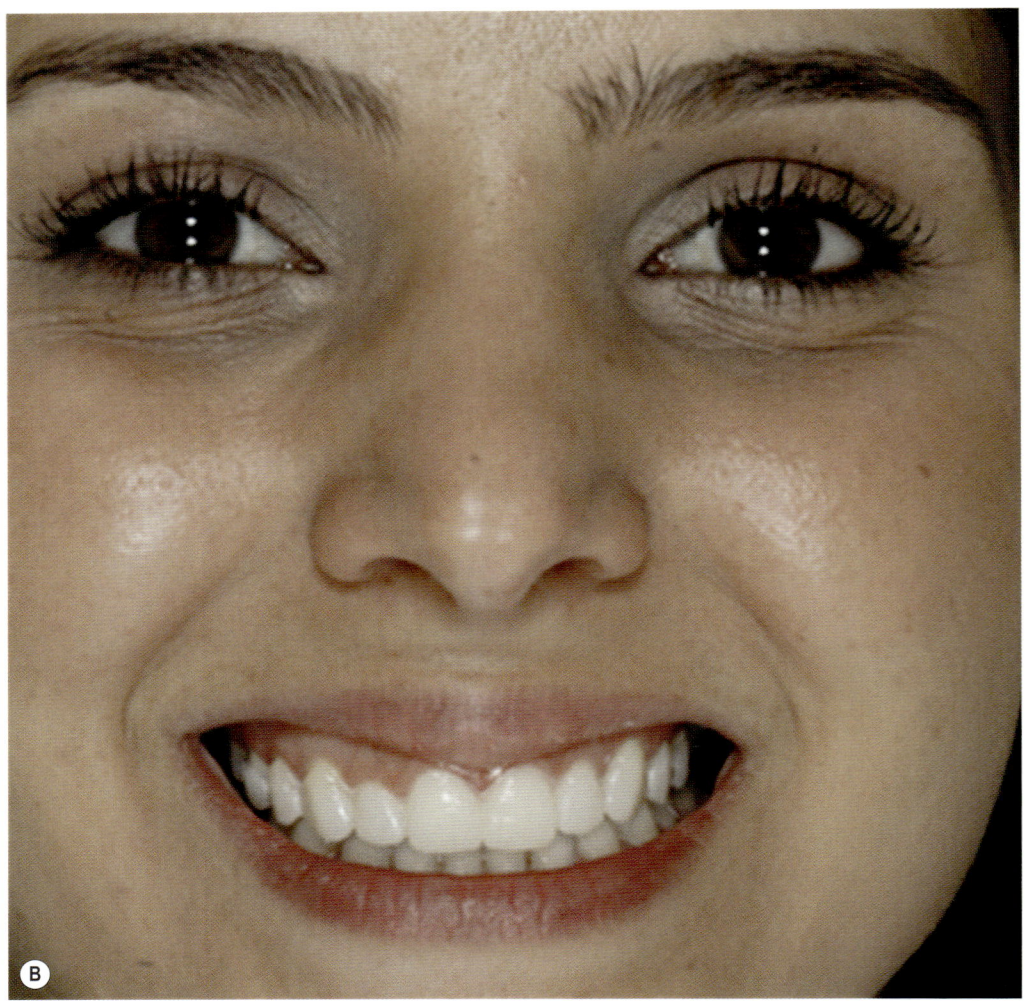

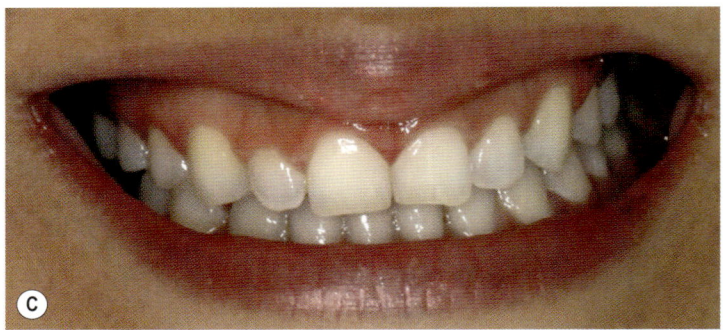

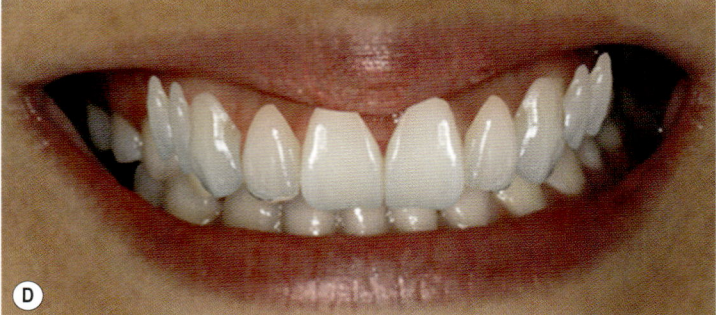

Fig. 9.9A–D *Continued*

HIGH-PERFORMANCE PLANNING WITH DIGITAL DESIGN

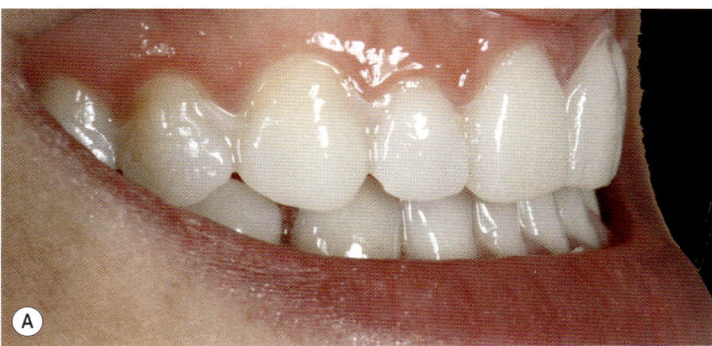
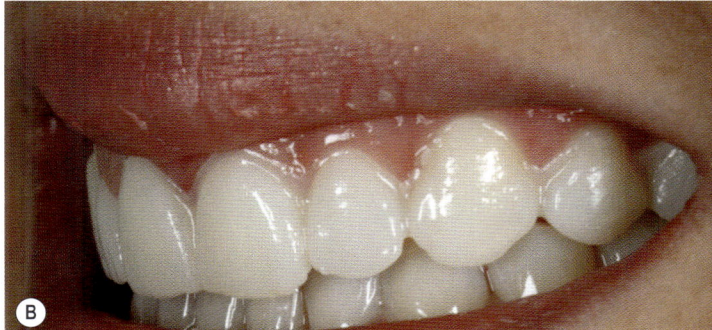

Fig. 9.10A,B The intra-oral mock-up, based on the digitally designed diagnostic wax-up

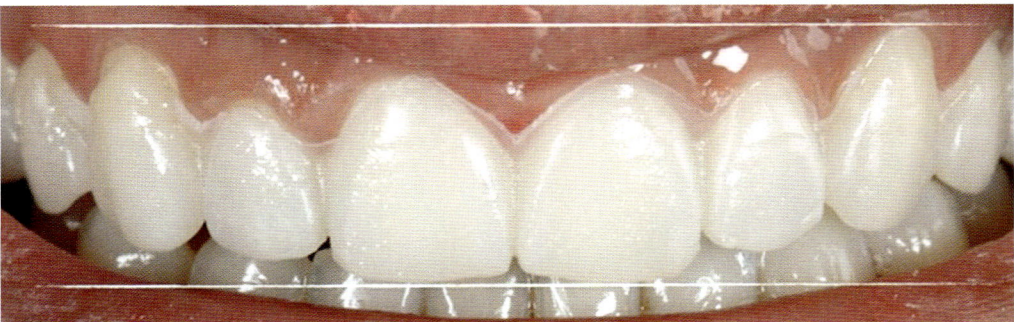

Fig. 9.11 Intra-oral mock-up.

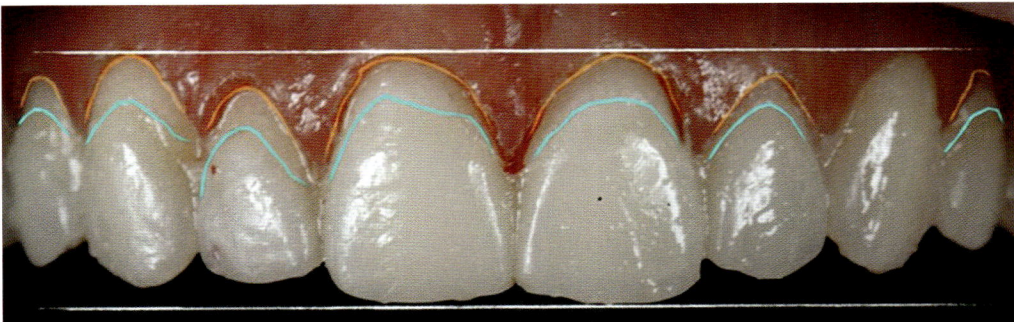

Fig. 9.12 The original and final zenith positions.

The gingival levels are corrected surgically, with the periodontist using the digital measurements as a guide. Figure 9.12 shows the original (turquoise) and final (orange) zenith positions, and Figure 9.13A–C shows how closely the gingival surgery followed the digital design.

Immediately following the gingival surgery, a new impression is obtained, a mock-up of the incisal changes is applied to the model itself, and a proper emergence profile is waxed for each tooth at the cervical region (Fig. 9.14).

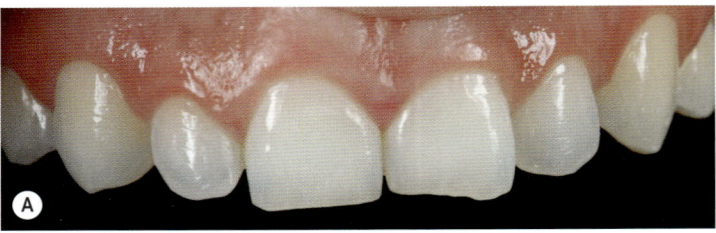
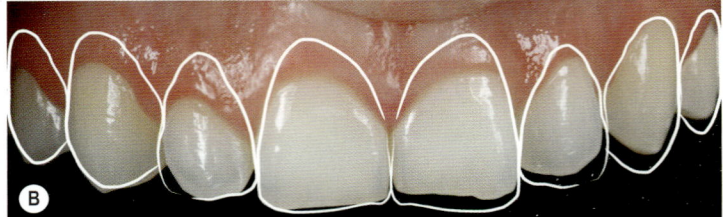
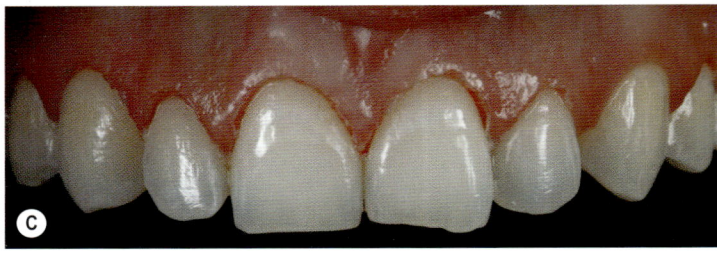

Fig. 9.13A–C Gingival surgery following the digital design.

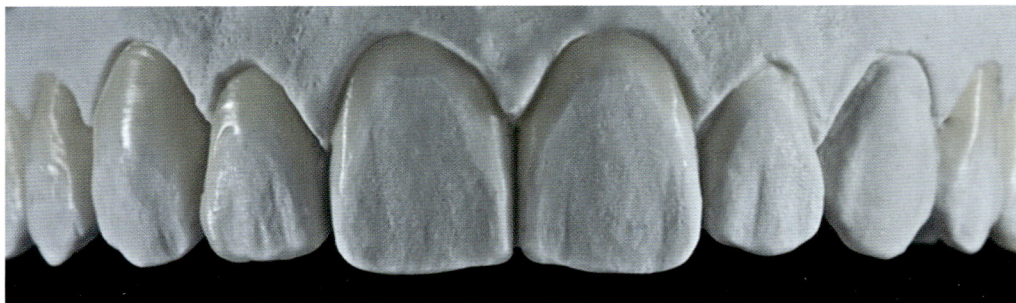

Fig. 9.14 Emergence profile with each tooth waxed at the cervical region.

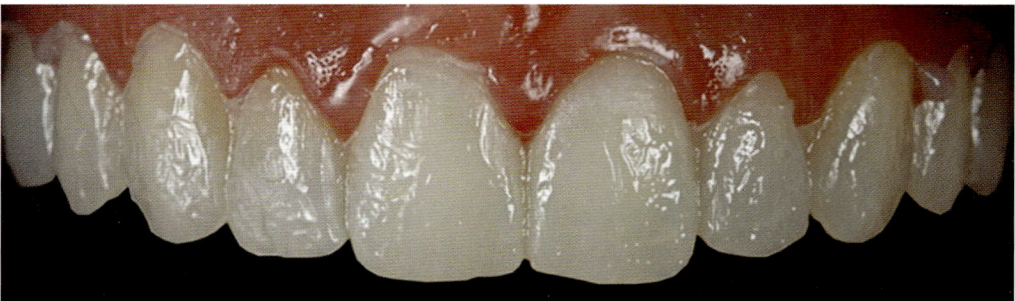

Fig. 9.15 A second mock-up is applied intra-orally.

After 4–6 weeks of healing, a second mock-up – now with corrected gingival zeniths – is applied intra-orally (Fig. 9.15). The Aesthetic Pre-Evaluative Temporary (APT) veneer preparation method (discussed in Chapter 8) is now used, with the veneers prepared directly through the mock-up. The APT technique allows us to be as non-invasive as possible, and the resulting preparations are

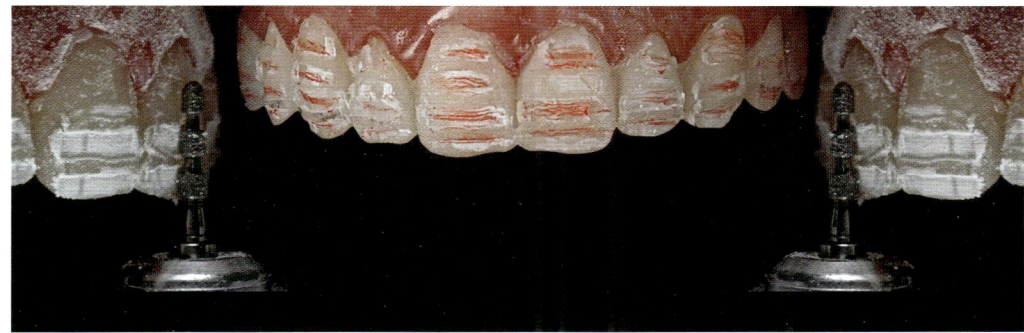

Fig. 9.16 The Aesthetic Pre-Evaluative Temporary method. Depth cuts made on the mock-up.

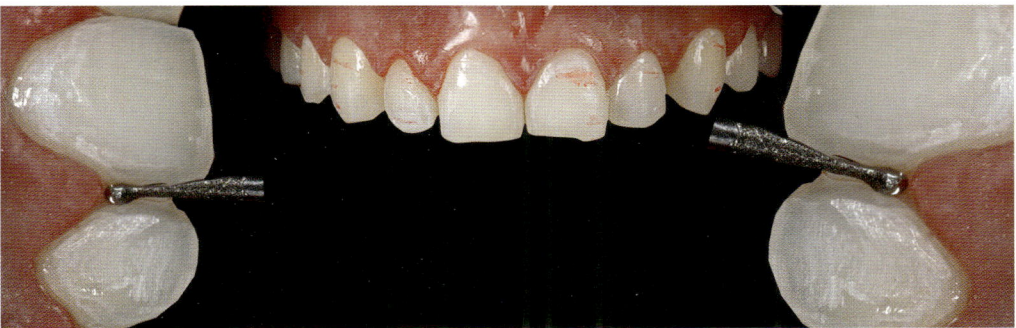

Fig. 9.17 Preparations in enamel.

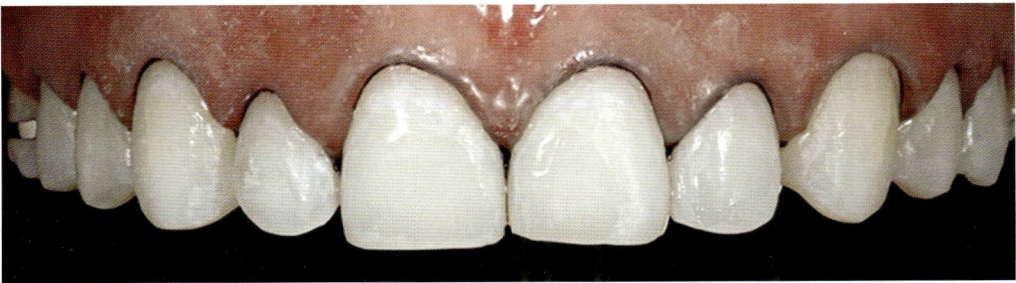

Fig. 9.18 The completed preparations (shown with retraction cord placed) are minimal and entirely in enamel. Note the acceptable, high-value starting shade. This is an excellent indication for 'contact lens' veneers, which are thin enough to transmit the underlying shade and give the restorations depth.

entirely in enamel (Figs 9.16–9.18). An impression is obtained and sent to the laboratory (Fig. 9.19).

LABORATORY TECHNIQUE

The working model is poured and waxed-up. We press it with IPS e.max HT Impulse O2, which is an ingot with an opalescence effect. The veneers in this case are referred to as 'contact lenses', wherein the underlying shade does not

LABORATORY TECHNIQUE

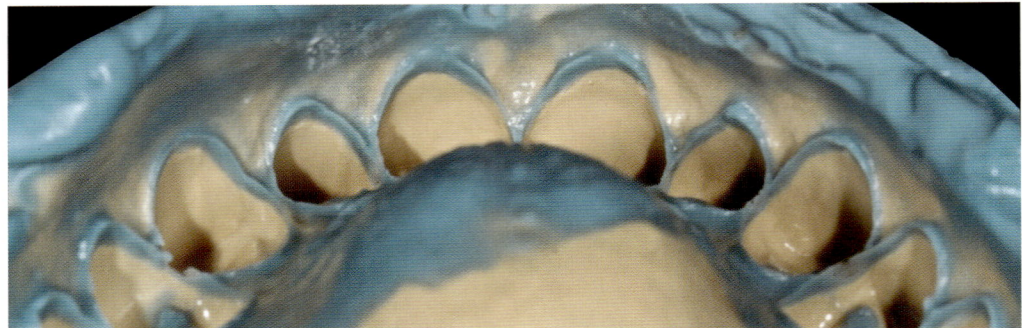

Fig. 9.19 An impression sent to the laboratory.

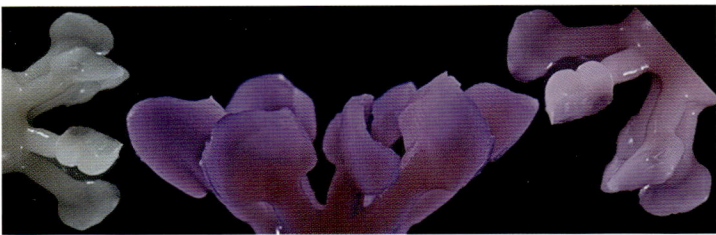

Fig. 9.20 Lithium disilicate is injected onto the ingots.

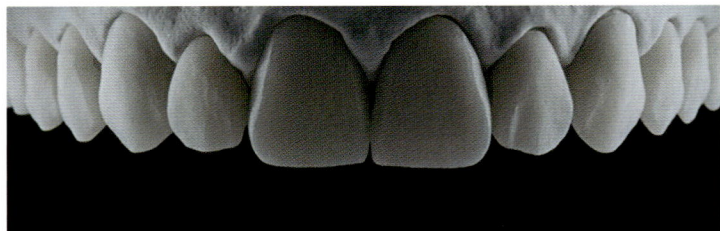

Fig. 9.21 Lenses are fitted onto the model.

need to be masked and is transmitted through the minimally thin (yet characterized) porcelain. If a tooth has a starting shade of A3 or darker, a contact lens style preparation would not be indicated. Instead, more preparation would allow for the blocking out of the undesirable stump shade.

The shade of the underlying tooth in this case is acceptable and of high value; therefore, the veneers will be 'contact lenses' and minimally thick (0.3 mm) in most areas.

After the lithium disilicate has been injected onto the ingots (Fig. 9.20), we fit the lenses onto the model (Fig. 9.21). We now start the cutting back, digging out the area where we will apply a minimal amount of ceramic. After the lithium disilicate has been cut back (Fig. 9.22), the artistic procedure begins, as mamelons, cracklines and internal paints are added (Fig. 9.23A–D). Thin layers of ceramic are used to create stratifications, opalescence effects, transparency, value effects and asymmetrical areas of shadow and light (Fig. 9.24).

We consider all micro- and macro-esthetic elements, including the texture, incisal line, size, shape, anatomy and, especially, emergence profile, which is the most important area for maintaining gingival health.

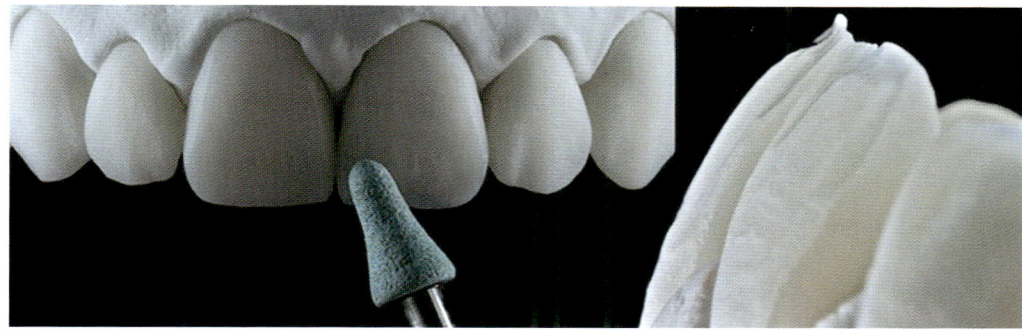

Fig. 9.22 The lithium disilicate is cut back.

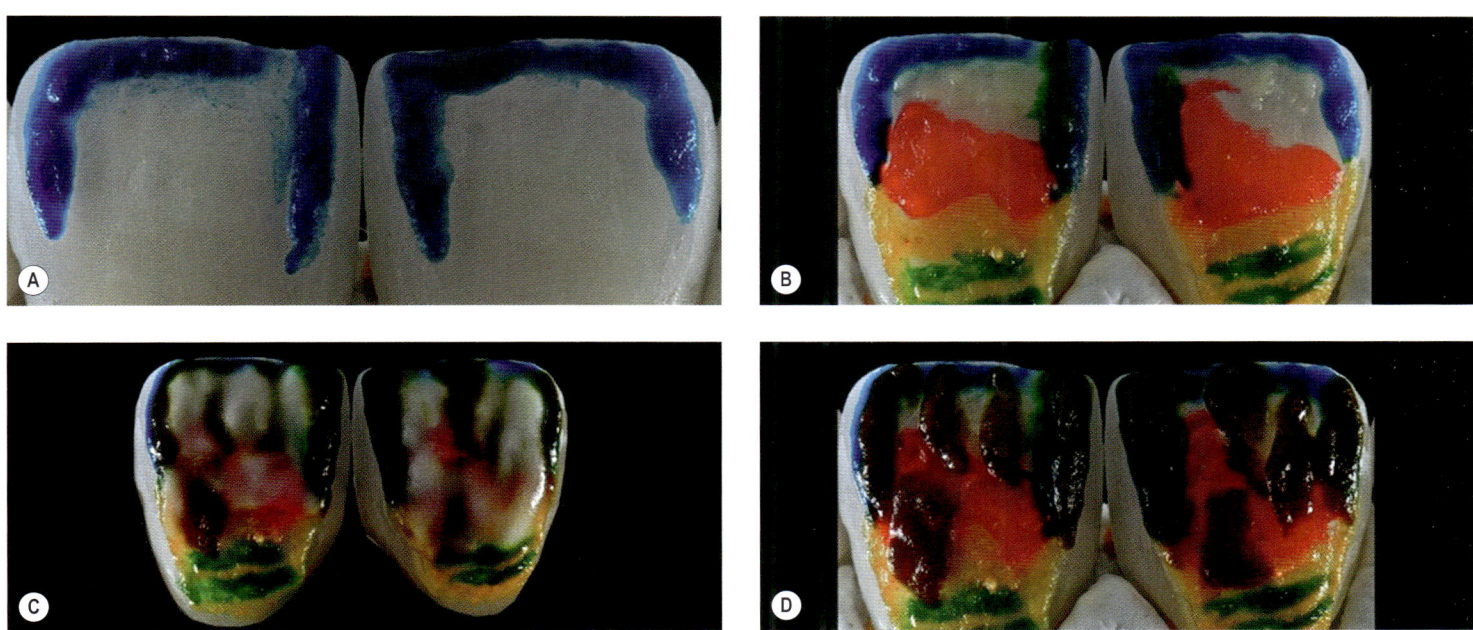

Fig. 9.23A–D Internal paints are applied to the cut back areas.

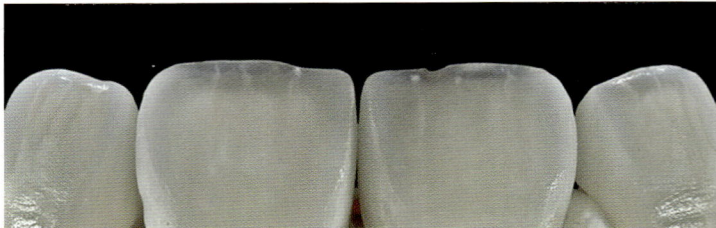

Fig. 9.24 Thin layers of ceramic are used to create stratifications, opalescence effects, transparency, value effects and asymmetrical areas of shadow and light.

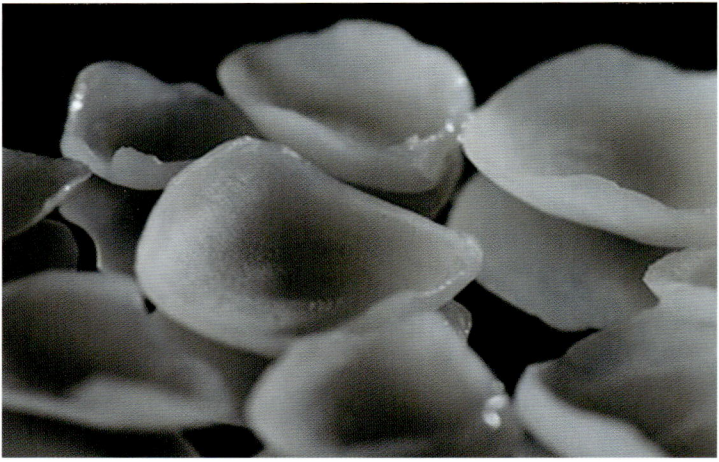

Fig. 9.25 Transparency.

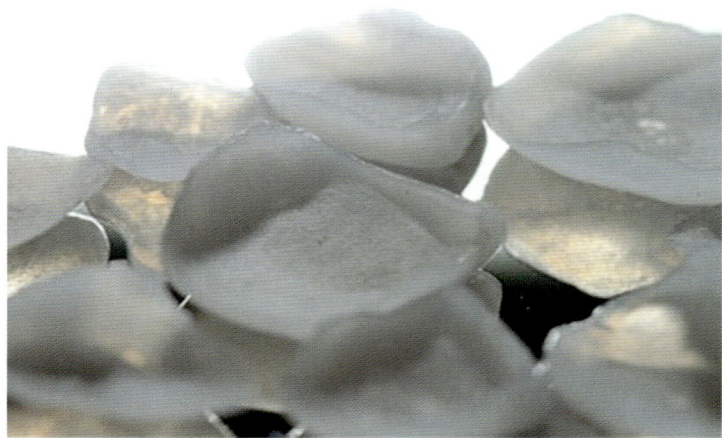

Fig. 9.26 Opalescence.

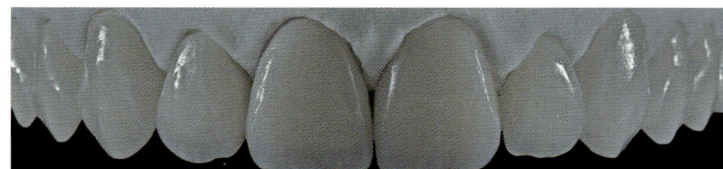

Fig. 9.27 The completed restorations.

Next we go through an optical checklist, analysing colour, brightness, value, transparency, opalescence and fluorescence. At this stage we start to play with light and shadow through the photographs, observing every optical detail described above (Figs 9.25 and 9.26). At the cementation appointment, the final veneers (Fig. 9.27) are delivered with 100% predictability and providing a natural smile in harmony with the patient's face (Fig. 9.28A,B).

HIGH-PERFORMANCE PLANNING WITH DIGITAL DESIGN

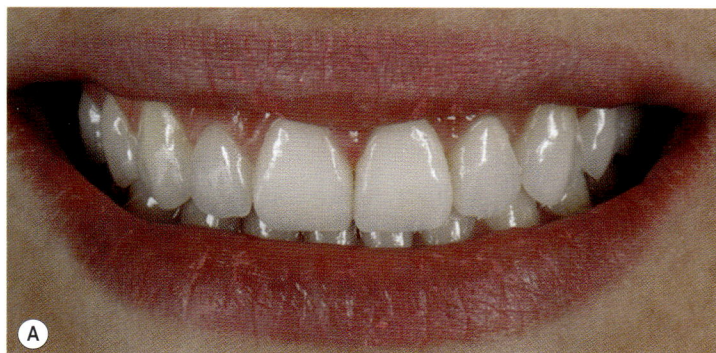
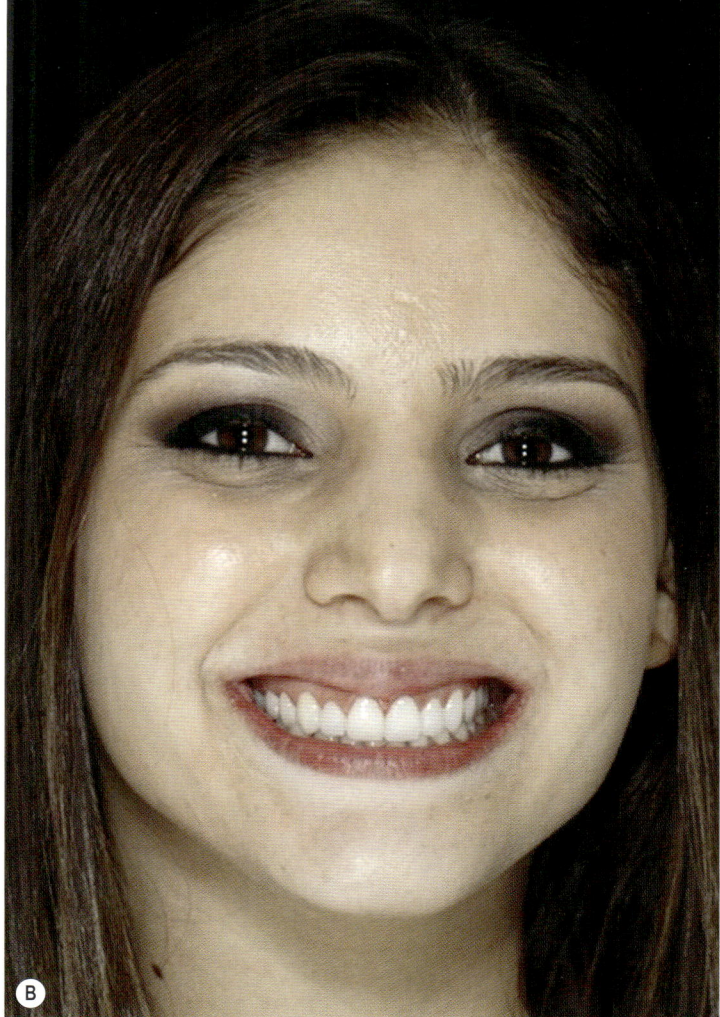

Fig. 9.28A,B (A) Dentofacial view of cemented restorations. (B) Facial view of cemented restorations.

CLINICAL CASE 9.1

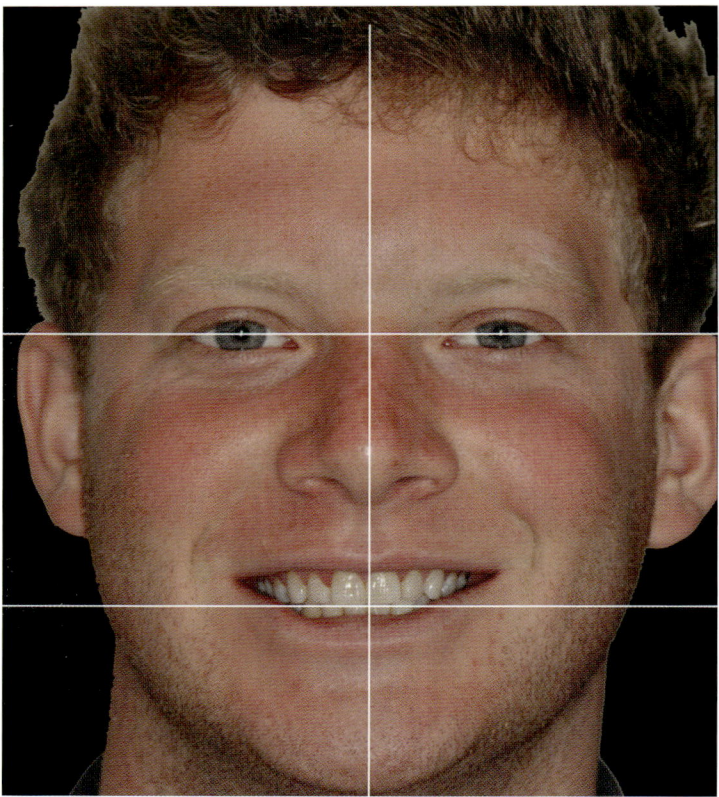

Fig. C9.1.1 The facial view with the head rotated so that the interpupillary line parallels the horizon and the ears are showing in the picture. The midline and incisal line are drawn as well.

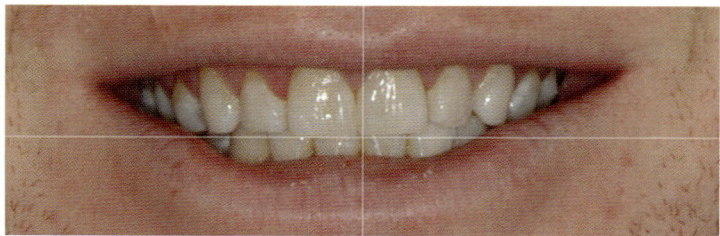

Fig. C9.1.2 The facial view is zoomed in upon to become the dentofacial view, and we can see the midline is 'off' and the incisal plane is canted.

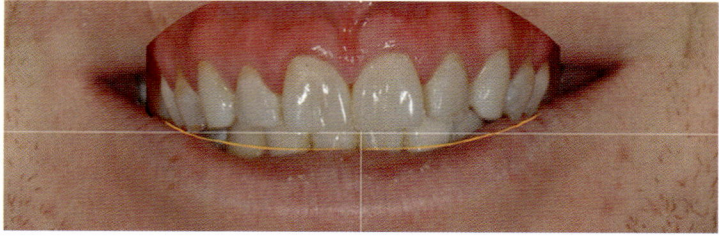

Fig. C9.1.3 The retracted view is laid over the dentofacial view and the lower lip line is traced.

HIGH-PERFORMANCE PLANNING WITH DIGITAL DESIGN

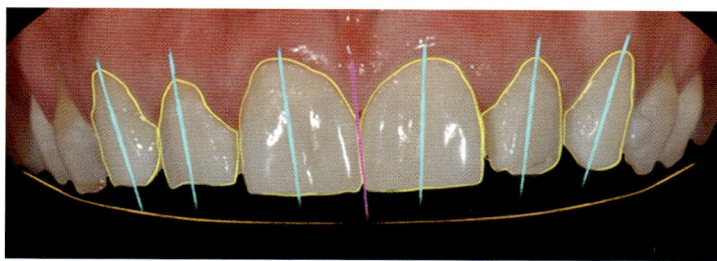

Fig. C9.1.4 The dentofacial view is removed, leaving a perfectly orientated retracted view and the tracing of the lower lip. The tooth forms are traced, as are the midline (note the cant) and axial inclinations of each tooth.

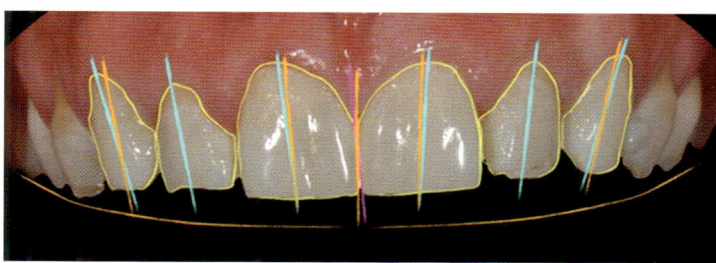

Fig. C9.1.5 Axial correction of the canines and central incisors as well as a corrected midline are drawn in orange.

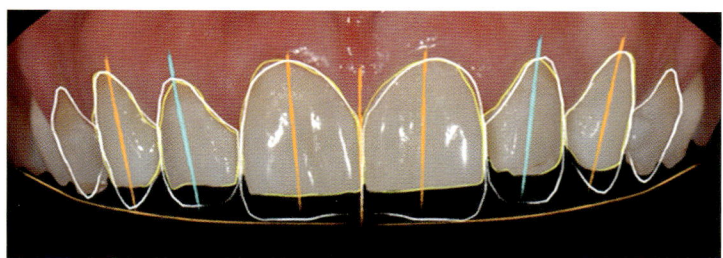

Fig. C9.1.6 New tooth forms are traced in white, bringing the incisal edges to follow the curve of the lower lip. In this particular case, the existing gingival levels will be maintained.

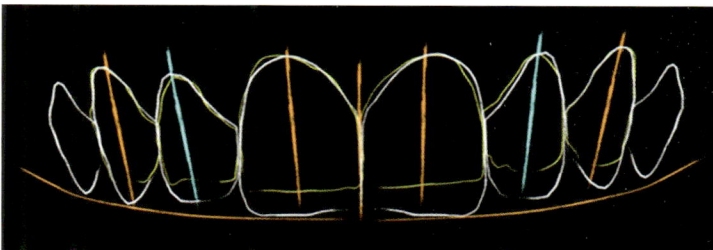

Fig. C9.1.7 The photo can be removed to clearly visualize the new tooth forms.

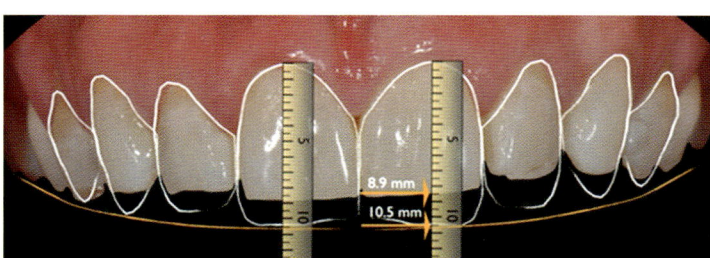

Fig. C9.1.8 Calibrated digital rulers are used to measure the new tooth forms. These measurements will guide the wax-up.

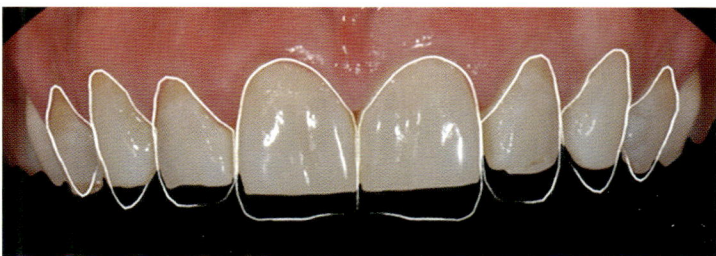

Fig. C9.1.9 The completed smile design.

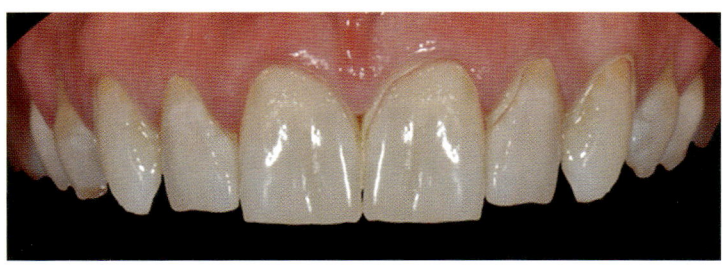

Fig. C9.1.10 Digital 'wax-up'.

CLINICAL CASE 9.1

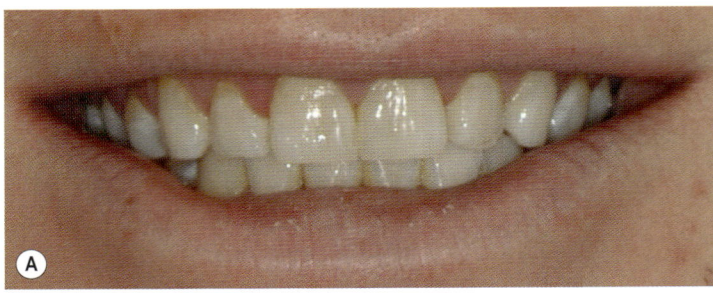
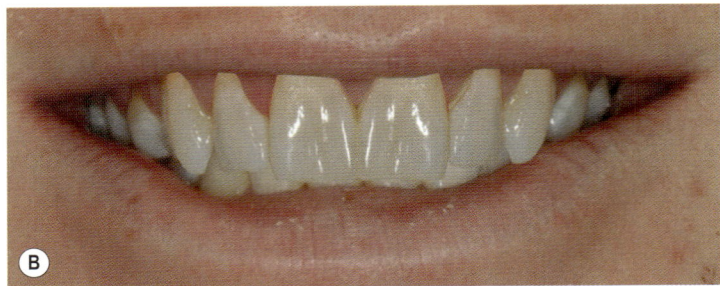

Fig. C9.1.11A,B A digital mock-up is shown to the patient for approval before wax-up fabrication. Prior to wax-up fabrication, the digital smile design can be tested virtually by simply cutting and pasting the new teeth into the patient's mouth. We observe the positioning of the lips, gingival zeniths and shapes and sizes of the teeth. Once both dentist and patient are satisfied, the wax-up can be fabricated according to this design and an intra-oral mock-up can be performed.

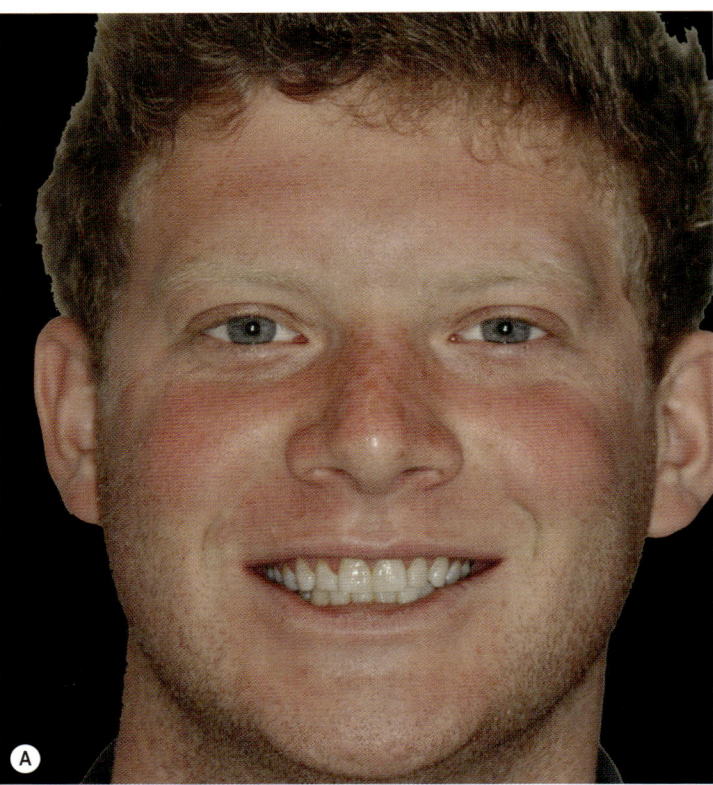
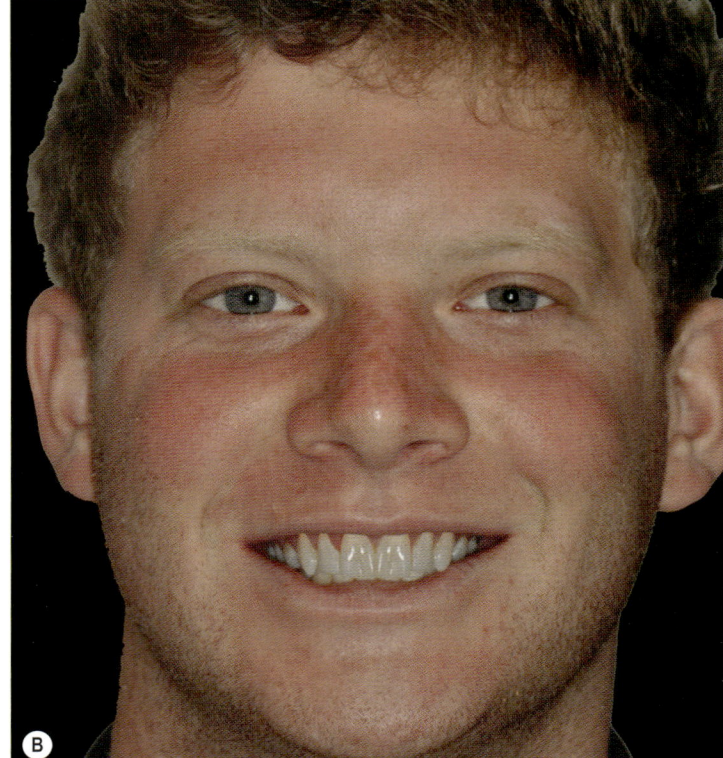

Fig. C9.1.12A,B Facial view of the digital mock-up.

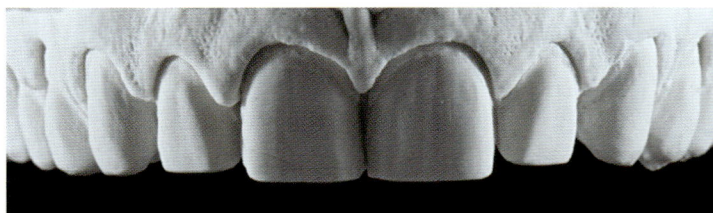

Fig. C9.1.13 Cast of the preparations displaying minimal (0.3 mm) proximal and labial reduction.

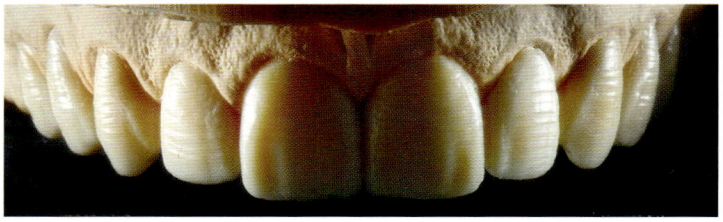

Fig. C9.1.14 Wax-up for final IPS e.max restorations.

HIGH-PERFORMANCE PLANNING WITH DIGITAL DESIGN

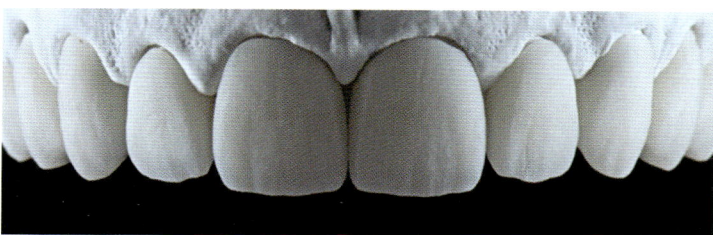

Fig. C9.1.15   IPS e.max pressed and on the cast.

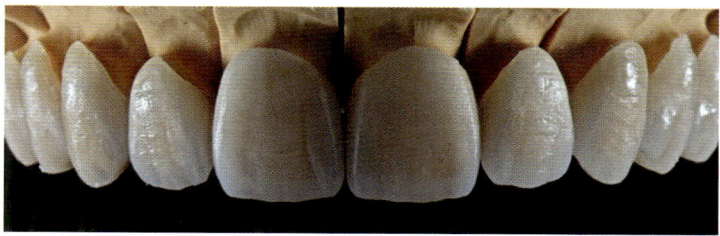

Fig. C9.1.16   IPS e.max restoration layered with IPS e.max Ceram (fluorapatite veneering ceramic) by Ivoclar Vivadent.

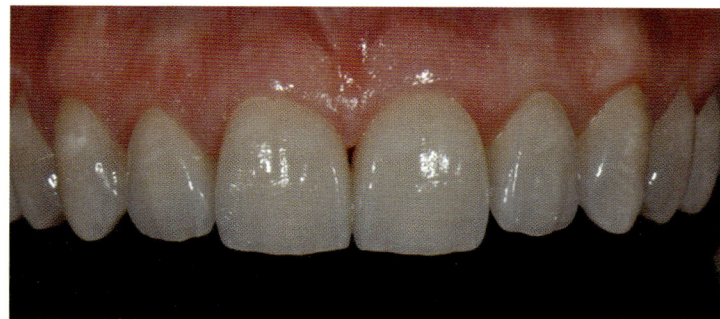

Fig. C9.1.17   Cemented final restorations (with lithium disilicate cut back and layered with feldspathic porcelain).

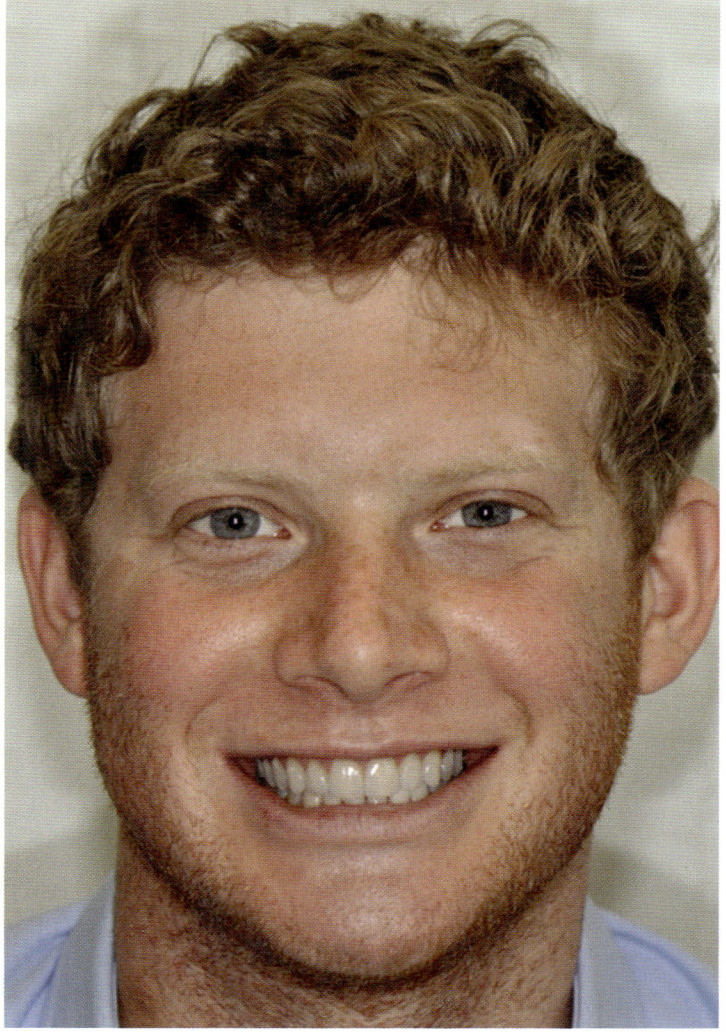

Fig. C9.1.18   Facial view of completed restorations.

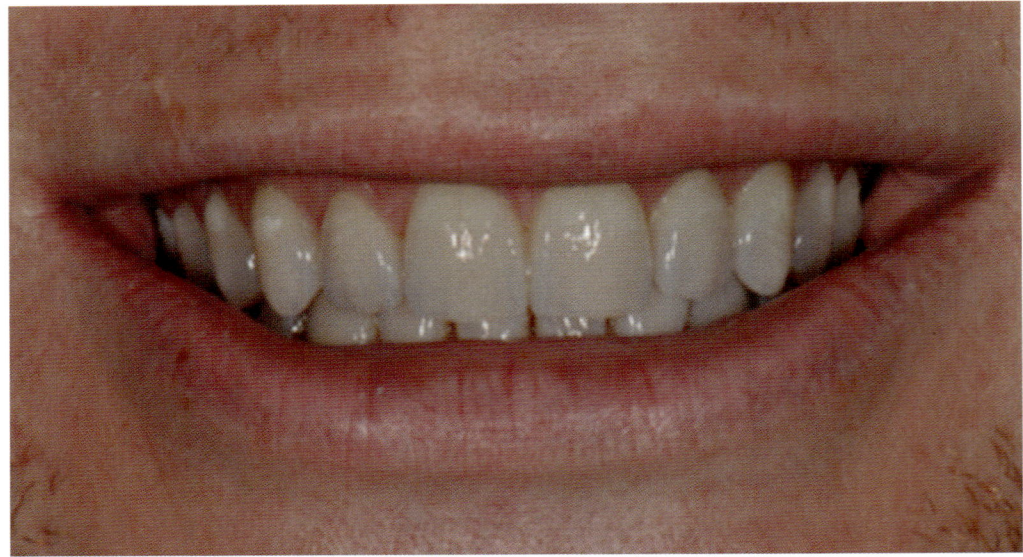

Fig. C9.1.19 Dentofacial view of completed restorations.

CLINICAL CASE 9.2

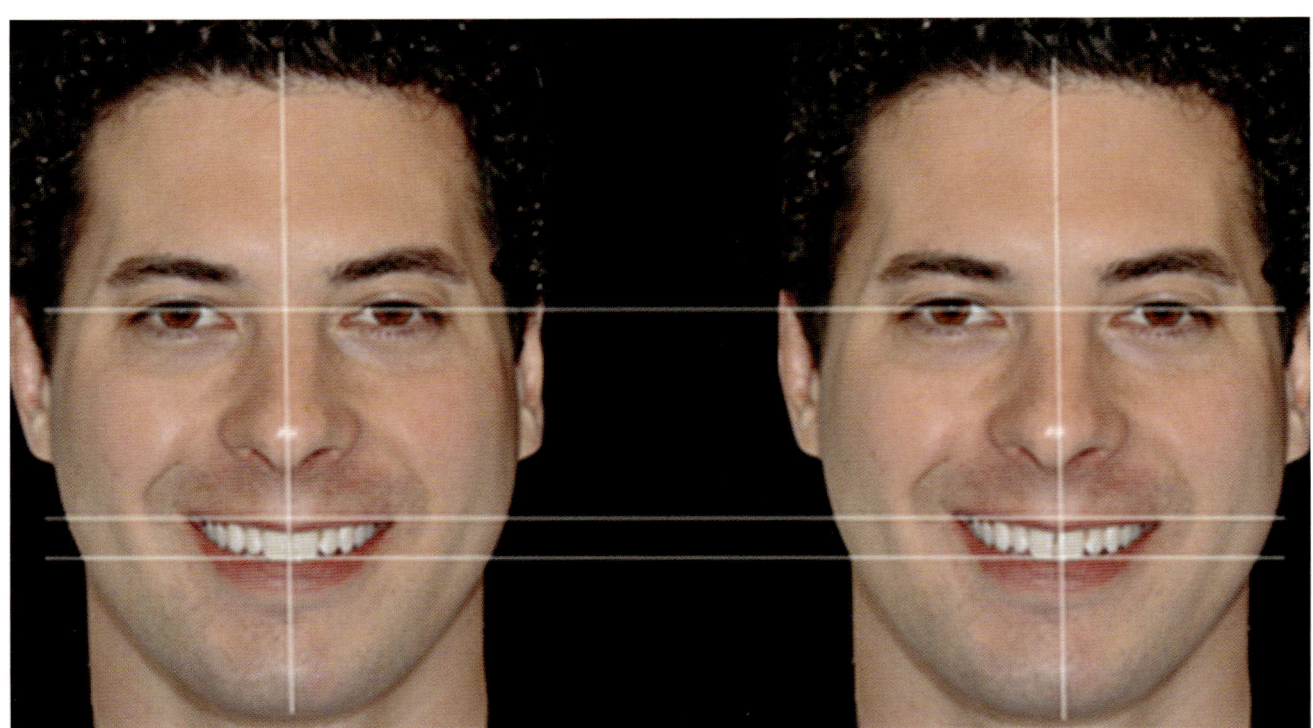

Fig. C9.2.1 The facial view is rotated so that the interpupillary line parallels the horizon.

CHAPTER 9

HIGH-PERFORMANCE PLANNING WITH DIGITAL DESIGN

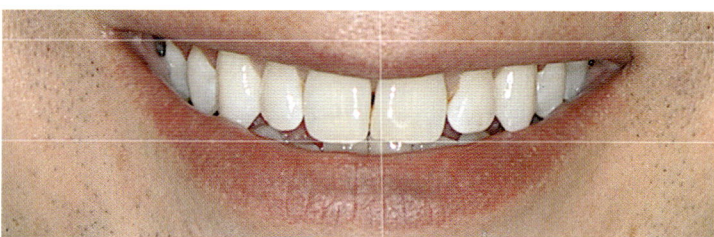

Fig. C9.2.2 The dentofacial view is zoomed in upon and the midline discrepancy is noted.

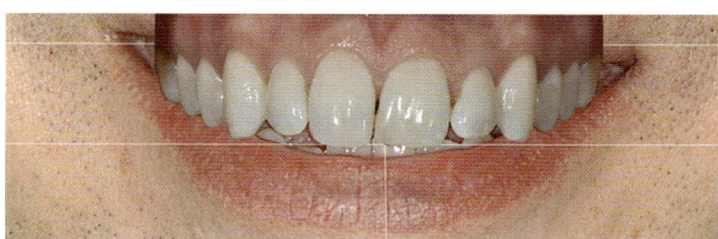

Fig. C9.2.3 The retracted view is overlaid over the dentofacial view in the exact same position and scale.

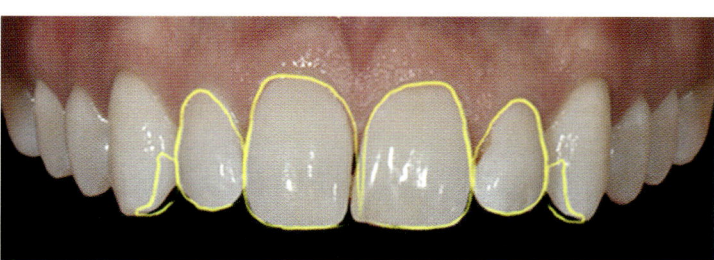

Fig. C9.2.4 The dentofacial view is removed and the new tooth forms are traced. Note that only small 'fragments' are added to the canines.

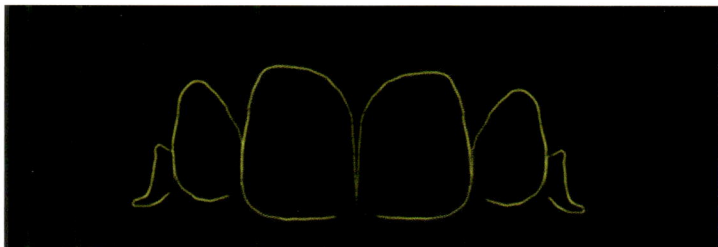

Fig. C9.2.5 The outline of our proposed changes.

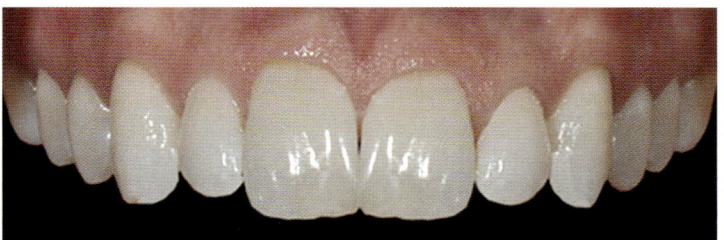

Fig. C9.2.6 A digital version of the proposed changes.

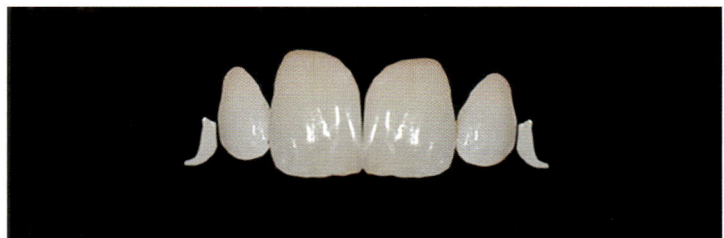

Fig. C9.2.7 The outline of our proposed changes with a tooth-coloured fill.

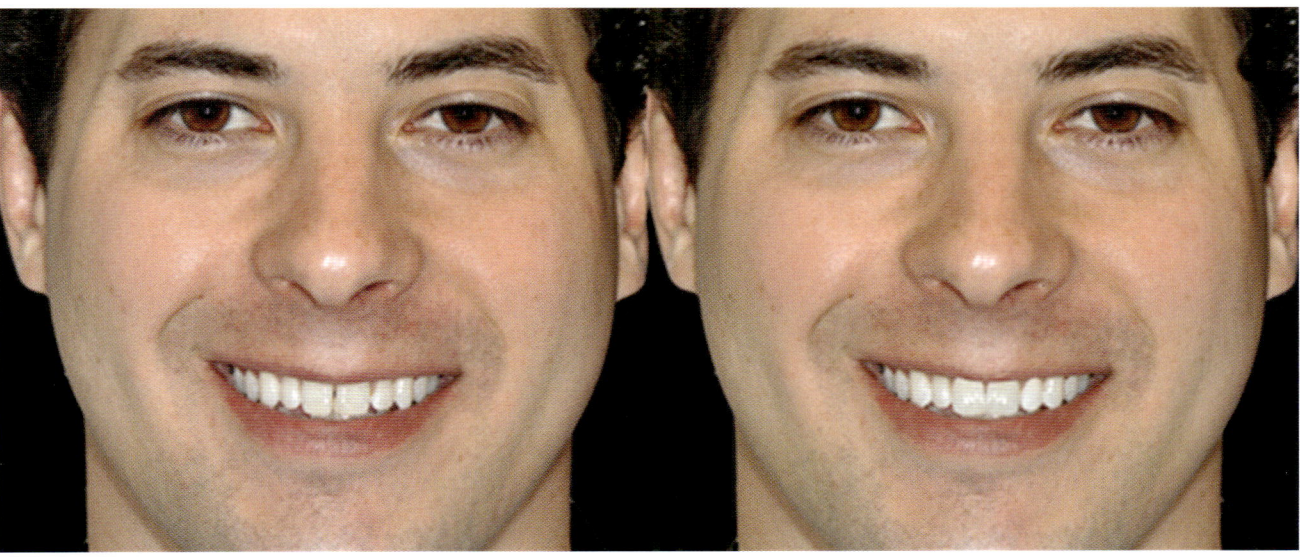

Fig. C9.2.8 A digital mock-up demonstrating the proposed changes.

293

CLINICAL CASE 9.2

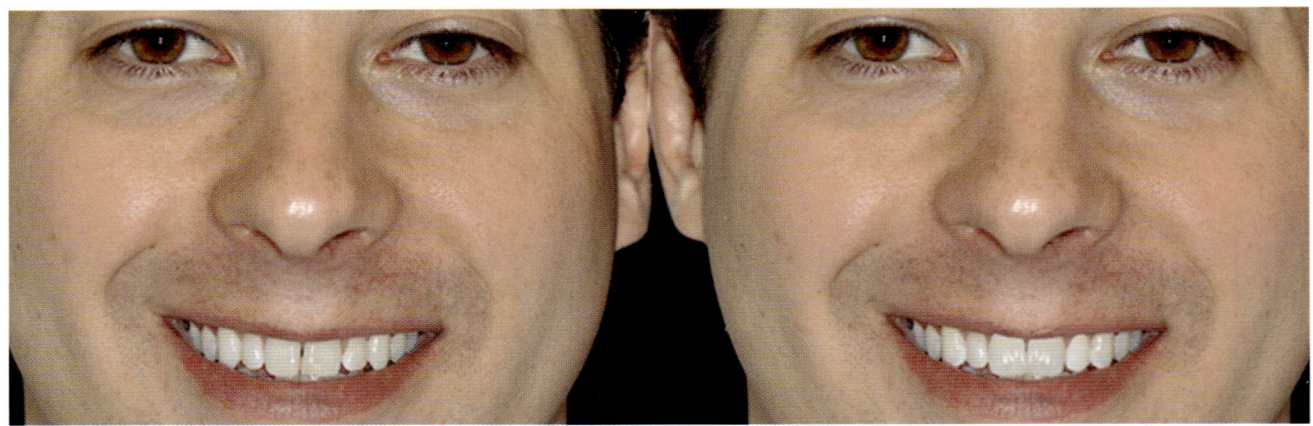

Fig. C9.2.9 A closer view of the digital mock-up.

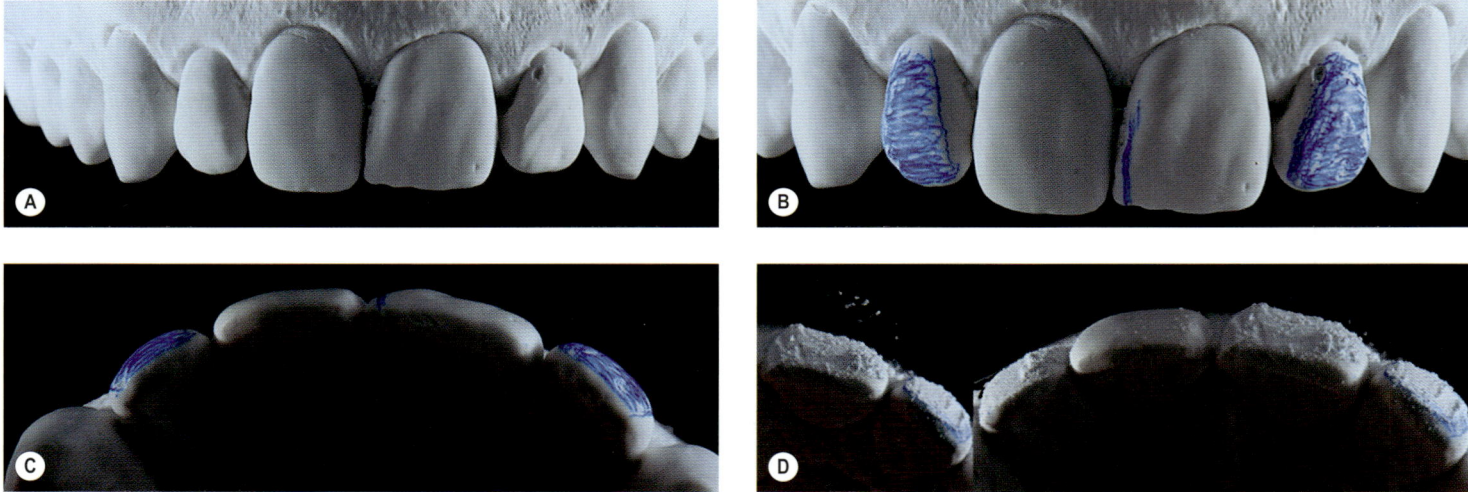

Fig. C9.2.10A–D Once the digital mock-up has been approved, a plaster model is prepared for the wax-up. Stone will be removed in the areas to be waxed.

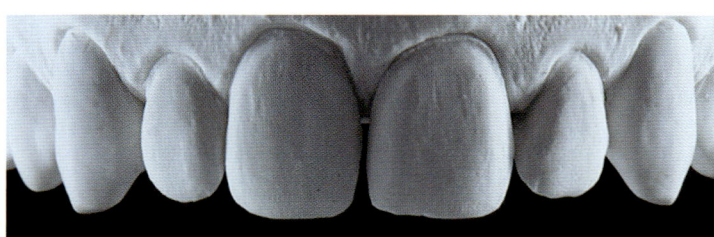

Fig. C9.2.11 The prepared plaster model ready to be waxed up.

HIGH-PERFORMANCE PLANNING WITH DIGITAL DESIGN

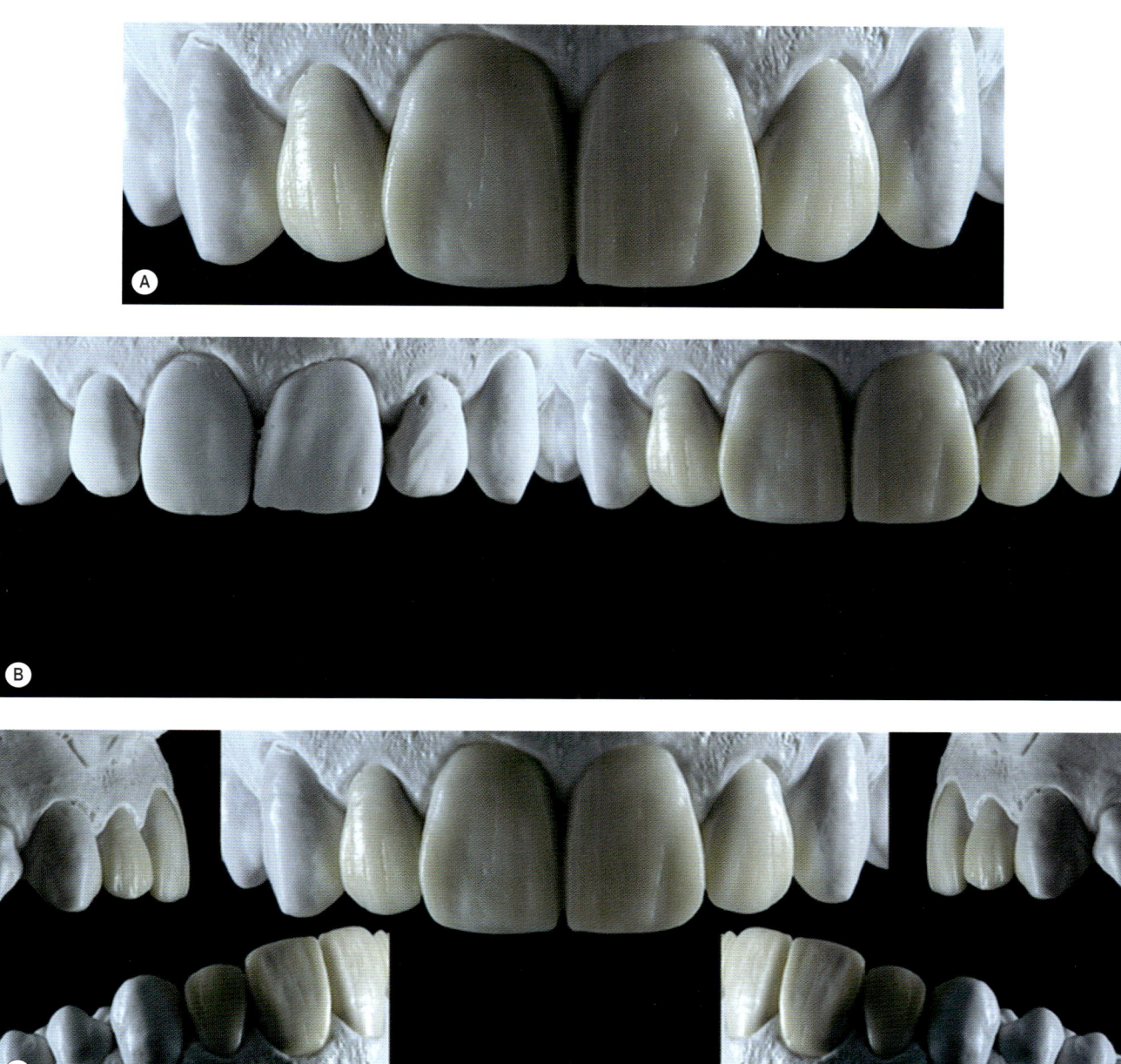

Fig. C9.2.12A–C The final wax-up demonstrating an improved midline and more symmetry. Note the incorporation of texture, which was a micro-esthetic element desired by this particular patient.

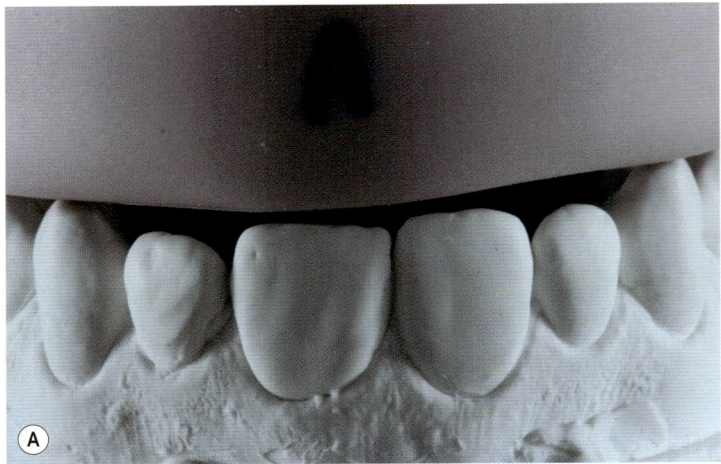
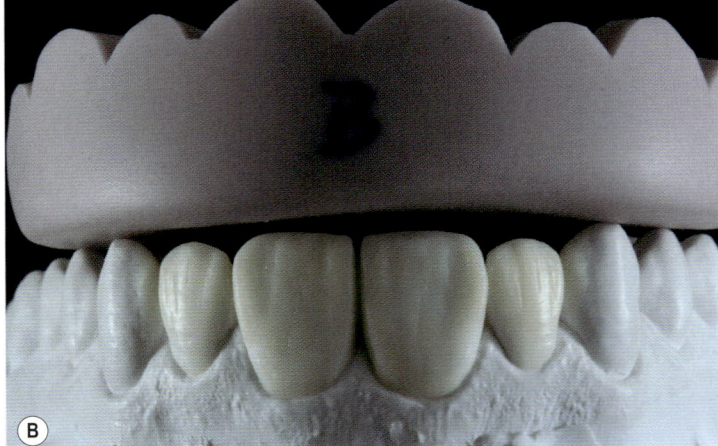
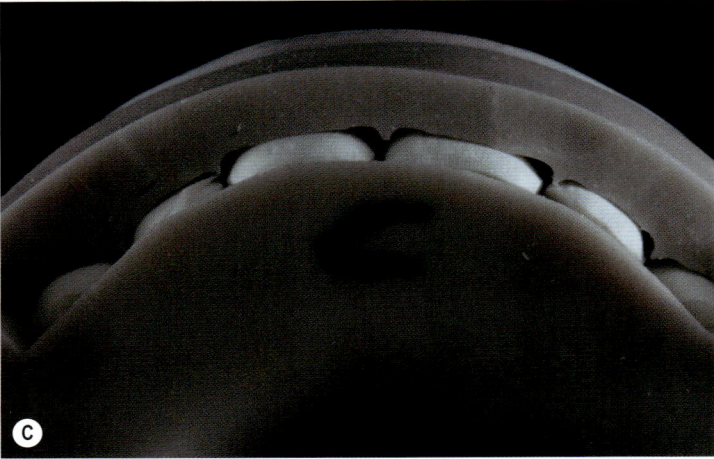

Fig. C9.2.13A–C Reduction guides. Once the photography, digital design and diagnostic wax-up are completed, reduction guides are fabricated and the clinician is set up for success.

CONCLUSION

High-performance planning is a reality when our technicians are located either close to us or thousands of miles away. We begin with the end in mind and work towards a visualized solution using the checklist approach of the Aesthetic Evaluation Form. With this information gathered chairside, the digital design helps the dental team (esthetic dentist, dental technologist, patient and other specialists) discover the esthetic issues and offers a digital solution that becomes a 3-dimensional diagnostic wax-up. Our clinical objective is esthetic predictability, with zero remakes and a very happy patient. High-performance planning takes the information from our Aesthetic Evaluation Form and creates a visual blueprint. Fewer remakes, happy patients and an excited dental team are the definition of high performance planning.

ESSENTIALS

- Digital smile design is a method used to further improve our laboratory, interdisciplinary and patient communication. Predictability as well as patient motivation is greatly enhanced.

- Digital smile design offers a clear advantage over traditional digital imaging systems, with the key difference being the use of a calibrated digital ruler. The digital smile design 'digital mockup' is grounded in real-world measurements, and thus the patient is shown only what is reasonably achievable.

- Just as outlined in Chapter 1, the digital smile design approach begins by analysing the following views: facial, then dentofacial and finally dental. The macro- and micro-esthetic elements of the Aesthetic Evaluation Form can be precisely assessed on a computer using lines and measurements.

- It is important to remember that although digital smile design is an incredibly powerful tool, it is only a supplement to our traditional diagnostics. The digital design must be translated into real-world dentistry, and thus must always be considered with respect to the biology and functional requirements of the masticatory system.

PATIENTS' FAQS

Q. Can I see how my smile will look before we begin any work?

A. Yes, the beauty of this digital smile design process is that it lets us preview one or even several different new smiles for you without even touching your teeth, and the simulation will be accurate enough to translate into a real-world design when you choose the look you like.

Q. How are you going to ensure the result is in harmony with my face and lips?

A. The digital smile design process is facially driven, meaning we look at your face and lips as a whole before we zoom in on your smile. We define the exact middle of your face, and assess the symmetry of your facial features. Thus, the smile we design for you will be harmonious and in balance with the rest of your face.

Q. Will my smile look artificial?

A. If you desire a more natural look, we will incorporate elements such as texture and translucency, and perhaps not select the whitest shade. Different patients request different degrees of naturalness, so this is an important conversation for you to be a part of.

Q. Can we make changes to the design?

A. Absolutely. The digital design process allows us to tweak each individual tooth's size, colour, shape and relative proportion. It is the dentist's responsibility to stay within the guidelines of what is achievable, but there is certainly room to adjust the design.

Q. Are you going to destroy my own teeth to accomplish this?

A. No! Thanks to the advanced digital planning methods and the materials we have today, we are able to be extremely conservative in our designs, meaning much less removal of tooth structure to achieve our goal.

ACKNOWLEDGEMENT

The authors would like to thank Dr Jonathan B. Levine for providing the Clinical cases in this chapter.

Further reading

Coachman C, Calamita M, Paolucci B. Visagism. Quintessence Dent Tech 2012;35:187–99.

de Andrade OS, Borges GA, Stefani A, Fujiy F, Battistella PA. Step-by-step ultraconservative esthetic rehabilitation using lithium disilicate ceramic. QDT 2010;33:114.

Hatjo J. Anteriores. Fuchstal: Teamwork Media; 2006.

Kina S, Bruguera A. Invisivel: restaurações estéticas cerâmicas. Maringa: Dental Press; 2008.

Ubassy G. Analysis. Fuchstal: Teamwork Media; 2002.

INDEX

Page numbers followed by '*f*' indicate figures, and '*b*' indicate boxes.

A

Accuracy of fit, in aligner therapy, 192
Adobe Photoshop, bleaching and, 91
Aligner therapy. *see* Clear aligner therapy
Anaesthesia, 248–255
Angulation, in dental photography, 104–105, 106*f*
Anorexia nervosa, 46
Anterior bonded restorations, 214–272
    APT preparation technique, 235–236, 235*f*–237*f*
    armamentarium for veneer preparation, 217–220
    clinical cases of, 259, 259*f*–271*f*, 261, 264–269
    continuous care, 255–258
    history, 216
    insertion and finishing, 248–255, 249*f*–257*f*
    material selection, 246–247, 247*f*
    posterior veneers, considerations for, 243–245, 245*f*
    provisionalization, 238–243, 240*f*–242*f*
    restoration of fractured and carious teeth with porcelain laminate veneer, 245–246, 246*f*
    retraction and impressioning, 236–238, 238*b*, 238*f*–239*f*
    shade selection, considerations for, 232–235, 234*f*
    veneer preparation
        guidelines for, 220–221, 220*f*
        step-by-step, 221–231
Anterior 'coupling,' between maxillary and mandibular incisors, 58
Anterior mandibular veneers, considerations for, 243, 244*f*
Aperture, in dental photography, 97–98
Apple's Keynote software, 276–277
Appliance
    delivery, in aligner therapy, 196
    'FEE'
        clinical case of, 79, 79*f*–80*f*
        for diagnosis, stabilization and visualization, 72–74, 74*f*
    fixed
        aligner therapy and, 186–187
        removable appliance *versus*, 185
    removable
        aligner therapy and, 186–187
        fixed appliance *versus*, 185
Assessment, psychological, 44–50
    guideline for evaluating patient's mental state in, 47–49
    psychological issues pertinent to esthetic dentistry and, 46–47
Attachments
    in aligner therapy, 188
    in ClinCheck, 192–196, 196*f*
    placement of, 197*b*
Auxiliaries, in aligner therapy, 192–196, 198*f*–199*f*, 208*f*
Axial inclination, 19, 20*f*

B

BDD. *see* Body dysmorphic disorder (BDD)
Binge eating, 46
Biologic model, 55–62, 56*b*, 56*f*–57*f*, 64–65
Biological width, 156–157
Bis-acryl mock-up, 235, 235*f*
    for diastema closure, 176*f*, 177*b*
Bite registration, 32–33
Bleaching, dental photography for, 91
Body dysmorphic disorder (BDD), 47
Bonding agent, application of, 253*f*
Buccal cusp, maxillary, 243
Bulimia nervosa, 46
Bur
    diamond, 219, 219*f*
    reduction
        self-limiting depth, 219, 219*f*
        two-grit gross, 219–220, 219*f*
'Button cutouts', 189, 192–196, 209*f*

C

Calibrated ruler, used in digital smile design, 279*f*, 289*f*
Caliper, digital, 228*f*, 266*f*
Camera, in digital smile design, 276
'Canine rise', 59–62
Casts, diagnostic, in three-step analysis, 31–33, 31*b*, 34*f*–35*f*
Cement, veneer
    injection of, 253*f*
    Variolink (Ivoclar), 251
Cemented restorations, 287*f*, 291*f*
Centric occlusion, 55
Centric relation, 56*f*
Ceramic, thin layers of, 284, 286*f*
Cheek retractors, for dental photography, 101, 103*f*
Chew positions, right and left, 59–62, 61*f*
Christian Coachman's Digital Smile Design protocol, 37–38
Class I gingival recession, 125
Class II gingival recession, 125
Class III gingival recession, 125
Class IV gingival recession, 125
Clear aligner therapy, 182–212, 201*b*
    accuracy of fit and, 192
    advantages of, 187–188
    age and, 201*b*
    aligner evolution and, 188–189
    clinical application of, 189–200, 190*f*
        appliance delivery, 196
        case progress in, 197–198, 197*f*–199*f*
        conclusion of active treatment in, 198
        initial visit in, 189–190

INDEX

Clear aligner therapy *(Continued)*
    orthodontic records in, 191–192
    patient preparation in, 191
    retention strategies in, 200, 200b, 203f–204f, 206f–207f
    virtual treatment in, 192–196, 195f–196f
  clinical cases in, 202, 202f–211f
  cost of, 201b
  duration of, 201b
  examples of, 185
  extraction and, 201b
  features of, 186–187
  fixed appliance *versus* removable appliance, 185
  manufacturing of aligner, 186, 192
  overview of, 184–185
  post-treatment considerations in, 200
  results in, 201b
  uniqueness of, 187
Clear silicone provisional matrix, 240f
ClinCheck, 191–196, 195f
  attachments and, 196f
Clinical photography, in esthetic dentistry
  basic principles of, 93–104
    depth of field in, 95, 96f–97f
    exposure in, 97–99, 98f
    illumination in, 100–101, 100f, 102f
    reproduction ratio in, 94–95, 95f
  clinical techniques for, 101b
  consent and medico-legal aspects, 91b, 92
  digital workflow and, 107
  equipment for, 92–93, 94f
    cheek retractors, 101, 103f
    contrastors, 103, 103f
    photographic mirrors, 103–104, 104f
  file types and, 107
  general technique for, 104–105, 105f–106f
  standard views for, 106–107
  uses of, 90–92, 96b
    for bleaching, 91
    for communication, 91
    for marketing, 91
    for treatment planning, 90, 90f
Close-up dental photographs, 117f
Communication
  with dental technician, dental photography and, 91
  triangle, in three-step analysis, 4f
Complete occlusion, 56–58, 56f, 58f–59f
Completed restorations, 286f, 291f–292f
Composite
  bonding, 80f
    in anterior bonded restorations, 216
  direct adhesive, for diastema, 165
  restorations, 80f
Computer imaging software, 37–38, 39f
Computer programs, aligner therapy and, 188
Concave profile, 12–13, 13f
Connective tissue (CT) graft, 126, 127b, 156
  subepithelial, 136b, 143, 143f–146f, 145b–146b
Consent, dental photography and, 91b, 92, 96b, 108b
Contact area, 23, 23f, 156–157
'Contact lenses', 283–284
Continuous care, in anterior bonded restorations, 255–258
Contour
  height of, 21, 22f, 24, 24f
  incisal edge, 25, 26f
Contrastors, for dental photography, 103, 103f
Convex profile, 12–13, 14f
Coronally advanced flap, 127b
  modified, 141f–143f, 142b
Crowding, 152, 152f, 160
  clinical case for, 171, 171f–175f, 172b, 175b
  treatment planning for, 163–165, 164f
Crown
  excessively long, compensation for, 162b
  excessively wide, compensation for, 160, 161b

  indications for, 170
  lengthening, planning on dental photograph, 90f
CT graft. *see* Connective tissue (CT) graft
Curing, full, 255f

D

DeLar wax bite registration, 32–33, 35f
Dental technician, communication with, dental photography and, 91
Dentition
  digital impression of, 192, 194f
  full, (retracted) view, 114f
    alternative, 114f
    faults in, 119f
    technique, 114f
  retracted view
    lateral, 115f
Dentofacial view, in dental photography
  lips at rest, 111f
  of smile, 111f
Dentolabial analysis, 159
Depth cuts, connecting and finishing, 229–231, 231f–233f
Depth grooves, for incisal reduction, 227f
Depth of field, in dental photography, 95, 96f–97f
Diagnostic and Statistical Manual of Mental Disorders, fifth edition (DSM-V), 46
Diagnostic casts, in three-step analysis, 31–33, 31b, 34f–35f
Diagnostic wax-up
  in crowding treatment planning, 165, 172b, 172f
  in diastema closure, 176f
  occlusal view of, 77f
  silicone putty of, 37f
  in three-step analysis, 3, 33–36, 35f, 36b
Diamond bur, 1 mm round, 219, 219f
Diastema, 152, 152f, 156–157, 160, 162–163
  closure of
    clinical procedures for, 176, 176f–178f, 177b
    correct *versus* incorrect preparation for, 227f
  treatment planning for, 165–170, 170b
    midline, 166
    spaces, larger, 166–167, 167f
Digital caliper, 228f, 266f
Digital mock-up, 290f, 293f–294f
  facial and dentofacial views of, 279f–280f
Digital record, 192, 194f
Digital smile design, 276–283, 276f–284f, 297b
  high-performance planning with, clinical case for, 274–298, 288f–292f, 297b
  laboratory technique for, 283–286, 284f–287f
  technique demonstration of, 292, 292f–296f
Digital workflow, and dental photography, 107
Direct adhesive composite, for diastema, 165
Direct frontal light, in photographs, 102f
Direct lateral light, in photographs, 102f
'Direct' provisionalization technique, 239–241
'Distalizing the defect' technique, 167, 168f
Documentation, dental photography for, 91–92
DSM-V. *see Diagnostic and Statistical Manual of Mental Disorders*, fifth edition (DSM-V)
Dual flash system, 100–101, 102f

E

Electrosurgery, 156, 266f
E.max HT Impulse O2, 283–284
E.max restorations, 291f
  wax-up for, 290f
Emergence profile, 281, 282f
Enamel erosion, 47
Enameloplasty, 217–220
  prepreparation, 221, 222f
Equipment, photographic, 92–93, 94f
Esthetic dentistry, psychological issues pertinent to, 46–47
Esthetic Evaluation Form, 3–25, 4b, 5f–7f, 55, 276
  effective questions in, 4–8, 8b, 9f
  facial, dentofacial and dental analysis, 8–17

INDEX

dental view (occlusal analysis and micro-elements), 16–17, 17f–26f, 20b
dentofacial view, 13–16, 14f–16f
facial view (macro-elements), 10–13, 10f–14f
Esthetic mock-up, 36–40
   intra-oral mock-up, 36–37, 37f–38f
   reductive mock-up, 37–40, 39f
Esthetic Pre-Evaluative Temporary preparation technique, 235–236, 235f–237f, 282–283, 283f
Esthetic predictability, 257b
Esthetics, 241
   integration of function and, 52–86, 74b–75b
      clinical case of, 76, 76f–78f, 82f–85f
   soft tissue, long-term maintenance of, 135–136, 136b
Etching, of teeth, 252f
Exposure, in dental photography, 97–99, 98f
   compensation settings, 99, 99f
Extraction, of teeth, 201b

F
Face, smile and, 74
Facial depth cuts, 229, 229f
Facial photos, 28f
Facial preparation, 229, 229f
Facial reduction, planes of, 230f
Facially directed treatment planning, 64
   concepts of, 64–65
'FEE appliance'
   clinical case of, 79, 79f–80f
   for diagnosis, stabilization and visualization, 72–74, 74f
FEE lines, seven, 69–71, 72f, 73b
Feldspathic porcelain, 247
File types, and dental photography, 107
Fixed appliance
   aligner therapy and, 186–187
   removable appliance versus, 185
Flap, coronally advanced, 127b
   modified, 141f–143f, 142b
Free gingival graft, 126, 127f–128f
F-stop, 95
Full curing, 255f
Full dentition (retracted) view, 114f
   alternative, 114f
   faults in, 119f
   technique, 114f
Full face view, in dental photography, 108f
   profile, with lips at rest, 110f
   technique, 108f
Full natural smile, in dental photography, 110f
   left lateral view, 112f
   right lateral view, 112f
   technique, 110f

G
Gingival embrasure, 156–157
Gingival graft, free, 126, 127f–128f
Gingival margin, 237f, 257b
   coronally placed, 155, 155f
   periodontal surgery and, 156
   placement of, 221–224, 222b, 223f, 224b
      different shade shift scenarios and, 223f
   variations in height, 156
Gingival recession, 124–126
   classification system for, 125
   connective tissue graft for, 126, 127b
   deep, 136, 137b, 137f–140f, 139b
   free gingival graft for, 126, 127f–128f
   multiple Miller I, 141, 141f–143f, 142b–143b
   treatment of, 125, 126b
Gingival surgery, following dental design, 281, 282f
Gingivectomy, 156
Gingivoplasty, 266f
Glass mirrors, 103
Gold crown, 153–154
Golden proportion, in treatment planning, 160

Graft
   connective tissue (CT), 126, 127b, 156
      subepithelial, 136b, 143, 143f–146f, 145b–146b
   free gingival, 126, 127f–128f
   pedicle soft tissue, for gingival recession, 125
'Gull-wing' effect, 19
Gum disease, 47

H
Hemodent-soaked cord, 250f

I
Illumination, in dental photography, 100–101, 100f
   direct versus indirect lighting for, 102f
   dual flash system for, 102f
Implant esthetics, 129–133
   implant position, 129–131, 129f–130f, 136b
   peri-implant mucosa, 131–132
   periodontal plastic surgery, for ridge defects in, 132–133
Implant position, 129–131, 129f–130f, 136b
Impressioning, 236–238, 238b, 238f–239f
   digital, 192, 194f
Incisal depth cuts, 222f, 229
Incisal edge contour, 25, 26f
Incisal edge lengthening, 159
Incisal edge position, 17–18, 18f
Incisal edge wear, upper and lower, clinical case of, 81f
Incisal embrasures, 23, 23f
Incisal reduction, 226–228, 227f–228f
Incisive position, 58, 60f
Incisors, maxillary
   central
      ideal width of, 159, 159f
      3-dimensional position of, 54, 54f
   'ideal' veneer preparation, 220f
   lateral, width of, 160, 161f
Indirect lateral light, in photographs, 102f
Insertion and finishing, in anterior bonded restorations, 248–255, 249f–257f
Integrated orthodontic-restorative approach, 162–163
Integration of function, and esthetics, 52–86
   clinical case of, 76, 76f–78f, 82f–85f
Intercuspation, maximum, 55
Interdental papilla, 133–135, 134f–135f
'Interferences', 58
Internal paints, digital smile design and, 285f
Interproximal bone, 156–157
Interproximal margins, 237f
   placement of, 224–225, 225f
Interproximal reduction, in alignment therapy, 196
Intra-oral mock-up, 36–37, 37f–38f, 281f
Intra-oral photography, 93–94
Intra-oral scanners, aligner therapy and, 192, 193f
Intracrevicular preparation, 221–224
Invisalign aligners, 185, 188, 202f–203f, 205f–207f, 209f
   cost of, 188
Invisalign Teen, 189
iTero intra-oral digital scanner, 192, 194f

J
JPEGs, 107

K
Kois Dentofacial Analyzer, 31, 34f

L
Laboratory technique, for digital smile design, 283–286, 284f–287f
Laser, 156
Lateral dentition, retracted view, 115f
Lateral facial photos, 30f
LCD. see Liquid crystal display (LCD)
Leaf gauge, for anterior stop, 34f
Left chew position, 59–62, 61f
Line angles, 21, 22f
Lingually locked teeth, restoration of, 165

INDEX

Lips
    anatomy of, 11
    close-up photographs of, 113f
    at rest, dentofacial view, 111f
    upper, range for, 63–64
Liquid crystal display (LCD), 92–93
Lithium disilicate, 284, 284f–285f
    veneers, 247, 247f, 263f

M

Macro-elements, facial view, 10–13, 10f–14f
Macro-esthetic elements, 10–13, 10f
Macro lens, for dental photography, 93, 94f
    reproduction ratio and, 94–95
Macrophotography, intra-oral, 93–94
Magnification, of digital SLRs, 93
Mandibular posterior teeth, preparation for porcelain laminate veneers, 243–244
Mandibular veneers, anterior, considerations for, 243
Marketing, dental photography for, 91, 91b
Mastication, muscles of, 66, 68f
Material selection, in anterior bonded restorations, 246–247, 247f
Maxillary buccal cusp, 243
Maxillary incisors
    central
        ideal width of, 159, 159f
        3-dimensional position of, 54, 54f
        'ideal' veneer preparation, 220f
        lateral, width of, 160, 161f
Maximum intercuspation, 55
Medico-legal aspects, dental photography for, 92
Memosil, 36
Mental state, guideline for evaluating patient's, 47–49
Metal mirrors, 103
Micro-elements, dental view of, 16–17, 17f–26f, 20b
Micro-esthetic dental analysis, for teeth measurement, 159
Micro-esthetic elements, 17–25
Miniscrews, aligner therapy and, 189, 210f
Mirror view, faults in, 119f
Mock-up
    bis-acryl, 235, 235f
    for diastema closure, 176f, 177b
    digital, 290f, 293f–294f
        facial and dentofacial views of, 279f–280f
    intra-oral, 36–37, 37f–38f, 281f
    reductive, 37–40, 39f
Modified coronally advanced flap, 141f–143f, 142b
Mouth, incisal silhouette of, 38, 39f
Multiple Miller I gingival recession, 141, 141f–143f, 142b–143b
Muscles, of mastication, 66, 68f

N

Nasolabial angle, 11–12, 12f, 64
Neutral zone, 62–65, 62b, 63f–66f
'Non-chewing' side, 59–62
'Non-working' side, 59–62

O

Oblique facial photos, 29f
Occlusal analysis, 56f, 66–69, 68f, 70f–71f
    dental view of, 16–17, 17f–26f, 20b
Occlusal plane, 65b
Occlusal stability, 154–155
Occlusal views, 116f
    technique
        lower, 117f
        upper, 116f
Occlusions
    centric, 55
    complete, 56–58, 56f, 58f–59f
    definition of, 62
Opalescence, digital smile design and, 286f
Orthodontic-periodontic-restorative procedures, 163

Orthodontic records, aligner therapy and, 191–192
Orthodontic treatment, 184–185
Orthodontics, role in restorative space management, 161–163
Overbite, anterior, overjet and, 56–58, 59f
Overcontouring, 167–169, 169f
Overeating, secretive, 46
Overexposed teeth, in dental photography, 97–98, 98f
Overjet, overbite and, 56–58, 59f

P

Panadent articulator, 31
Papilla
    levels of, esthetics and, 156–157
    proportions, 21, 22f
Parallel of curves, 25, 26f
Pedicle soft tissue grafts, for gingival recession, 125
Peri-implant mucosa, 131–132
Periodontal architecture, and restorative space management, 155–157, 155f
Periodontal factors, 122–148
    gingival recession, 124–126
    implant esthetics, 129–133
    interdental papilla, 133–135, 134f–135f
    long-term maintenance of soft tissue esthetics, 135–136, 136b
Periodontal plastic surgery
    for gingival recession, 125
    postoperative complications associated with, 128b
    for ridge defects, 132–133
    for root coverage, 136b
Periodontal surgery, gingival margins and, 156
Periodontium, biology of, RSM and, 157–158
Phonetics, 15–16, 15f–16f
Photographic mirrors, 103–104, 104f
Photography
    see also Clinical photography, in esthetic dentistry
    and video, in three-step analysis, 27, 28f–33f
Plaque, bone loss and, 135
Plaster model, 294f
Plastic surgery, periodontal
    for gingival recession, 125
    postoperative complications associated with, 128b
    for ridge defects, 132–133
    for root coverage, 136b
Polyvinyl siloxane, 74
    impression material index, 77f
    putty, 217–220
Porcelain laminate restoration, 165
Porcelain laminate veneer, 220
    diastema closure and, 166
    restoration of fractured and carious teeth with, 245–246, 246f
Porcelain veneer, 216, 258b
    process, 267f
    technique, 216
Posterior contacts, 58
Posterior veneers, considerations for, 243–245, 245f
Post-orthodontics, 79f
Power ridges, 188
'Precision cuts', 189, 192–196, 209f
Pre-orthodontics, 79f
Preparation guides, for crowding treatment planning, 165
Profile view, of tooth, 25, 25f
Provisional veneer, 238, 240f–241f, 257b–258b
    process, 267f
    removal of, 248f
Provisionalization, 238–243, 240f–242f
Psychological assessment, 44–50
    guideline for evaluating patient's mental state in, 47–49
    psychological issues pertinent to esthetic dentistry and, 46–47

Q

Questions, effective, in Esthetic Evaluation Form, 4–8, 8b, 9f

INDEX

R

RAW image format, 107
Records, in three-step analysis, 27–33
    diagnostic casts, 31–33, 31b, 34f–35f
    photography and video, 27, 28f–33f
Reduction bur
    self-limiting depth, 219, 219f
    two-grit gross, 219–220, 219f
Reduction guides, 217–220, 217b, 257b
    polyvinyl siloxane, 218f
Reductive mock-up, considerations for, 37–40, 39f
Refinement, in aligner therapy, 198, 199b
Removable appliance
    aligner therapy and, 186–187
    fixed appliance versus, 185
Reproduction ratio, in dental photography, 94–95, 95f
Resolution, of digital camera, 93
Restorations
    anterior bonded. see Anterior bonded restorations
    cemented, 287f, 291f
    completed, 286f, 291f–292f
    composite, 80f
    E.max, 291f
    of fractured and carious teeth, with porcelain laminate veneer, 245–246, 246f
    of lingually locked teeth, 165
    need for, 153–155
Restorative space management, 150–180, 152b, 170b, 178b
    clinical considerations for, 153–158
    crowding treatment planning in, 163–165, 164f
    dentogingival structural compromises in, 157–158, 158b
    diastema treatment planning in, 165–170, 166f–170f, 170b
    esthetic parameters in, 158–160
    goals of, 153
    need for restoration, 153–155
    orthodontic role in, 161–163
    periodontal architecture and, 155–157, 155f
Retention, in aligner therapy, 200, 200b, 203f–204f, 206f–207f
Retracted view
    of full dentition, 114f
        faults in, 119f
    of lateral dentition, 115f
Retraction, 236–238, 238b, 238f–239f
Retractors, cheek, for dental photography, 101, 103f
Rickett's E-plane, 12–13, 12f–14f
Ridge defects, periodontal plastic surgery procedures for, 132–133
Right chew position, 59–62, 61f
Ring flash, in dental photography, 100–101, 100f
Root coverage
    complete, 128b, 136b
    free gingival graft for, 126
Rubber dam, 250f
Rubber tip instrument, 254f
Rubber wheels, 220
Ruler, calibrated, used in digital smile design, 279f, 289f

S

Secretive overeating, 46
Shade selection, considerations for, 232–235, 234f
Shame, in patients seeking esthetic enhancement, 47–48
Shutter speed, in dental photography, 97–98
Silicone putty, 36, 37f
Single-lens reflex (SLR) camera, 93, 108b
'Slice prep', 224
    closing diastema, 226f, 257b
SLR camera. see Single-lens reflex (SLR) camera
Smile, 75
    dentofacial, 111f
    digital design, 276–283, 276f–284f, 297b
        high-performance planning with, clinical case for, 274–298, 288f–292f, 297b
        laboratory technique for, 283–286, 284f–287f
        technique demonstration of, 292, 292f–296f
    evaluation of, 54
    face and, 74
    full natural, in dental photography, 110f
        left lateral view, 112f
        right lateral view, 112f
        technique, 110f
    healthy, 75
    line analysis, 159
    post-treatment, displaying esthetics and function, 80f
    types of
        'clean, healthy and natural', 8, 9f
        'straight, white and perfect', 8, 9f
        'white and natural', 8, 9f
    variety of, photographs of, 109f
Smoking, bone loss and, 135
Soft tissue
    esthetics, long-term maintenance of, 135–136, 136b
    grafts, pedicle, for gingival recession, 125
    profile analysis, 64–65
    symmetry, 18, 19f
Split-full-split flap incisions, 142f
Standard views, for dental photography, 106–107, 108b
Stent, vacuum-style
    classic, 217f
    clear, 217–220
Subepithelial connective tissue (CT) graft, 136b, 143, 143f–146f, 145b–146b
Subgingival preparation, rule of thumb for, 222b
Symmetry, soft tissue, 18, 19f

T

Teeth (tooth)
    complete occlusion, 56–58, 56f, 58f–59f
    extraction of, 201b
    fractured and carious, restoration of, 245–246, 246f
    lingually locked, restoration of, 165
    malalignment, restorative correction of, 157
    minimal reduction of, 258b
    natural position and form of, 54–55
    overexposed, in dental photography, 97–98, 98f
    texture of, 24, 24f
    underexposed, in dental photography, 97–98, 98f
    upper anterior
        faults in view of, 119f
        frontal view of, 118f–119f
        lateral view of, 118f
Texture, of tooth, 24, 24f
Three-step analysis, 2–3, 3b, 3f–4f, 40b–41b
    diagnostic wax-up in, 33–36, 36b
    Esthetic Evaluation Form, 3–25, 4b, 5f–7f
        effective questions, 4–8, 8b, 9f
        facial, dentofacial and dental analysis, 8–17
    esthetic mock-up, 36–40
        intra-oral mock-up, 36–37, 37f–38f
        reductive mock-up, 37–40, 39f
    records in, 27–33
        diagnostic casts, 31–33, 31b, 34f–35f
        photography and video, 27, 28f–33f
Through the lens (TTL), 92–93
    exposure metering, 98–99
Tooth contacts, ideal, 57f
Tooth preparation, for diastema closure, 167–169, 169f
Tooth proportion, 19, 21f
Tooth-to-tooth proportion, 20, 21f
Transparency, digital smile design and, 286f
Treatment planning
    crowding, 163–165, 164f
    dental photography in, 90, 90f
    for diastema, 165–170, 170b
        midline, 166
        spaces, larger, 166–167, 167f
    facially directed, 64
        concepts of, 64–65
Trigonal shapes, 19, 19f

INDEX

'True vertical' line, 63–64, 67f
TTL. *see* Through the lens (TTL)
Tubulicid, 252f
Two-grit gross reduction bur, 219–220
    connects depth cuts, 230f

U

Ultrasonic bath, 251f
Underexposed teeth, in dental photography, 97–98, 98f
Unrounded labial-incisal angle, 231
Upper anterior teeth
    faults in view of, 119f
    frontal view of, 118f
        with contrastor, 119f
        technique, 118f
    lateral view of, 118f
        technique, 118f

V

Vacuum-style stent
    classic, 217f
    clear, 217–220
Variolink veneer cement (Ivoclar), 251
Veneer
    anterior mandibular, considerations for, 243, 244f
    cement, injection of, 253f
    foods and, 258b
    lithium disilicate, 247, 247f, 263f
    porcelain, 216, 258b
        process, 267f
        technique, 216
    posterior, considerations for, 243–245, 245f
    provisional, 238, 240f–241f, 257b–258b
    restorative material for, 246–247
Veneer-onlay laminate veneer, 246, 246f
Veneer preparation, 257b–258b
    armamentarium for, 217–220
    guidelines for, 220–221, 220f
    ideal mandibular anterior, 244f
    ideal mandibular posterior, 245f
    ideal maxillary posterior, 245f
    step-by-step, 221–231
        depth cuts, connecting and finishing, 229–231, 231f–233f
        facial preparation, 229, 229f
        gingival margin placement, 221–224, 222b, 223f, 224b
        incisal reduction, 226–228, 227f–228f
        interproximal margin placement, 224–225, 225f
        prepreparation enameloplasty, 221, 222f
Video, photography and, in three-step analysis, 27, 28f–33f

W

Wax-up, diagnostic
    in crowding treatment planning, 165, 172b, 172f
    in diastema closure, 176f
    occlusal view of, 77f
    silicone putty of, 37f
    in three-step analysis, 3, 33–36, 35f, 36b
Wear, incisal edge, upper and lower, clinical case of, 81f

Z

Zenith points, 169, 170f, 221–224, 281f